P9-EJU-461

Bottom Line's
HEALTH
BREAKTHROUGHS

2021

BottomLine**Books**

BottomLineInc.com

Copyright © 2020 by Bottom Line Inc.

All rights reserved. No part of this publication may be reproduced, scanned, distributed or
transmitted in any form, by any means, electronic or mechanical, without
permission in writing from the publisher.

10 9 8 7 6 5 4 3 2 1

ISBN 0-88723-841-6

Bottom Line Books® publishes the advice of expert authorities in many fields.
These opinions may at times conflict as there are often different approaches to solving problems.
The use of this material is no substitute for health, legal, accounting or other professional services.
Consult competent professionals for answers to your specific questions.

Telephone numbers, addresses, prices, offers and websites listed in this book are accurate
at the time of publication, but they are subject to frequent change.

Bottom Line Books® is a registered trademark of Bottom Line Inc.
3 Landmark Square, Suite 201, Stamford, Connecticut 06901

BottomLineInc.com

———————————————————

Bottom Line Books is an imprint of Bottom Line Inc., publisher of print periodicals,
e-letters and books. We are dedicated to bringing you the best information from the most
knowledgeable sources in the world. Our goal is to help you gain greater wealth,
better health, more wisdom, extra time and increased happiness.

———————————————————

Printed in the United States of America

Contents

Contents

Contents

Contents

15 • NATURAL HEALERS

16 • PAIN RELIEF

17 • RESPIRATORY HEALTH AND ALLERGIES

Contents

18 • WOMEN'S HEALTH

Preface

We are proud to bring you the all-new *Bottom Line's Health Breakthroughs 2021*. This collection represents a year's worth of the latest health news and scientific discoveries in a broad spectrum of fields.

When you choose a Bottom Line book, you are turning to a stellar group of experts in a wide range of specialties—medical doctors, alternative practitioners, renowned nutrition experts, research scientists and consumer-health advocates, to name a few.

We go to great lengths to interview the foremost health experts. Whether it's cancer prevention, breakthrough arthritis treatments or cutting-edge nutritional advice, our editors talk to the true innovators in health care.

How do we find all these top-notch professionals? Over the past 40 years, we have built a network of leading physicians in both alternative and conventional medicine. They are affiliated with the world's premier medical institutions. We follow the medical research and bring the latest information to our readers. We also regularly talk with our advisers in teaching hospitals, private practices and government health agencies.

Bottom Line's Health Breakthroughs 2021 is a result of our ongoing research and contact with these experts, and is a distillation of their latest findings and advice. We hope that you will enjoy the presentation and glean helpful information about the health topics that concern you and your family.

As a reader of a Bottom Line book, please be assured that you are receiving reliable and well-researched information from a trusted source. But, please use prudence in health matters. Always speak to your physician before taking vitamins, supplements or over-the-counter medication…changing your diet…or beginning an exercise program. If you experience side effects from any regimen, contact your doctor immediately.

The Editors, Bottom Line Books, Stamford, Connecticut.

CHAPTER 1

Aging Well

Reinvent Yourself at Any Age: How to Find the Path to Your Passion

Sadly, many people have a very narrow view of old age—none more so, perhaps, than those who are aging themselves. We can get so caught up in what we're losing that we fail to see how much we gain as we age, often even more than we have lost. *With life expectancy growing and the science of aging continually expanding, it's time for a different perspective…*

THE BRAIN IMPROVES WITH AGE

While there are many jokes about senior moments, I believe that older brains have enormous potential because of the aging and learning process. How so? Seniors make better decisions… are more at peace with themselves…and have more informed perspectives on life. I think aging allows for a more mature way of thinking in that older people are able to draw on a greater history of experience when analyzing situations and tend to be less emotionally reactive. Pulling from a broad store of memories and experiences also allows older people to problem-solve more creatively.

Taken all together, aging can be a jumping-off point for a renewed sense of purpose and growth if you are willing to explore some new directions…

•**Try a more creative approach.** Part of problem-solving comes from being able to think divergently, along different pathways. As the brain matures, we get better at doing this and our solutions become more creative. In real terms, this means that if you find yourself facing a challenge, such as being unable to stand for long periods of time or unable to hold your hand steady, you usually can find a work-

Marc Agronin, MD, board-certified geriatric psychiatrist and chief medical officer of MIND Institute at Miami Jewish Health. He is author of six books on aging, including most recently, *The End of Old Age: Living a Longer, More Purposeful Life*. MarcAgronin.com around—maybe one that is even better than the original way you had of doing things.

Example: The famous French painter Matisse almost died from an intestinal ailment in the early 1940s. Miraculously, he survived, but certainly not in the same physical condition. He could no longer stand and paint the big canvases that he was used to. So he had a choice to make. He either had to give up his career or find a new way of doing it. In the end, he found a new way of doing it that revolutionized the art world. From his wheelchair, he cut shapes from vividly colored sheets of paper and instructed his assistant on how to paste them up on the wall. He captivated the world with these images and his bold use of colors. Much of what Matisse is best known for comes from the last 10 years of his life, at a point when many people would've said, "It's time to give up and stop creating."

•**Find ways to reinvent yourself.** I work with a lot of people who have lost a longtime spouse or a partner. That can be very difficult, but it also can be a moment for reinvention.

Example: One woman, after facing losses, decided that she wanted to work with people facing similar challenges. She thought about being a psychologist or a social worker, but at that point in her life, she didn't want to return to school. Instead, she received training in a hospice program and started working with other individuals who were facing the death of a loved one. It allowed her to heal herself in many ways while helping others to heal as well.

Try this: Volunteer opportunities are everywhere. They are a good way for you to dip a toe into something to see if you might want to spend more time doing it.

•**Think of yourself as liberated.** We tend to think that liberation and experimentation are the domain of the young, but that's not true. With age comes fewer inhibitions. In my experience, older people often feel less encumbered by previous approaches, ideologies and ways of thinking than they did when they were younger. It's time to shake up the stereotypes we have about aging and realize that we can take a leadership role in terms of doing things differently. You even have the freedom to reinvent the type of relationships you have with people in your family—especially the younger generation.

•**Take stock of all your personal assets.** Think of your life as you would a financial portfolio. What are your assets? They are different for everyone. And remember, it doesn't have to be the ability to cure cancer.

Example: One woman, Mary, continued to make amazing Italian dinners for her family every Sunday. She was the glue that held the family together, and Sunday dinner gave their week a sense of rhythm. I don't think Mary would ever think her meatballs were some great, wise approach to life, but they really were. And I promise you that someday when her grandchildren are older, they will make those same recipes and the feeling of warmth and love will return to them.

It could be sewing…it could be your ability to set up and maintain a budget…it could be that you still are a very good driver. Talking to people about your list of unique skills and assets will help to redefine how you see yourself and how you can define your future. This is what I call "re-aging," because then you can start pursuing some of these new activities.

•**Be open to new directions.** Are you happy with the roads you have pursued so far? Do you want to continue on the same path? Look back, and ask yourself, *What were some of the most challenging experiences in my life?…How did I get through them?…What pushed me forward?* The answers to these questions give individuals a sense of their purpose, and this may drive ideas for what you can do going forward. Just because you have always been an accountant doesn't mean that you now can't pursue your

Make a "Chuck It" List

Don't just have a bucket list. Also create a "chuck it" list of things you want to stop doing. Free yourself of stuff you've always thought you must do, and focus on what's important to you.

Nancy Collamer, career coach, speaker and founder of MyLifestyleCareer.com, Old Greenwich, Connecticut, and author of *Second-Act Careers*.

passion for gardening. It's not too late. Make a list of the things you want to do now. This is not a traditional bucket list of travel destinations. It's about how you want to live the coming years… and the legacy you want to leave behind.

New Tech for Staying Safe and Independent at Home

Laurie Orlov, tech-industry analyst and founder of Aging in Place Technology Watch, a market research company that provides research and analysis about tech designed to help seniors continue to live safely in their homes. AgeInPlaceTech.com

---

New high-tech products, ranging from devices that predict falls to those that provide computer-generated reminders, are making it safer and easier for more people to remain independent as they grow older. *Here are some of the notable new tech devices that can help seniors continue to live safely in their homes and communities, including some that are not yet available but will be soon…*

VIRTUAL CAREGIVING

These days, living alone doesn't have to mean there's no one around to help. A number of new tech products can provide some of the oversight and support traditionally supplied by a caregiver when no one else is around—and they can do so without the loss of privacy that comes with an in-home caregiver. *Examples…*

•**CarePredict Tempo** is a behavior-monitoring device that is worn like a wristwatch, but it uses sophisticated pattern-recognition technology to identify the wearer's nascent health issues before they escalate. The system closely monitors the person's movements inside the home—walking speed, the amount of time spent in bed or in the bathroom and the amount of time spent eating, for example—then identifies changes to these patterns that could potentially presage a developing health or fitness concern. When the device spots a troubling change, it notifies loved ones via text and/or e-mail, often before the situation becomes dire. According

to the company, a pilot study conducted in assisted-living facilities reduced falls by 25% by identifying the early stages of movement and balance problems. CarePredict Tempo costs $449 and $69/month for monitoring services. CarePredict.com

•**LifePod from LifePod Solutions, Inc.,** is comparable to "virtual assistants" Alexa and Siri, but it's designed specifically to provide support to people of advancing age. LifePod can be programmed to ask its user how he/she is feeling at predetermined intervals, and it reports appropriate replies to loved ones via text message. Caregivers (or seniors themselves) can ask LifePod to provide reminders, such as "It's 10:00—did you take your morning pills?" or "It's your grandson Tommy's birthday—don't forget to call him." Like other smart speakers, it also can respond to verbal requests to play music, read audiobooks, check the weather and more. $49/month or $432 for one year. LifePod.com

FALL DETECTION

Each year, around 25% of people 65 and older suffer falls. Wearable devices that can summon assistance in these situations have been around for decades, but the latest generation of fall-detection tech even can identify a fall and call for help on its own when the wearer is unconscious. *Among the options…*

•**Apple Watch Series 5** can detect that its wearer has fallen and notify a preselected emergency contact if that wearer is unresponsive. Its Emergency SOS feature lets users quickly and easily call 911 and/or notifies emergency contacts via text message when the wearer requires help in other situations. This watch, which is designed to work in conjunction with an Apple iPhone, can monitor heart rate—it even generates electrocardiograms for viewing the results on the watch itself—and serves as an activity and sleep tracker. Non–health-related functions include streaming music, providing maps and directions and making and receiving phone calls and texts. Its price starts at $399 (or $499 for a version that has built-in cellular capabilities so that it can function when the user's iPhone is not nearby). Apple.com

•**MyNotifi** is a fall-detection device that can be worn either as a wristband or with a belt clip.

Like the Apple Watch, MyNotifi sends a text to preselected emergency contacts when it detects a fall (unless the wearer dismisses the fall as a false alarm)—but it does not include the other health-monitoring features of the Apple Watch. It costs $199 for a version that works in conjunction with your smartphone…$229 for a version that does not require a smartphone. MyNotifi is compatible with iOS and Android. MyNotifi.com

MEDICATION MANAGEMENT

•**MedMinder Pharmacy** ships prefilled, presorted weekly pill trays to patients, so they don't need to sort out pills on their own…and so they never have to worry, *Did I remember to take my pills this morning?* The prefilled disposable trays are placed in the company's automated pill dispenser—when it's time to take medication a light flashes in the compartment containing the appropriate pills. If pills are not taken on schedule, the device beeps. If that doesn't work, the patient and/or his/her loved ones receive an alert via phone, text or e-mail. MedMinder Pharmacy does not charge extra for this pill-sorting service. It accepts most insurance and Medicare Part D plans, and your co-pays typically are the same as they would be at a pharmacy. There is a monthly fee for the high-tech pill dispenser—prices start at $49.99 per month—but if you want to avoid the added cost, presorted "weekly pill packs" that are designed to be used on their own, without the dispenser, also are available at no additional charge. MedMinder.com

HEARING ASSISTANCE

•**Oticon Opn and Opn S hearing aids** also serve as wireless Bluetooth headsets for making and receiving smartphone calls when paired with an accessory called ConnectClip. This accessory clips to the hearing aid wearer's clothing and includes a microphone so that its user can be heard clearly by callers. It works with both Apple and Android smartphones. ConnectClip also can be used to stream music and other audio directly to these Oticon hearing aids…and it can be used as a remote microphone—place ConnectClip directly in front of the person you are speaking with to hear him better in a noisy environment. Connect-

Clip tends to sell for around $400, while Opn and Opn S hearing aids generally cost $2,000 or more per ear from an audiologist. (The Opn S is the latest generation of the Opn and fares somewhat better in tests of speech understanding.) Oticon.com

Heart Drugs May Increase Risk of Falls

Frederik Dalgaard, MD, cardiovascular researcher at Herlev and Gentofte Hospital, Hellerup, Denmark, and leader of a study published in *Journal of the American Geriatrics Society.*

Taking A-fib drugs may increase risk for falls and fainting in older patients.

Latest finding: Amiodarone (Nexterone and Pacerone) was associated with fainting and falls in older people with A-fib, in part because it can lead to bradycardia (slow heartbeat). Use precautions—such as rising from a seated position slowly—especially in the first two weeks after starting the medication.

Other A-fib drug previously linked to falls: Digoxin (Lanoxin).

High Doses of Vitamin D Don't Help Bone Health

There was no difference in bone strength between people who met the recommended dietary allowance (RDA) of 600 International Units (IU) of vitamin D and people who took 4,000 IU or 10,000 IU supplements—but there was density loss in the tibia with higher doses. For bone health, current findings don't support supplementing over the RDA if you do not have a deficiency.

David A. Hanley, MD, is professor emeritus of medicine, oncology and community health sciences at University of Calgary, Canada, and coauthor of a three-year trial of people ages 55 to 70, published in *JAMA.*

What's Really to Blame for Your Balance Problems

Victor M. Romano, MD, a board-certified orthopedic surgeon in private practice in Oak Park, Illinois, where he specializes in sports medicine. He is also a clinical affiliate faculty member at Midwestern University Chicago College of Osteopathic Medicine and a clinical assistant professor at Loyola University in Chicago. He is author of *Finding the Source: Maximizing Your Results—With and Without Orthopaedic Surgery.* RomanoMD.com

If you feel a little wobbly on your feet, you may chalk it up to the fact that you're simply growing older. After all, when your muscles, joints and vision don't work as well as they once did, it can destabilize you—making a fall more likely.

No one wants to break a hip and end up using a walker or living in a nursing home, so you're probably doing your best to prevent a disabling fall. But are you doing all you can to address the underlying causes of poor balance?

To learn about these hidden culprits, we spoke with Victor M. Romano, MD, a board-certified orthopedic surgeon who diagnoses and repairs ailing bones, joints and muscles. In his practice, he has learned about unexpected issues that can sabotage balance.*

THE MISALIGNMENT PROBLEM

The medical community has almost entirely ignored two scientific papers published just over a decade ago in *Practical Pain Management,* which uncovered a missing link in the role that chronic pain and muscle weakness play in causing poor balance.

The problem: If a joint (where two bones connect) is out of correct alignment, the body unconsciously compensates to restore stability. For example, if one of the joints in the right foot is out of alignment, the body unconsciously overuses the left foot. This "compensation" causes left knee pain, weaker muscles on the right side—and poorer balance. Because there are more than 300 joints in the human body, it can be challenging to find a misalignment—even for an orthopedic surgeon!

*Check with your doctor before starting this—or any new—exercise program.

Dr. Romano's solution: A series of simple stretches that I have developed and successfully used in my practice over the past five years—called the Romano Stretches—prevent or correct nearly every misalignment that can cause balance problems. By doing these stretches, you will help restore your balance, relieve aches and pains, improve strength and flexibility—and, in turn, prevent falls.

THE ROMANO STRETCHES

The following stretches address the most common areas where misalignment occurs in the human body, leading to balance problems. *Do the stretches daily—you can complete them all in just a few minutes…*

•**Pelvic stretch.** Restoring pelvic balance improves your side-to-side balance and range of motion of your shoulders. You will feel this stretch in the lower back and buttocks.

What to do: While lying flat on your back, grab your right knee with your left hand and bring your knee across your body toward the left side of your chest. At the same time, stretch your right arm and shoulder to the right, keeping them on the floor. (See above.) Turn your head to the right for an additional stretch if you desire. Hold for five to 10 seconds. Next, do the exercise on the other side, grabbing your left knee with your right hand, and stretching your left arm and shoulder to the left while turning your head to the left if you desire. Repeat twice on each side of your body.

•**Hip stretch.** This stretch helps restore alignment in the back and neck—and is excellent for reversing loss of balance and restoring mobility of the hip. You should feel this stretch in the top of your thigh, particularly toward the hip.

What to do: While standing about six to 12 inches in front of a chair, bend your right leg at the knee so that your foot (toes pointed) and a few inches of your shin rest on the seat of the chair. Lean back to feel a stretch in your right groin. Then slowly bend your left knee slightly to get a deeper stretch. Hold the stretch for five to 10 seconds and return to an upright position. Then do the same stretch with your left leg on the chair behind you, bending your right knee. Repeat twice on each side.

If you feel unstable while doing this stretch: Use a chair with arms and hold onto them as you lean back or stand next to a sturdy counter or desk to steady yourself.

•**Rib stretch.** A misalignment in the ribs can cause pain and weakness in the upper back, neck, shoulders, hands and elbows—all of which can contribute to poor balance. You should feel this stretch in your upper back and ribs.

What to do: While standing, bend your arms to a 90-degree angle and bring your elbows out to your sides, parallel to the ground and just below shoulder level. Forcefully and quickly, pull your elbows backward in two short bursts and repeat two to three times.

•**Back stretch.** This stretch is excellent for relieving upper and lower back pain. Patients with this problem have impaired balance when moving their heads up or down or turning side to side. This stretch should be felt in your lower back.

What to do: While standing, put your fists against the small of your back and arch your back as far as you can for five to 10 seconds. Relax and slowly exhale while stretching. Repeat two to three times.

Senior Communities That Have It All!

Brad Breeding, CFP, president of myLifeSite, which helps consumers research continuing-care retirement communities. Based in Raleigh, North Carolina, he is author of *What's the Deal with Retirement Communities?* MyLifeSite.net

Most people prefer to stay in their homes as long as they can as they age—even after they can't take care of all the things they used to. But that can be socially isolating and physically difficult. It's also stressful for family members who, at some point, will have to help maintain the older person's home, make sure that he/she eats properly and scramble for medical care and housing if the person develops new health problems or the person's abilities erode.

One alternative that has grown in popularity—a continuing-care retirement community (CCRC) that lets seniors age in place as their abilities and needs change. There are more than 2,000 CCRCs in the US now, and their signature attribute is that they essentially are hybrids. Able singles and couples live independently but have the option of sharing communal services such as dining halls and daily social activities. Within the same campus, residents have access, should it become necessary, to assisted-living services such as daily dressing and bathing support, a skilled-nursing home and sometimes even special facilities for dementia and/or hospice care.

In a well-run CCRC, no one has to live less independently—or more independently—than makes sense. Residents can maintain a continuum of comfort and connections no matter what happens.

If there's a downside, it's that these communities require a big financial commitment, typically six-figure fees up front. (See "What CCRCs Cost" on page 7.) Those who choose to deploy their money this way, though, look at it as a worthwhile expense. *Here's how to figure out whether a CCRC would be a good choice for you (or a loved one) and how to evaluate and compare them...*

HOW CCRCS WORK

There are CCRCs in every state. (For a list, go to CCRCS.com.) To apply, you typically need to be at least 62 years old and able to live independently. A community may be a mix of physically adjacent buildings, such as garden apartments or townhomes spread across a campus setting. In more urban areas, there might be a single high-rise building. Upscale amenities are the drawing card for many CCRC residents. These can include on-campus walking trails, gyms, activity centers, golf courses, excursions to mu-

Will Your CCRC Be Around for the Rest of Your Life?

About 80% of CCRCs are nonprofits, and some were started decades ago by churches or charitable organizations to serve their aging members. But you still want to make sure that any CCRC you consider has the financial reserves, income and cash flow to meet its long-term obligations to you. Although fewer than 2% of these communities have filed for bankruptcy protection over the past 10 years, a CCRC that runs into financial trouble could mean residents lose any refundable entry fees, or it could be bought out by a new owner, resulting in changes to amenities and services.

What to do to protect yourself…

•**Check for an occupancy rate of around 90% or higher.** CCRCs can't afford many ongoing vacancies if they want to maintain their staff and services and continue to make improvements and upgrades.

•**Find out whether your CCRC is in good standing with state regulators.** CCRCs often are regulated by the state's insurance commissioner or the department of health or aging and are required to meet certain criteria for financial stability. But 11 states and Washington, DC, have no special oversight of CCRCs, so the vetting process falls more heavily on residents in those places. The 11 states are Alabama, Alaska, Hawaii, Mississippi, Montana, Nebraska, Nevada, North Dakota, Utah, West Virginia and Wyoming.

Request a copy of the CCRC's audited financial records, also known as disclosure statements, for the past five years. It's a red flag if the CCRC doesn't offer complete transparency about its finances. Consider hiring an elder-law attorney or CPA if you don't feel qualified to evaluate these documents. Look for anything unusual, such as a large amount of debt, failure to meet bond obligations or evidence of liabilities assets, or expenditures exceeding operating income.

seums, theaters and stores, and fairly posh dining halls. *How to evaluate a CCRC…*

•**Make sure that the place meets your practical needs.** Country club–like amenities are nice, but you need to be comfortable with the age range and mix of residents, how attentive the staff is and whether the meal schedule and food selection work for you if you choose communal dining. Most CCRCs have guest suites. Plan to visit and live there for several days. Examine the list of weekly activities. Is there enough to engage you and help expand your social circle? If you are considering giving up your car, what kind of transportation is available?

•**Evaluate the quality of care.** Check with your state's long-term-care ombudsman, who advocates for residents of adult-care facilities, to see whether there are any complaints on file (TheConsumerVoice.org/get_help) and, if so, how serious they are. Also, use the "Nursing Home Compare" tool at Medicare.gov, which rates nursing-care facilities and compares important statistics such as the total number of licensed-nurse staff hours devoted to each resident per day.

WHAT CCRCS COST

Residents typically are charged a onetime "buy-in," or entry fee, which can range from less than $100,000 to more than $1 million, and a monthly recurring fee generally ranging from $2,000 to $5,000 for singles ($3,000 to $6,000 for couples) that covers the communal amenities including meals, your rental housing unit and utilities. Only a tiny percentage of CCRCs allows residents to purchase their homes or become co-op owners. Expect monthly fees to increase at a rate of 3% to 4% annually.

The exact amount of your entry fee and monthly fees are determined by the type of contract you sign with the CCRC.

Most common: A fee-for-service contract is a pay-as-you-go option that offers low entry and monthly fees for independent living—but if you need assisted-living services or the nursing home in the future, you pay the CCRC's going rate at that time, which is tacked on to your regular monthly charges. According to extensive documentation on pricing from CCRCs in all states in which they are regulated, this type of contract would cost a single person in an independent studio unit around $90,100 for the entry fee and a monthly charge of around $2,100. A couple in a two-bedroom unit would pay around $203,600 for an entry fee and a monthly charge of around $3,900, though these figures vary greatly by region and type of amenities. Moving up to advanced-level care in the future could easily double your monthly charges. Consider the fee-for-service contract if you have long-term-care insurance or if you are in good physical health and think you'll have enough assets in the future to cover the cost of advanced health care.

A life-care contract has much higher entry and ongoing monthly fees, but there are no additional costs for advanced health care. An individual would pay around $159,700 as an entry fee and monthly charges of around $2,450…a couple, around $289,450 for an entry fee and a monthly charge of around $4,750. A life-care contract means that you essentially prepay for long-term care that you may not end up needing, but it provides financial security and peace of mind by limiting the risks of those costs skyrocketing in the future.

Important: CCRCs do not provide or cover doctor's visits, most medication or hospitalization. These are costs that may be covered if you have long-term-care insurance or by Medicare or supplemental Medicare insurance for those age 65 and older.

Before signing a CCRC contract…

•**Consult a financial adviser.** Whether it's wise to choose a CCRC is not only about your lifestyle but also a long-term financial decision that will depend in part on your age, existing assets, your ability to absorb future cost increases and your health status. Most CCRCs require a prospective resident to have total assets equivalent to at least twice the entry fee and monthly income that is at least 1.5 times the monthly fees.

•**Check the refund policy pertaining to residents who leave the community.** Most CCRC contracts allow a full refund of entry fees to you or your heirs if you and your spouse move out or if either of you dies during a specified time period, which might be two years or more. After that, the refundable portion of your fee may decline for each year that you stay.

If Your Voice Is Shaky and Weak, Here's the Checkup You Need

Lesley Childs, MD, associate professor of laryngology, neurolaryngology and professional voice at University of Texas (UT) Southwestern Medical Center in Dallas. She also serves as the associate medical director of the Clinical Center for Voice Care at UT Southwestern. Dr. Childs is a classically trained soprano.

With age, our vocal cords tend to thin and lose flexibility, often causing us to develop chronic hoarseness and/or a weak, shaky voice. But you don't have to live with this. With the right checkup, you can get the treatment you need to improve (or even correct) the problem. *Voice symptoms that should be investigated…*

•**Your voice is hoarse or your sound quality has changed for two weeks or more—regardless of your age.** For example, if your voice is raspy, breathy or shaky or you notice a change in pitch—to a lower or higher range—you should find out what's going on.

•**You feel pain or discomfort when you talk or sing.** Some people with such symptoms are straining their neck muscles to produce sounds.

•**Your voice grows weaker or strained over the course of a day.**

UNRAVELING THE PROBLEM

If your voice problems aren't linked to an obvious cause, such as laryngitis, consider seeing an ear, nose and throat specialist (an otolaryngologist).

If possible, it's even better to seek out a laryngologist, an otolaryngologist who specializes in voice, airway and swallowing disorders. Such doctors often work as part of teams, along with speech therapists, at specialized voice centers. To find a laryngologist near you, consult the American Academy of Otolaryngology—Head and Neck Surgery, ENTnet.org.

When you go for a checkup, you'll be asked to describe what's bothering you. When doing so, mention what—if anything—seems to help or make matters worse. Also describe how you use your voice. Are you a salesperson who is on the phone several hours a day? A teacher in a noisy classroom? Providing this information will help in evaluating your problem.

Your vocal cords will then be examined using a scope equipped with a video camera that passes through your nose or mouth to your larynx (voice box). This test is called laryngoscopy.

The gold standard version includes stroboscopy, an exam in which a strobe light is combined with the camera on the scope. The stroboscopy, which is available at most voice centers, allows for visualization of the vocal cord vibrations, so it provides more detail.

You will be asked to speak so that the camera can capture and record video images of your vocal cord vibrations when you make sounds.

Voice problems can be symptoms of many different conditions, including…

•**Noncancerous growths, such as nodules, polyps and cysts, on the vocal cords.** These often result from trauma caused by using your voice too much or incorrectly without adequate rest. This occurs more often in singers, teachers, ministers and other people who use their voices in their work.

•**Allergies and/or postnasal drip** can irritate the throat, leading to voice changes.

•**Chronic throat clearing and coughing are both traumatic to the vocal cords** and expose the delicate vocal cord tissue to undue wear and tear.

Helpful: Try sipping water instead of throat clearing or coughing.

•**Laryngopharyngeal reflux, in which stomach acid washes up into the larynx.** The condition often improves with weight loss (when needed)…not eating right before going to bed…and other lifestyle changes.

•**Neurological conditions such as a vocal tremor.** However, vocal tremors are not necessarily a sign of a systemic neurological condition, such as epilepsy or Parkinson's disease.

•**Cancerous growths.** If your doctor sees something suspicious on the vocal cords or in the voice box, a biopsy will be performed to determine whether a malignancy is present.

•**Stress and anxiety are sometimes felt in the throat.** For example, someone who is on the verge of tears may feel tightness in the throat.

GETTING THE RIGHT TREATMENT

The cause of your voice problem will determine which treatment is most appropriate. *Treatment options…*

•**Speech therapy.** If your problems are caused by misuse of your voice, a speech therapist (ideally, one with special training in the voice) can teach you techniques that will help. By pairing sound production with diaphragmatic breathing, for example, most people speak more efficiently and without straining.

Note: People who are unhappy with the way their voices have changed with age also can work with speech therapists. Over time, changes occur to the vocal cord tissues and the respiratory system, which affect the quality of the sound. Voice therapy helps us optimize how we are producing sound to better adapt to changes that occur over time.

•**Vocal pacing.** This involves being aware of how much you are using your speaking and singing voice in a day. Reducing your "vocal dose" and pacing your vocal demands, such as resting the voice for five minutes for every 30 minutes of use, can help prevent injury to the vocal cords.

Also helpful: Teachers, fitness instructors and other public speakers may be urged to try a personal amplification system for the voice—basically, a microphone that helps them be heard without raising the volume of their voices.

•**Hydration/vocal hygiene.** Water is the best choice for hydration because it helps thin the mucus that then lubricates and protects your vocal cords as they vibrate.

Best practice: Consume 64 ounces of water daily, drinking it throughout the day to keep the vocal cords hydrated.

Important: Avoid too much caffeine and alcohol—both are drying. If you consume these fluids, match with an equal amount of water—in addition to the daily recommendation of 64 ounces.

Also: Chronic use of decongestants is drying, and certain inhaled medications, such as inhaled corticosteroids to treat asthma and chronic obstructive pulmonary disease (COPD), can be irritating to the vocal cords.

• **Surgery.** People with vocal cord lesions may benefit from surgery to remove them. Oftentimes, however, voice therapy is recommended as a first step as most voice-related vocal cord abnormalities are reversible to an extent. If vocal cord surgery is needed, it is usually performed through the mouth with a microscope and under a general anesthetic. If vocal cord cancer is to blame, treatment for the malignancy typically includes surgery and another therapy, such as radiation.

• **Laser treatment.** Some specific types of vocal cord lesions benefit from laser treatments. These can be performed both in the operating room and in the office.

• **Filler injections.** People whose voices have become weaker due to age-related vocal cord atrophy or who have vocal cord weakness may be offered a procedure in which temporary fillers are injected into the vocal cords to help them vibrate more effectively. Often, insurance covers these procedures, which are usually performed in the office. All fillers are temporary and can last up to 12 months, depending on the material used.

• **Botox.** Neurological voice disorders, such as vocal tremors and spasmodic dysphonia, cause the vocal cords to spasm, resulting in a choppy-sounding voice. For these individuals, a vocal cord injection with botulinum toxin (Botox) can be used. The treatment can ease spasms that interfere with smooth speech. The effects from these injections in the vocal cords typically last about two to three months. Insurance usually covers these injections, which are performed in the office.

Fast Walkers Live Longer

Thomas E. Yates, PhD, professor of physical activity, sedentary behavior and health at University of Leicester, UK, and a lead author of the study using data from 475,000 people, published in *Mayo Clinic Proceedings*.

Researchers found that women who walked at a brisk four-miles-an-hour pace lived about 15 years longer—to age 87—than slow walkers. For men, it was nearly 20 years longer—to age 86. This was regardless of weight or waist circumference, showing that physical fitness may be a better indicator of longevity than body mass index (BMI).

6 Most Common Problems of Aging Feet

Jonathan D. Rose, DPM, a podiatrist in private practice in Baltimore. He is coauthor of *The Foot Book: A Complete Guide to Healthy Feet*. PodiatryAssociates.org

On average, most people will have walked about 50,000 miles by the time they reach age 50. Active people will have walked or run even more. So it's not surprising that up to 25% of older adults complain of assorted types of chronic foot pain. Here are six common problems and the simple things you can do to keep your feet healthy...

PROBLEM: Thinning of the fat pads in the ball of the foot. The fatty padding under your feet naturally wears away over time, which can lead to pain and inflammation in the soles of the feet, a condition known as metatarsalgia. By age 50, many people have lost half of their natural padding. Fat pad atrophy (FPA) affects men and women equally.

What to do: To prevent the fat pads from thinning, wear comfortable walking shoes. Frequent use of high-heeled shoes can cause FPA as well as conditions such as rheumatoid arthritis. If you must wear heels for an event, limit the distance you walk in them. Excess weight also can have an impact on FPA. Staying within a normal body mass index (BMI) range can help maintain your foot padding. Once thinning has begun, you can add gel pads or inserts into shoes to substitute for the loss of your natural padding. If that doesn't do the trick, remove the shoe's existing insert and replace it with a cushioned orthotic insert.

Alternate solution: If the pain persists or gets worse, ask your podiatrist about injections of steroids or, in more extreme cases, a nerve block to relieve the pain.

Not recommended: Injections of fat or synthetic products to repad the sole. These treatments offer only temporary relief and are unproven.

PROBLEM: **Corns and calluses.** Corns are areas of thickened skin that develop on the tops or sides of the toes, usually due to friction or pressure from wearing shoes that are too tight. Calluses are broader areas of thickening that develop on the bottom of the feet. They're also usually due to friction or pressure, or they can occur in areas where there isn't a lot of fat padding.

What to do: You've probably already tried the corn and callus cushion pads at your local drugstore—possibly with limited success—but the best thing you can do is simply buy new shoes. Corns and calluses often go away on their own if you stop the offending friction and pressure caused by wearing a shoe that squeezes your toes or a shoe that's too small. You may not realize this, but there's a chance you need a larger size shoe at age 60 than you did at 30, as the ligaments and tendons in your feet lose their elasticity, making your feet expand. Choose shoes with soft uppers and wide toe boxes, so your feet don't rub against the shoe.

Tip: Go shoe-shopping late in the day when your feet will be at their widest. Bring the socks with you that you intend to wear with those shoes to make sure they don't rub.

Alternate solution: Rub a pumice stone over the hardened area after taking a shower. Moisturize afterward. And be patient—these types of skin issues can take several months to heal.

Note: Avoid over-the-counter products that contain salicylic acid to eat away corns and calluses—they often take healthy tissue with them. Likewise, don't shave corns and calluses your-self. See a podiatrist if you think the area needs to be exfoliated.

Important: Don't manage corns and calluses or other foot problems yourself if you have diabetes, rheumatoid arthritis or cancer. That can lead to infection.

PROBLEM: **Bunions and hammertoes.** You usually inherit bunions and hammertoes. Poor shoe choice, however, can increase the speed that the deformity develops. Rheumatological conditions or injury also can contribute to bunion or hammertoe deformities. Despite its appearance, a bunion is not a growth on the joint—rather, it reflects movement of the big toe toward—or over or under, in severe cases—the second toe.

What to do: Ditch the high heels and pointy-toed shoes. You can buy gel and silicone toe separators, splints, wraps or guards for both bunions and hammertoes. Splints are better for bunions at night. Guards, toe separators or pads are helpful for bunions when people are wearing shoes. Pads cushion the deformities, while splints attempt to delay the progression. Avoid overwearing flip-flops and clogs, which increase the risk for hammertoes because they encourage curling of the toe to grip the shoe.

Alternate solution: Use paper tape to gently push down your hammertoe. Apply the tape around the toe to pull it down, and tape it to the bottom of the foot so that it doesn't rub against your shoe. You may be able to get some relief with products such as YogaToe GEMS that spread toes apart to stretch weak ligaments. Surgery is a last-resort option, done to correct a deformity that causes you severe pain and functional limitations and that cannot be relieved by other treatments.

PROBLEM: **Toenail thickening.** Toenails tend to become thicker with age, which can make them difficult to cut. It doesn't help that, for many elderly people, bending down to reach the nails becomes increasingly difficult.

What to do: It seems obvious, but many people don't do this—go to a podiatrist or have regular professional pedicures if you are too stiff or inflexible to easily cut your toenails your-self. Using nail softeners also may help make it easier to cut your nails. Cut nails straight across or take small snips in them to prevent painful ingrown toenails. Smooth the ends with an emery board. Clean under the toenails regularly with a nail file.

PROBLEM: **Nail fungus.** Age can make toenails more prone to nail fungus, an unsightly nail infection that is caused by dampness and spread in gyms, pools and public showers. Three-quarters of people over age 60 have had nail fungus at some point in their lives. It is very difficult to treat successfully once you have a fungus—the available drugs and lasers take a long time to work and aren't effective for everybody.

What to do: The best defense is a good offense—wear rubber sandals in public showers, pools and gyms to prevent picking up fungus. If you have machine-washable shoes, wash them with bleach and water to disinfect them. Change to fresh socks every day (or multiple times a day if your feet sweat). Wear acrylic socks that wick away moisture instead of cotton socks. A home remedy to treat nail fungus that you can try is to apply Vicks VapoRub to the affected nail daily for six to 12 months.

PROBLEM: **Dry skin.** The skin on the feet gets drier as you age. When severe, skin fissures can occur.

What to do: Keep things simple. Just wash feet daily, and pat dry. Showering is best. Soaks in the tub are too drying. Regular twice-a-day moisturizing is essential. Apply a moisturizer that contains urea, which helps slough off the dead skin and keeps skin hydrated. Apply at night, and then sleep with socks on. If severe, you can also wrap the foot in plastic wrap at night to increase penetration of the lotion.

Important: Don't apply moisturizer between toes where fungus or bacteria might grow.

EASY EXERCISES FOR FOOT HEALTH

The right exercises can help keep your toes and feet limber and strong.

EXERCISE #1: **Pick up marbles.** This will strengthen muscles in the bottom of your feet and may help prevent plantar fasciitis. Place marbles on the floor. Pick up one marble at a time with your toes, and drop it into a nearby bowl or cup. Repeat with your other foot.

EXERCISE #2: **Grasp a towel with your toes.** This exercise encourages you to do toe curls that will strengthen the tops of your feet. Sit in a straight-back chair with a small towel at your feet. Use the toes of one foot to scrunch the towel and pull it toward you. Repeat with the other foot.

EXERCISE #3: **Trace the alphabet.** This exercise helps ankle mobility. Sit down and extend your leg. Trace the alphabet in the air with your big toe. Repeat with the other foot.

EXERCISE #4: **Do toe raises.** This exercise helps to strengthen the Achilles tendon and the arch of the foot. Stand with your hands resting on the back of a sturdy chair, and slowly rise up on your toes and come back down. Toe raises can be done in three sets of 10. Repeat two to three times a week.

Note: Toe raises are not recommended for people suffering with plantar fasciitis. Instead, you want to stretch the calf by bringing the toes and feet upward toward the shin.

Bladder Not Cooperating?

Jill Rabin, MD, professor of obstetrics, gynecology and women's health at the Donald and Barbara Zucker School of Medicine at Hofstra/Northwell in Hempstead, New York. Dr. Rabin is coauthor, with Gail Stein, of *Mind Over Bladder*.

We've all heard of overactive bladder—that "gotta-go" feeling that so often strikes at the worst possible times. It's annoying—especially when it leads to embarrassing dribbles (incontinence). But there could be a hidden side to this problem that you and your doctor are overlooking.

For some people, those too-frequent trips to the bathroom occur because of "underactive bladder," in which sufferers don't empty their bladders completely when they urinate, so they soon make additional trips to the toilet.

About half of women and one-third of men in the US suffer from underactive bladder at some point in their lives. *Key facts to know…*

WHAT GOES WRONG

Under normal conditions, urine, which is made by your kidneys around the clock, trickles into your bladder all the time. A well-functioning bladder stores the fluid until it gets full enough to send a "time to go" signal to your brain.

Ideally, you heed that sensation and get to a toilet. Then your brain sends signals back to the bladder, causing it to contract and squeeze out urine. At the same time, the brain tells several sets of sphincter muscles to relax, allowing urine to pass through the urethra. The process is the same in men and women, even though the anatomy is slightly different. *When the waterworks do not work, symptoms of underactive bladder might include...*

•**Feeling that you need to go again right after you pee,** resulting in frequent trips to the toilet.

•**Weak urinary stream.**

•**Urges to strain, push and bear down to empty your bladder.**

•**Swelling, tenderness or pain below your belly button.**

If the problem becomes chronic, partial emptying of your bladder may allow urine to collect bacteria, leading to recurrent urinary tract infections.

FINDING THE ROOT CAUSE

Underactive bladder is largely due to two main culprits—obstructions and impaired bladder contractions.

Some causes of obstruction...

•**Prostate enlargement.** For men, this is the most common cause. With prostate enlargement, this walnut-shaped gland surrounds the urethra at the neck of the bladder and grows as a man ages.

•**Constipation.** In both men and women, hard, impacted stools can press on the bladder and urethra, interfering with the bladder's ability to empty.

•**Weak pelvic floor muscles.** These muscles may be weak in men due to prostate removal. In women, multiple vaginal deliveries can damage or weaken pelvic structures and nerves, leading to a sagging bladder and/or uterus, which can interfere with bladder function. After menopause, the decline in a woman's estrogen levels causes the pelvic floor to thin and weaken.

Note: Research on supplemental estrogen has been mixed. Kegel exercises that strengthen pelvic muscles can help women—and men—who need to build up these muscles to improve their bladder control.

If Kegels are new to you, here's the basic idea: While sitting or standing, tighten the muscles you would use to stop your stream of urine and those used to keep from passing gas for three seconds (without clenching your abdomen or buttocks), then relax for three seconds. Repeat in sets of five, starting with just a few sets at a time. Slowly work up to 10 sets of five per day.

•**Fibroids.** These benign tumors in the uterus can obstruct the neck of the bladder.

Among the causes of impaired bladder contraction...

•**Years of holding in your urine.** This was once called "schoolteacher's bladder," because schools used to forbid teachers to take bathroom breaks except at lunchtime. As a result, the bladder can "forget" how to function.

•**Conditions that involve nerve damage, such as stroke, Parkinson's disease, diabetes and multiple sclerosis.**

•**Medications,** including muscle relaxants, sedatives, antihistamines, tricyclic antidepressants, such as *amitriptyline* (Elavil), and decongestants.

HOW TO GET RELIEF

If your no-go symptoms haven't become so severe that they are significantly interfering with your life, just improving a few bathroom habits can help. *Here's what to try first...*

•**Urinate at least every two to three hours during the day,** even if you do not feel the urge.

Helpful: Use a smartphone timer to remind yourself to go on this schedule. If you feel much more frequent urges, try to stretch out your bathroom visits by at least 15 minutes at a time, which will train your bladder to wait.

•**Do your best to find private bathrooms if you are prone to "bashful bladder,"** which occurs when you need to urinate but aren't able to do so in the presence of another person.

•**Don't push or strain to urinate…but try shifting your position.** For example, some women and men find that it helps to lean forward or press a hand gently against the lower abdomen to help push urine out of the bladder.

•**Try double voiding.** Urinate, then wait a minute and go again. That can help drain the bladder and prevent the feeling that you need to go again the minute your pants are zipped.

TO GET MORE HELP

If you're still struggling after trying the steps described above, talk to your doctor, and be clear about what's bothering you. A good work-up will include a lab check of your urine to ensure that you don't have a urinary tract infection…and—after you return from giving your urine sample—a simple ultrasound test to see how much urine is left in your bladder. There will always be some, but more than 100 to 150 milliliters, depending on your age, indicates a problem.

Be sure to ask your doctor if any of your medications could be contributing to your problem.

Important: Never discontinue a prescribed drug without checking with your doctor.

If you have a medical condition that increases your risk for underactive bladder (such as those mentioned earlier), be sure to get proper treatment for it. In other cases, you may have an underlying cause that requires surgery, such as pelvic floor reconstruction for a sagging bladder. Or the doctor may refer you to a physical therapist or other professional who will help you with behavior changes that give you more control over your bladder function.

Also helpful: In some cases, you may be asked to try using a disposable strawlike catheter to empty your bladder several times a day. It's easier than you might think and is sometimes the best way to get on with a normal life.

What You Don't Know About Night Sweats

Adam Perlman, MD, MPH, director of Integrative Health and Wellbeing at Mayo Clinic in Jacksonville, Florida. He is board-certified in internal medicine.

You wake up drenched…pajamas sopping wet, sheets clammy beneath you…and it's not the first time. But the bedroom is relatively cool, and you aren't dressed too warmly—in other words, all that heat is coming from you.

Contrary to popular opinion, menopause isn't the only cause of night sweats. But if you're a man or a woman not affected by menopause, you may be scratching your head at the same time you're mopping your brow. Why are you getting these nightly soakings?

LITTLE-KNOWN CULPRITS

Menopause is the main cause of chronic night sweats, but for women and men, other health conditions and factors can be to blame for excessive sweating that occurs at night (and sometimes during the day). *These include…*

•**Medications.** Various drugs, used long term or even for just a few days, are a lesser recognized cause of night sweats. These include anti-depressants…pain relievers including aspirin, *acetaminophen* (Tylenol) or opioids…niacin/vitamin B-3, often taken to help lower cholesterol…*tamoxifen* (Nolvadex) to reduce breast cancer risk…steroids…*hydralazine* (Apresoline) to lower blood pressure …nitroglycerin for angina pain…and erectile dysfunction drugs such as *sildenafil* (Viagra).

•**Thyroid problems.** An overactive thyroid, in which the gland produces too much thyroid hormone (hyperthyroidism), can rev up metabolism, triggering night sweating. But paradoxically, night sweats also can stem from an underactive thyroid (hypothyroidism) or cancer (see next page) of the thyroid gland.

•**Low testosterone.** This one is a men's issue. Drops in testosterone, dubbed "manopause," prompt hot flashes and night sweats that are similar to those that plague menopausal women. Hormone treatment for prostate cancer also can be to blame.

•**Other hormone problems.** In addition to thyroid and sex hormone fluctuations, various hormone disorders might be at play. These include *carcinoid syndrome*, which results in the overproduction of chemicals, including serotonin, in the presence of a rare, slow-growing cancer that may occur in the lung or digestive tract…or a type of adrenal gland tumor that ramps up hormones called catecholamines.

•**Infections.** If you've had the flu, you may have felt the wrath of night sweats on top of classic symptoms such as fever, cough and achiness. But many infections can soak your sheets, including urinary tract infections (UTIs)…abscesses in the skin, tonsils, gut or appendix…and less commonly, tuberculosis…HIV…and heart valve inflammation known as endocarditis.

•**Low blood sugar.** Among people with diabetes, those taking insulin or pills to help control blood sugar sometimes experience drops in blood sugar during sleep that trigger sweating.

•**GERD.** Gastroesophageal reflux disease (GERD), a common cause of heartburn, can trigger night sweats.

•**Neurologic disorders.** While an unusual trigger for night sweats, brain conditions such as Parkinson's disease, stroke or autonomic neuropathy (a condition that damages nerves controlling involuntary body functions such as digestion) may be the culprit.

•**Cancer.** Night sweats are an early symptom of certain cancers—particularly lymphoma and leukemia. But in this less common scenario, other symptoms are usually also present, including fever and unexplained weight loss. Chemotherapy to treat certain cancers can cause night sweats as well.

•**Food.** Certain foods may provoke sweating at night. Spicy foods, caffeine and alcohol are among the most common triggers. However, these foods are more likely to cause hot flashes right after eating them than night sweats.

•**Stress or anxiety.** These largely overlooked triggers can greatly contribute to night sweats by promoting the release of additional epinephrine, the body's "fight-or-flight" hormone.

•**Excess body weight.** People who are overweight or obese are more likely to suffer night sweats than those of normal weight—due, in part, to body fat acting as insulation that traps heat and raises the body's core temperature.

PINPOINTING THE CAUSE

Unless it's a clear case of menopause, night sweats should never be dismissed. That's because they're a symptom of something else, so it's crucial to see a doctor to get to the bottom of it.

Important: If you're a menopausal woman suffering from night sweats, work with your primary care doctor and gynecologist to ensure that the symptom is due to menopause and not one of the conditions described earlier.

To find the cause, your doctor should…

•**Take a thorough medical history,** including a travel history, to determine if you visited a region where tuberculosis is prevalent.

Other questions may include: What medications, vitamins or supplements are you taking? Were you ill recently? Are any other unexplained symptoms occurring? This step is key because it tells the doctor how aggressively to pursue additional testing.

•**Perform a complete physical exam,** checking weight and for signs of disease such as nodules on the thyroid or loss of muscle mass in a male, which might indicate low testosterone.

•**Order blood tests to check hormone levels or rule out various infections or certain types of cancer.**

•**Perform other tests,** such as a Mantoux tuberculin skin test for tuberculosis and, when appropriate, evaluate for certain cancers, such as leukemia, through blood work.

•**Order imaging tests,** such as X-rays or a CT or MRI scan, to rule out malignancies such as thyroid cancer.

•**Review your medications.** Because certain drugs, including those described earlier, can trigger night sweats, it's important for your doctor to review all medications and supplements you're taking. In some cases, a different drug can be prescribed.

Caveat: After exhausting every possible avenue to figure out why the waterworks turn on while you sleep, it's possible that your doctor may find…nothing. In this case, night sweats are deemed a case of idiopathic hyperhidrosis, which means your body sweats too much at night for no identifiable medical reason.

Important: If a cause is not determined and night sweats continue, be sure to report any new symptoms, such as weight loss and/or fever.

HOW TO GET RELIEF

If there's an underlying medical cause, treating that condition should eliminate night sweats. But if that's not the case, you'll want to take the obvious steps to get some relief, such as using fans, dressing in easy-to-peel-off layers and lowering the temperature in your bedroom. *Beyond that, try these additional strategies…*

•**Invest in newer high-tech bedding or nightwear.** These products include quick-drying or moisture-wicking sheets or pajamas and are available online.

Note: A device called BedJet includes a fan that is installed beneath the bed to blow cool (or warm) air into the bedding.

•**Freeze an icy gel pack during the day… and place it under your pillow at bedtime.** You can flip the pillow periodically during the night to sleep on the chilled side.

•**Try stress-busting techniques, such as acupuncture, meditation, deep breathing and/or yoga.**

Smart idea: Do these close to bedtime, when it's helpful to quiet down the nervous system prior to going to bed.

•**Consider taking vitamins and other supplements believed to combat night sweats.** These include B-complex vitamins, vitamin E, black cohosh, red clover and evening primrose oil.

Important: Get your doctor's advice on which supplement(s) would be most appropriate for you—some may interfere with medications you're taking.

•**Decrease sugar in your diet.** This advice is ideal for overall health, of course, but is believed to also reduce inflammation in the body, which may contribute to hot flashes and night sweats.

•**Ask your doctor about medications to battle night sweats if all else fails.** This may include off-label use of a low-dose antidepressant, such as *paroxetine* (Paxil)…or the blood pressure drug *clonidine* (Catapres).

Blue Light Accelerates Aging

Study by researchers at Oregon State University, Corvallis, published in *Aging and Mechanisms of Disease.*

Blue light from screens may accelerate aging. Fruit flies exposed to 12 hours of blue light and 12 hours of darkness lived significantly shorter lives than those kept in total darkness or exposed to light with blue wavelengths filtered out. Blue-light–exposed flies had damaged retinal cells and brain neurons and developed difficulty climbing the walls of their enclosures. Human blue-light exposure is increasing quickly through widespread use of LED lighting and electronic devices.

Car Exhaust Linked to Eye Damage

Suh-Hang Hank Juo, PhD, researcher, Graduate Institute of Biomedical Sciences, China Medical University, Taichung, Taiwan.

Recent finding: People exposed to high levels of the pollutants carbon monoxide or nitrogen dioxide, major components of automobile exhaust, were 84% and 91%, respectively, more likely to develop the potentially blinding condition age-related macular degeneration (AMD) than those exposed to the lowest levels, according to a study of nearly 40,000 men and women ages 50 and older.

If you live in a heavily trafficked area: Avoid the outdoors during peak traffic time.

Protecting Your Eyes in a Screen-Focused World

Marc Grossman, OD, LAc, doctor of optometry and licensed acupuncturist in New Paltz and Somers, New York. He is coauthor of *Natural Eye Care: Your Guide to Healthy Vision & Healing*. A holistic eye doctor, his multidisciplinary approach uses nutrition, lifestyle changes and Traditional Chinese Medicine to tackle eye problems. NaturalEyeCare.com

The good news is that, as part of the brain, our eyes share in our brain's innate adaptability. The not so great news is that modern demands on vision, especially our constant focus on close-up screens, is causing our eyes to make unhealthy adaptations. But there's more good news—you can do something about that! *Here's how…*

For millennia, humans spent most of their time focused on distance—such as scouting the horizon for dangerous predators, weather, food and shelter. Today, we spend our days primarily staring at objects only 18 inches (or less!) from our eyes—smartphones, tablets, iPads, e-books and the like. Constantly focusing on near objects and not looking off into the distance is a main cause of myopia (nearsightedness). And while wearing eyeglasses or contact lenses may seem like an easy solution, nearsightedness is about more than blurry distance vision.

Before the age of technology, nearsightedness was found primarily among professions that required a lot of reading, such as accountants, lawyers and college professors, and hardly ever found among, for instance, farmers. Now nearsightedness is reaching epidemic proportions. For example, in China and Japan up to 90% of students (teenagers and older) are nearsighted…while in parts of Africa and among other cultures that don't spend extended periods of time doing close work far fewer people are nearsighted.

WHY EYEGLASSES AREN'T THE ANSWER

Nearsightedness is associated with other ocular problems, such as higher risk for glaucoma, cataracts and macular degeneration…and increased likelihood of developing those conditions at an earlier age. There is evidence, in fact, that our near-focus habit is damaging our eye tissue and aging our eyes faster. Studies have linked computer overuse to glaucoma risk… while other research links exposure to blue light (the kind of light emitted by our electronic devices) to macular degeneration and cataracts.

Eyeglasses, contact lenses and surgery, including Lasik and PRK, can bring distant objects into focus, but these don't address the other ocular problems. *Technology is not going away, nor would we want it to…but following these 10 steps can keep your eyes healthier in a near-focused world…*

1. Use smartphones the smart way. Smartphones strain eyes more than do computer screens or tablets. Smartphones are typically held closer to eyes and the font is smaller, both of which concentrate focus, making eye muscles have to work harder.

Solution: Hold your phone as far away as you can to comfortably read the screen.

2. Get outdoors. Being outdoors changes what you're looking at (that is, not a screen and something farther away), and also gives you a chance to exercise your peripheral vision.

Tip: As you walk around, keep your eyes forward but maintain awareness of your whole visual field rather than focusing on a particular object. Do this effortlessly—don't strain!

3. Take breaks. Rest your eyes periodically by letting them wander and rest on the horizon.

Rule of thumb: For every 20 minutes of close work, rest two minutes…for every 30 minutes of close work, rest five minutes…and for every hour of close work, rest 10 minutes.

4. Blink, breathe…and smile! People unconsciously blink less and breathe more shallowly when looking at a screen. Your eyes need to blink to maintain a healthy tear film and protect against dry eye. Taking deep breaths keeps blood flowing so that sufficient oxygen gets to your eyes.

Try this: Blink rapidly six times…then close your eyes and take two slow, deep breaths. Repeat four times.

Easy way to prevent eyestrain: Make a small smile. When you smile you can't put strain on your eye muscles.

5. Try rose water. Rose water is especially good for your eyes, as it has a relaxing effect and helps tired eyes feel more hydrated. Spray rose water around your head and eyes (close your eyes first).

6. Watch TV from a safe distance. Ideally, the distance between your eyes and the screen should be at least seven times the width of the screen. For a 40-inch screen, that would be about 23 feet away. If the ideal distance isn't practical, even half that distance is still better than sitting two feet away from the screen.

7. Keep neck muscles loose. Tense muscles in the neck and shoulders can affect nerves at the back of the neck that lead to eye pain. Neck strain also can cause ocular headaches.

What helps: Do neck rolls, put warm compresses on your neck…and avoid hunched postures!

8. Avoid extremes of light/dark contrast. In darkness, your pupils dilate to let more light into your eyes so you can see better…and in bright light, the pupils contract to keep light out. When you look at a bright screen against a dark background it gives the eyes a mixed message. Try to keep screen brightness at 50% for smartphones, tablets, laptops and monitors. Avoid looking at brightly lit screens against total darkness—such as watching TV with all the lights turned off.

9. Lounge "consciously." Avoid slouching in bed or on the couch to watch TV, read or work on a laptop. Instead, sit up and have what you're focusing on at a comfortable level for your eyes—ideally 20 degrees below eye level. Use a lap desk to elevate a laptop, book or tablet.

10. Look up! Looking up from near work and into the distance relaxes your eyes' extraocular muscles (the muscles that move your eyes to the left, right, up and down) and ciliary muscles (which help the eyes to focus) and helps those muscles stay flexible.

Can You Treat Cataracts with an Eyedrop?

Marc Grossman, OD, LAc, doctor of optometry and licensed acupuncturist in New Paltz and Somers, New York. He is coauthor of *Natural Eye Care: Your Guide to Healthy Vision.* A holistic eye doctor, his multidisciplinary approach uses nutrition, lifestyle changes and Traditional Chinese Medicine to tackle eye problems. NaturalEyeCare.com

Cataract surgery is now so streamlined and commonplace, it can almost seem like an inevitable part of aging. However, the procedure isn't risk free—and some people can't have the surgery. Wouldn't it be wonderful if cataracts could be treated with something as simple as an eyedrop? That may be more than wishful thinking!

About 20% of people over age 60 and 80% over age 75 have cataracts. It's the leading cause of blindness worldwide, largely because cataract surgery, the only approved treatment, requires highly trained surgeons and high-tech surgical equipment that are not available in many parts of the world. In the US, however, cataract surgery is a simple, painless, outpatient procedure that is usually covered by insurance. (*Note*: Certain kinds of corrective implantable lenses may not be covered.) However, the procedure can have complications, especially for patients with other eye conditions, such as macular degeneration or glaucoma. Even without other eye conditions, while most of the time one procedure is sufficient, it's not uncommon to need additional surgeries to adjust vision.

CATARACTS 101

Cataracts form when oxidative stress—such as from sun exposure, diabetes, high blood pressure, smoking or simply aging—damages protein molecules in the lens of the eye, causing them to clump together. Normally, the protein molecules are arranged in a way that lets light pass through. When the molecules clump, they cloud areas of the lens…and as the clumps grow, larger areas of the lens cloud, making it harder and harder to see.

Antioxidants can reduce or prevent cell damage caused by oxidative stress. One antioxidant in particular, N-acetylcarnosine (NAC), is a strong antioxidant that occurs naturally in the heart, muscles and brain. Human studies have demonstrated that NAC eyedrops can improve cataracts.

WHAT THE RESEARCH SHOWS

Most of the research on NAC eyedrops for cataracts has been done in Russia, and the most impressive study comes from Helmholtz Research Institute of Eye Disorders in Moscow and was published in *Journal of Anti-Aging Medicine*. For the study, 49 patients (average age 65) with cataracts received either NAC eyedrops or placebo eyedrops twice daily. After 24 months, 90% of the NAC group had significant improvement in their cataracts...compared with significant progression of their cataracts in nearly 90% of the placebo group. The researchers found that adding an acetyl molecule to NAC allowed it to be absorbed through the front (anterior chamber) of the eye, where it could counteract oxidative stress in the eye lens.

The FDA will need more research, such as large studies, before approving NAC eyedrops for treating cataracts. However, eyedrops approved as moisturizing drops that contain 1% NAC, the same strength used in the study, are available now without prescription. People with cataracts—and some eye doctors—have been treating cataracts with the drops and reporting good results. Brands include Can-C, which contains the same formula that was used in the Russian trials, and OcluMed, which contains additional nutrients that are beneficial for treating cataracts.

SHOULD YOU TRY NAC EYEDROPS?

It's important to note that NAC drops are most effective for nuclear cataracts—age-related cataracts that form in the center of the lens—that are still at an early stage. The drops will not improve cataracts present at birth...subcapsular cataracts (cataracts that form at the back of the lens, often from diabetes or taking high doses of steroid medications)...or cortical cataracts (cataracts that form at the edges of the lens). While NAC drops may slightly improve advanced cataracts, they are unlikely to improve vision enough to avoid the need for surgery.

The usual treatment is one drop twice a day and can be continued as long as there is vision improvement. The only side effect experienced by some people is a few seconds of slight stinging when applying the drops, especially if eyes are dry. People who wear contact lenses should wait 15 minutes after applying the drops before putting on contacts.

Check with your eye doctor before using this or any other kind of eyedrops. As there are no known risks, medical condition warnings or other contraindications, NAC drops may be worth trying, particularly if your cataracts are at an early stage. If the drops are going to help, you should see an improvement within the first three months. Even if your cataracts aren't completely reversed, NAC drops may at least keep them from progressing...or slow their progression so that you can hold off longer on surgery. Taking oral supplements of glutathione, n-acetyl cysteine, alpha-lipoic acid and vitamin C also can help slow down the progression of cataracts.

Besides NAC eyedrops, remember that healthy vison also depends on a healthy lifestyle...

- **Don't smoke.**
- **Wear sunglasses.**
- **Eat plenty of fruits and vegetables to get more antioxidants.**
- **Work with your doctor to control diabetes and/or high blood pressure.**
- **Limit alcohol.**

Statins May Reduce Glaucoma Risk

Louis Pasquale, MD, site chair of the department of ophthalmology and professor of ophthalmology at Icahn School of Medicine at Mount Sinai Hospital, New York City, and coauthor of the study published in *JAMA Ophthalmology*. MountSinai.org

Glaucoma-free people age 40 and older who took statins for five years or longer were 21% less likely to develop the most common form of glaucoma than were people who never used statins. This might be due to statins' ability to affect enzymes that play a role in blood flow to the eye.

Help for Under-Eye Circles

The herb arnica can do more than just ease sore muscles and reduce bruises. Apply a thin swipe of arnica (gel or cream) under the eyes to combat puffiness and dark circles. *Caution:* Avoid getting it in your eyes.

Andrew Rubman, ND, founder and medical director, Southbury Clinic for Traditional Medicines, Southbury, Connecticut. SouthburyClinic.com

Natural Tricks for More Youthful Skin

Anthony Youn, MD, FACS, board-certified plastic surgeon. Named a "Top Plastic Surgeon" by U.S. News & World Report, Dr. Youn is assistant professor of surgery at Oakland University William Beaumont School of Medicine in Rochester, Michigan. He is author of *The Age Fix: A Leading Plastic Surgeon Reveals How to Really Look 10 Years Younger.* DrYoun.com

I am enthusiastic about the boost in self-esteem that patients gain from cosmetic surgery, but I encourage my patients to try preventive measures first and view surgery as a last resort. *A number of natural methods can delay or reduce wrinkling and other signs of aging of the face and body with techniques that not only are simple but also inexpensive...*

•**Train your muscles to contract less—without Botox.** Repeated contractions of the facial muscles lead to a creased appearance of the skin. I would never advise someone to smile or laugh less often—those lines are evidence of a life well-lived. But there is no reason to go out of your way to make repetitive movements you don't need. Repeatedly furrowing your brow, for example, etches lines over time.

Instead, do the opposite—train your muscles to contract less. Isolating the small muscles involved in forehead furrows, crow's feet or frown lines is challenging but gets easier with practice. If you ever learned to roll your tongue or flare your nostrils as a child, you already have experience in the type of concentration needed.

While breathing slowly and gently, imagine the muscles of your face softening and widening, even melting. Do this for one to two minutes at least five times a day and whenever you think of it.

Helpful: Frownies (available at Frownies. com or Amazon.com) are lightweight patches that you wear overnight or while relaxing at home to help smooth wrinkles. You stick the patch gently over the lines on your forehead or around your lips, and it acts as a kind of splint, preventing you from contracting those muscles. It also makes you more aware of what happens when you engage the small muscles, so that after a few weeks, you learn to contract them less, even when you are not wearing the patch.

Note: Working out your facial muscles will not stave off sagging and wrinkles. Aging faces droop because they are losing collagen and elastin—two proteins that are the skin's major building blocks—not from lack of exercise. In fact, overexercising your face can cause more wrinkles.

•**Sleep on your back.** You may have noticed creases on your face the morning after you slept on your stomach or your side. Skin creases are the result of gravity pulling your facial muscles downward as your skin presses against the pillow. Sleep wrinkles are temporary, but over months or years, repeated pressure from your face against the pillow can make these creases permanent, especially as the elastin in your skin diminishes with age, reducing its ability to "bounce back" to shape.

In contrast, when you sleep on your back, gravity works in your favor. If back-sleeping feels awkward, try using a cervical neck pillow to cradle your neck and keep your head gently in place. A memory foam mattress also may help you feel more comfortable by conforming to your body shape and providing extra support.

Important: Put a pillow under your knees to prevent lower-back strain.

If you cannot fall asleep on your back, invest in a silk pillowcase. They're available on Amazon.com for around $25. Silk doesn't cling to the skin the way cotton or synthetic fabrics do, so you will have less creasing.

An option for side sleepers is the JuveRest pillow, $160 (JuveRest.com). It is designed to reduce skin compression by minimizing contact with the face.

• **Lower the water temperature.** A long, hot shower or bath may feel comforting in the winter, but hot water dries out the skin, whether you are bathing or washing your face. Keep water lukewarm, and don't stay in too long.

• **Lighten sunspots with homemade lemon-juice ointment.** Dark spots from sun exposure on the hands, face and arms will make anyone look older. To lighten those spots, mix equal parts soy milk, lemon juice and honey. The mixture should have a pasty consistency so that it does not drip when applied to your face and body. Apply the mixture to your skin, and leave it on for 20 to 30 minutes. Rinse off with lukewarm water. Use daily until you see improvement.

Why it works: Lemon juice contains citric acid, a natural skin lightener, while proteins in soy milk inhibit the skin's production of the darkening pigment melanin. Honey binds the two ingredients and is a good moisturizer.

Important: Soy milk spoils quickly, so only mix as much of this blend as you will use right away. Start with one teaspoon of each. Note that lemon juice can irritate skin and cause photosensitivity, so wear sunscreen.

• **Wear sunglasses—even on winter days.** You know you should wear sunscreen to protect your skin from premature aging and skin cancer, but your eyes are at risk, too, and the skin around your eyes is too delicate for sunscreen. Protect the area with sunglasses that filter out UVA and UVB rays. By keeping you from squinting, sunglasses—especially those with wraparound frames—also delay and reduce wrinkling.

• **Smooth out crow's feet with a mayonnaise mask.** For a quick eye-lift, use your fingers or a cotton ball to apply a small amount of mayonnaise to your crow's feet. After 30 minutes, wash off gently with lukewarm water. Apply in the morning to look better all day.

Why it works: Mayonnaise contains eggs and oil. The albumin in eggs tightens skin almost immediately, and oil moisturizes it. This treatment won't banish crow's feet forever, but it will make a noticeable difference for a day or so.

• **Mix your own chemical peel at home.** Chemical peels refresh the skin's appearance by removing the top layer of dead or dying skin cells and stimulating the body to produce new cells more quickly. Older skin looks duller than younger skin because this natural process of skin-cell turnover simply slows down with age.

Instead of going to the doctor's office for costly chemical peels, create your own gentle exfoliant by mixing three tablespoons of apple juice, two tablespoons of milk and one egg white. Apply the mixture to your face, and gently rinse off with water after 15 minutes.

Why it works: The malic acid in apple juice and the lactic acid in milk help to remove dead skin. Egg white tightens the skin.

Caution: Exfoliating too often irritates skin and can cause it to age faster, so don't do it every day. If you have normal skin, you can apply this treatment two or three times a week. If your skin is sensitive or if you notice redness after the treatment, don't exfoliate more than once a week.

• **Avoid foods that age you.** One of the worst offenders is sugar, including refined starches such as white bread and white rice, which turn to sugar. Sugar molecules bind to collagen and elastin through a process called glycation, making these skin proteins stiffer and leading to premature wrinkles and sagging. Although avoiding sugar can't reverse damage that has already occurred, it can help slow further aging.

The other major offender is fat—specifically, saturated and trans fats, which increase inflammation. Opt for monosaturated fats, found in olive oil and most nuts, and for omega-3 fatty acids, found in salmon and other cold-water fish, flaxseed and tofu. Over time, these fats calm inflammation and improve the skin's elasticity, and they even may reduce the damage from sun exposure.

Note: You also can add a collagen supplement to your daily regimen.

Your Blood Could Combat Hair Loss

Amelia K. Hausauer, MD, director of dermatology at Aesthetx, a plastic surgery and dermatology practice, Campbell, California, and lead author of a study published in *Dermatologic Surgery*. Aesthetx.com

Platelet-rich plasma therapy is an established treatment for joint injuries—platelets from patients' blood are injected into joints.

Recent finding: When platelets are injected into the scalp, hair regrows, particularly when treatments begin within five years of hair-loss onset. Treatments are performed monthly for three months, then every three to six months thereafter and cost around $1,000 each.

Beyond Wrinkles... Top Treatments for Thinning Skin

Abigail Waldman, MD, instructor of dermatology at Brigham and Women's Hospital and Harvard Medical School, both in Boston. She is also director of Mohs surgery at VA Boston Healthcare System.

Wrinkles may get most of the attention, but thinning skin is another age-related skin issue you'll want to pay attention to. Thinning skin not only makes you look older but can cause other skin problems as well.

Fortunately, there are some exciting new advances as well as some effective well-established treatments that can help make your skin thicker and restore its smoothness and elasticity.

WHY SKIN GETS THIN

Skin is composed of a scaffold called the extracellular matrix, which is made up of proteins including collagen and elastin. This matrix is what gives durability and resilience to skin, allowing it to "snap back" and keeping it from being easily damaged.

As we age, some of the components that make up the extracellular matrix break down. Eventually, fibroblast cells within the skin no longer make enough collagen...and the old, "worn out" proteins that make up the extracellular matrix don't get replaced. The result is skin that is thinner and more fragile, which can look saggy, crepey and wrinkled, especially on the face and hands.

SUN EXPOSURE, GENDER AND MORE

In addition to age, a main cause of thinning skin is UV radiation from sun exposure. UV radiation causes oxidative damage to DNA, skin proteins and the extracellular matrix. People who have had a lot of sun exposure are at increased risk of having thinner skin at an earlier age.

At greater risk: People with very pale skin have less protection from UV radiation, so they are more susceptible to thinning skin. Smoking—another powerful source of oxidative damage—also increases the risk for thin skin.

At less risk: On average, men's skin is thicker than women's because men have a higher testosterone-to-estrogen ratio, which helps stimulate collagen production and other skin proteins. So while men's skin is susceptible to the same factors as women's skin, it will take longer to be affected.

Risky medication: Prescription-strength topical corticosteroid creams also can thin the skin where they're applied, and long-term use of oral steroids can cause thinning as well—and the thinning can be permanent. Areas of special concern are places where the skin is already thin, such as the face, or areas that absorb medication more easily, such as in the armpits or groin. Always follow a doctor's instructions when using a prescription corticosteroid.

Note: Over-the-counter (OTC) hydrocortisone cream is generally safe and not a risk for thinning skin.

TO IMPROVE THE LOOK OF YOUR SKIN

While you can't regain the skin of your 20s, there are more options than ever for turning back the clock...

My top advice: Hydrate! The outer layer of skin (the stratum corneum) acts as a kind of brick wall to prevent water from leaving the body. As we get older—and if you have skin damage from the sun or cigarette smoking—

that brick wall gets holes in it, which makes it harder for the skin to retain moisture, resulting in a dry, sallow appearance.

Water is the best all-around hydrator, but any liquid you drink counts, even coffee and tea. It's a myth that the diuretic effect of caffeine offsets hydration. Of course, you'll want to avoid soda and other sweet drinks.

To help trap water in skin, I advise an emollient ointment, such as petroleum jelly or Aquaphor (if you prefer not to use a petroleum-based ointment, look for a glycerin-based ointment)…or a product that contains hyaluronic acid, a natural compound that preserves moisture. Many drugstore products containing hyaluronic acid (such as Neutrogena Hydro Boost Water Gel) are as effective as more expensive creams.

•**Use this topical, cream, serum and/or supplement.** As with any skin-care regimen, the key is consistency and patience. Your skin didn't thin overnight—it could take weeks or even months before you see a difference when using these therapies…

Topical retinoids are chemical compounds derived from vitamin A. They have been shown to boost the activity of the extracellular matrix, increasing production of collagen and elastin and making the skin measurably thicker. Topical retinoids are available by prescription or OTC (Retinol).

Note: A retinoid can cause irritation, so begin by using it for just two to three nights per week until the skin adjusts.

Glycolic acid creams and vitamin C serums increase collagen by combating oxidative stress. Many OTC creams and face washes contain glycolic acid, including Glytone. For vitamin C serums, look for brands that contain vitamins C and E and ferulic acid.

Note: Use these products in the morning if you are also using a retinoid, as the combination can be irritating.

Newest treatment: Nicotinamide, a form of vitamin B-3. Research has shown that nicotinamide can actually reverse sun damage that causes skin cancer. A typical dose to combat skin damage from UV radiation is 500 mg of OTC nicotinamide, taken orally, twice a day.

Check with your doctor before taking this (or any) supplement.

•**Try skin treatments.** There are a wide variety of treatments available to help thinning skin. A board-certified dermatologist or plastic surgeon can evaluate your condition and recommend the most appropriate treatment based on your skin and discuss possible risks. Some treatments could be painful, so pain medication or anesthesia may be advised, and you may require more than one treatment to achieve desired results. All treatments should be performed by or under the supervision of a board-certified dermatologist or plastic surgeon.* *Examples…*

•Laser treatments use pulses of light to remove damaged skin, correct imperfections and stimulate production of collagen. Different lasers and frequencies are used for different problems. For example, some lasers target areas of skin discoloration…others correct surface wrinkling…and others penetrate more deeply to correct heavy wrinkles.

•Microneedling works to stimulate collagen production via tiny needles that poke minuscule holes in the skin.

•Ultrasound uses high-frequency sound waves to boost collagen. The result is tighter skin in areas where the ultrasound is used.

•**Guard against injury.** People who have thin skin do tend to bruise more easily, especially on the tops of the hands. The greatest risk is when the fragile skin tears open, leaving it vulnerable to infection. These tears should not be covered with an adhesive bandage—removing it may cause more injury. Instead, I advise applying an emollient ointment several times a day to keep the tear moist until it heals.

•**Wear sunscreen.** To avoid further sun damage, be sure to use a sunscreen with an SPF of at least 30 every day…and wear a wide-brimmed hat when outdoors. Also, avoid being out in the sun during the warmest part of the day (10 am to 2 pm).

*Check with your doctor for costs—they will vary depending on your location.

The Truth About Body-Sculpting Treatments

Anthony Youn, MD, FACS, board-certified plastic surgeon and assistant professor of surgery at Oakland University Beaumont School of Medicine, Rochester, Michigan. He is author of *The Age Fix*. DrYoun.com

As we age, some pockets of fat on the body are extremely difficult to eliminate—even with a very healthy lifestyle. Noninvasive treatments such as CoolSculpting and SculpSure promise fat loss in specific areas without dieting, exercise or surgery, and in my experience, they generally do provide modest results.

Both are FDA-approved for basically the same areas—the abdomen, including "love handles," inner and outer thighs, back and double chin—and in studies have been shown to reduce fat by about 25%. With CoolSculpting, an applicator freezes fat cells underneath the skin…and with SculpSure, a laser (heat) disrupts fat cells. In both treatments, the fat cells are naturally eliminated from the body.

These procedures can be mildly uncomfortable but are not typically painful. Swelling and/or bruising is common afterward, but goes away quickly. To date, few serious side effects have been reported. It costs about $1,500 to $3,000 for either treatment, depending on where you live in the US, and it takes about a half hour.

Note: SculpSure can treat up to four small areas at the same time.

It can take two to three months to see the final result, but the result should be permanent provided the patient maintains a healthy lifestyle.

Consult a board-certified plastic surgeon to see if you're a good candidate. Treatments should be performed by a trained technician who could be a doctor, nurse or aesthetician.

Keto Diets Are Risky for Older People

Roundup of experts on diet, reported at AARP.org.

Keto diets can deprive the body of the protein it needs to build and maintain muscle mass. The diets often limit protein to 15% of calories consumed, with the rest of the diet consisting of about 75% fat and 10% carbs. But older people tend to need more protein than these diets allow to avoid frailty, falls and fractures. Keto diets also have effects on people of all ages that may be more serious for older adults, including increasing risk for kidney stones, renal damage and elevated LDL cholesterol. The diets can be difficult to maintain—even with professional assistance, half the people using a keto diet to fight diabetes dropped out within a year. And the evidence of whether the diets work is inconclusive.

CHAPTER 2

Brain Health

Beware of Popular Drugs Linked to Dementia

If there were more than 50 prescription and over-the-counter (OTC) medications that had been linked to an increased risk for Alzheimer's disease and other related dementias, you'd think that everyone would avoid those drugs—especially when safer alternatives are often available. But that's not happening.

Sobering new finding: When medications known as anticholinergics are taken for three or more years, previous research has linked them to about a 50% higher risk for dementia, but a new finding shows that these medications are still being widely used to treat conditions ranging from the common cold, allergies and incontinence to Parkinson's disease, motion sickness and muscle pain. *To protect yourself and your loved ones...*

WHAT ARE ANTICHOLINERGICS?

More than 10 million Americans, age 65 and older, use anticholinergic drugs. The medications block the action of acetylcholine, a neurotransmitter (brain chemical) that activates many key body functions involving muscles, the heart, digestive system, lungs, urinary tract and blood vessels. These drugs, which include medications from various drug classes, also have effects on the brain and are used to treat dizziness, nausea, epilepsy and depression.

Well-documented side effects from these drugs include dry mouth and constipation. Because these medications also affect the brain, they can cause confusion and memory loss. Older adults are at highest risk for dementia from these drugs because they tend to take

Malaz Boustani, MD, MPH, Richard M. Fairbanks Professor of Aging Research at Indiana University School of Medicine in Indianapolis and research scientist at the Regenstrief Institute, Regenstrief.org, an Indianapolis-based research organization that focuses on informatics and health-care research. Dr. Boustani created and validated the Anticholinergic Cognitive Burden (ACB) Scale.

more of them than younger adults. Older adults also are at increased risk for dementia due to their age—in part, because acetylcholine production declines as people grow older.

NEW STUDY SOUNDS THE ALARM

In the study mentioned earlier, which was published in *JAMA Internal Medicine*, the medical records of about 225,000 patients (ages 55 to 100) who had not been diagnosed with dementia were compared with those of about 60,000 dementia patients to see how many in each group had taken a prescription-strength anticholinergic drug during an 11-year period.

The researchers found that 57% of the dementia patients and 51% of the non-dementia patients had been prescribed at least one of the 56 anticholinergic drugs included in the study. The most commonly used drugs were prescribed to treat depression, dizziness, nausea, vomiting and bladder spasms. *Other key findings…*

•**Greater exposure, bigger risk.** Patients who took an anticholinergic on a daily basis for three years had a 49% higher risk of being diagnosed with dementia than patients with no exposure. Those who took one of the drugs for less than three months had a 6% increased risk.

•**Some drugs are riskier than others.** The highest-risk anticholinergics included antipsychotics, such as *olanzapine* (Zyprexa) or *quetiapine* (Seroquel)…overactive bladder medications, including *tolterodine* (Detrol) and *oxybutynin* (Ditropan)…anti-parkinsonian drugs, such as *benztropine* (Cogentin)…antiepileptics, including *carbamazepine* (Tegretol) and *oxcarbazepine* (Trileptal)…and antidepressants, such as *amitriptyline* (Elavil) and *paroxetine* (Paxil).

Even though these findings are observational (that is, they do not prove cause and effect), they are consistent with earlier research. For this reason, the researchers recommend that doctors carefully weigh the risks and benefits of prescribing these drugs for patients who are middle-aged and older and strongly urge the use of other effective drugs, that are not anticholinergics, whenever possible.

Omega-3 Boosts B Vitamins for the Brain

Take an omega-3 supplement to boost B-vitamins' brain benefits.

Background: People with high blood levels of the amino acid homocysteine are at increased risk for Alzheimer's disease.

An underreported finding: In the VITA-COG study, people who took homocysteine-lowering B vitamins (B-12, folate and B-6) for two years had less brain atrophy and slower cognitive decline—but only if they had adequate blood levels of omega-3.

If you're concerned about cognitive decline and have elevated homocysteine: Ask your doctor about taking an omega-3 supplement along with a B-complex.

Richard Podell, MD, MPH, clinical professor, Rutgers Robert Wood Johnson Medical School, New Brunswick, New Jersey.

WHAT SHOULD YOU DO?

To avoid the potential harms of anticholinergics, you should know which medications have been linked to the greatest dementia risk.

To get a clearer picture of the risk associated with the most widely used anticholinergic drugs on the market, consult the Anticholinergic Cognitive Burden (ACB) Scale, which ranks both prescription and OTC anticholinergic drugs, according to their degree of risk (see page 38).

If you are taking a prescription drug that appears on the list, talk to your doctor. Ask if you can stop taking the drug…or if there is a suitable substitute that is safer for you. For example, if you are taking an antidepressant on the ACB Scale, *sertraline* (Zoloft) or *citalopram* (Celexa) may be a safer choice, since each has minimal anticholinergic effects.

Caution: Never stop taking a medication that your doctor has prescribed without consulting him/her.

It's also worth noting that many OTC anticholinergics are considered high risk. Among the most widely used are the antihistamines *diphenhydramine* (Benadryl) and *chlorpheniramine* (Chlor-Trimeton)…the cold and allergy medicine *brompheniramine-PPA* (Dimetapp)… and the motion-sickness drug *dimenhydrinate* (Dramamine).

If you take an OTC anticholinergic frequently (one pill for 60 days in a 12-month period), ask your doctor or pharmacist if you really need it. You can also ask if there is a substitute drug that is not an anticholinergic.

Important: Dementia risk linked to these drugs is added to any other risk factors you may have, such as older age…high blood pressure…diabetes…inactivity…a family history of dementia…and smoking. For this reason, your entire risk profile should be considered when discussing the use of these drugs with your doctor.

Mushrooms: The Brain Food That Fights Dementia

Study titled "The Association between Mushroom Consumption and Mild Cognitive Impairment: A Community-Based Cross-Sectional Study in Singapore" by researchers at the National University of Singapore, published in *Journal of Alzheimer's Disease.*

B lueberries, salmon, walnuts and other well-known brain-healthy foods are the go-to foods for people who want to keep their minds sharp.

But there's another food that should be added to that list, according to a study published in *Journal of Alzheimer's Disease.*

"It seems that a commonly available single ingredient could have a dramatic effect on cognitive decline," said Lei Feng, MD, PhD, lead author of the study and assistant professor in the department of psychological medicine at the National University of Singapore.

WHAT IS THIS BRAIN-FRIENDLY FARE? IT'S MUSHROOMS!

Here's how the research unfolded…

In the first phase of the six-year study, scientists gave 663 adults, age 60 and older, neuropsychological tests to assess whether they showed any mild cognitive impairment (MCI), a form of cognitive decline—beyond normal aging—that often progresses to Alzheimer's disease.

The study participants were also interviewed to find out about their medical history, lifestyle and dietary habits. When the testing was complete, the researchers collated the data to determine whether there were any associations between MCI and consumption of mushrooms.

The researchers were particularly interested in the study participants' intake of mushrooms because an earlier study had found that people with MCI have significantly lower levels of an amino acid known as *ergothioneine* (ET), whose mainly dietary source is—you guessed it!—mushrooms.

Study findings: The participants who ate more than two servings (a total of one-and-a-half cups) of cooked mushrooms each week were half as likely to have MCI as those who ate them less than once a week. This association was independent of age, gender, physical and social activities, and other medical conditions. The mushrooms identified in the study were golden, oyster, shiitake and white button mushrooms, as well as dried and canned mushrooms.

Good news: Even one ¾-cup portion of mushrooms per week contributed to better brain health in this study.

ET is a specific compound found in almost every type of mushroom. It has anti-inflammatory and antioxidant properties that seem to promote brain health. In addition, there are other phytonutrients in mushrooms that may play a role in preventing cognitive decline, so the authors plan to test additional compounds found in mushrooms to determine which ones have a positive effect. That way, they may be able to identify other foods that have the same benefits as mushrooms on the aging brain.

Bottom line: Because MCI has been shown to increase risk for Alzheimer's disease, a simple dietary habit, such as consuming mushrooms, is a smart move. They are low-calorie, low-fat and delicious. To help your brain age like a champ's, consider adding button mushrooms to a pizza…shiitakes to a stir-fry…or whatever mushroom dish strikes your fancy.

Caution: Do not eat wild mushrooms unless they have been approved by a mushroom-identification expert, warns the National Capital

Poison Center. Mushroom poisoning is common—and can be fatal.

Test for Alzheimer's

Nature Medicine

Alzheimer's disease could be predicted up to 16 years before symptoms occur with a new blood test.

Implication: The experimental test detects a protein that's released by damaged neurons and could identify people who will develop clinical symptoms.

How Gum Disease Is Linked to Alzheimer's

Sim Singhrao, PhD, senior research fellow, School of Dentistry, University of Central Lancashire, UK.
Study titled "Porphyromonas gingivalis in Alzheimer's disease brains: Evidence for disease causation and treatment with small-molecule inhibitors," by researchers at Cortexyme, Inc., South San Francisco, Jagiellonian University, Poland, et al., published in *Science Advance*s.

Finding the cause of Alzheimer's—and hopefully, a cure—has long seemed like the search for the Holy Grail. But new breakthrough research may be uncovering a critical clue to this debilitating neurodegenerative disease.

Hint: The elusive clue may be hiding in our mouths.

Researchers have suspected that brain infection is at the root of Alzheimer's disease. For one thing, people who have died with the disease show inflammation in their brains similar to the kind caused by infection. People with Alzheimer's also frequently have chronic periodontitis, a gum infection, which is known to also affect other parts of the body, such as the heart. But it has not been clear whether gum disease causes Alzheimer's...or if the poor oral hygiene common among Alzheimer's patients causes gum disease.

In a new study, researchers from the US, Europe, New Zealand and Australia looked for *Porphyromonas gingivalis*, a bacterium that causes gum disease, and toxins released by P. gingivalis in brain samples from people who had died with Alzheimer's.

They found the toxins in nearly all (up to 99%) of the brain samples...with the highest concentrations in samples that had the most beta-amyloid plaques and tau tangles, classic hallmarks of Alzheimer's.

The researchers had also looked at brain samples from people without Alzheimer's and found that while some had P. gingivalis and beta-amyloid proteins, they were at low levels. Since plaques and tau tangles accumulate in the brain for years before Alzheimer's symptoms appear, the new research may have found the evidence that P. gingivalis may cause Alzheimer's...rather than be the result of the disease.

To test that theory, the researchers gave P. gingivalis gum infections to mice—and found that the infection did spread to their brains... and also led to beta-amyloid plaques, tau tangles and neurodegeneration similar to what is seen in brains with Alzheimer's.

While these findings are exciting and potentially a major breakthrough, Alzheimer's is a complex disease. For instance, there is evidence that genes may play a role in development of the disease. Many questions remain unanswered and more research is needed to fully understand these new results and how best to use them.

Promising: This study, which was sponsored by Cortexyme, a San Francisco–based biotech company, also looked at whether it was possible to block the toxic effects of P. gingivalis. They found that antibiotics, a common treatment for people who have gum infections, had no effect on brain infection in the mice. But an oral drug the researchers developed specifically for the study not only blocked the gingipain toxins—it also halted the brain degeneration. The drug specifically inhibits the different types of gingipains enzymes secreted by P. gingivalis by irreversibly binding to the active catalytic site of the gingipains enzymes, permanently inhibiting their activity. Phase 2 and 3 clinical trials to test the drug on people with mild to moderate Alzheimer's are ongoing..

In the meantime, it doesn't hurt to be vigilant about oral hygiene. Not only will your teeth thank you, so will the rest of your body—and you just may be protecting your brain from getting Alzheimer's.

Dementia May Be Linked to Marital Status

Married people are less likely to develop dementia as they age—and divorced people are twice as likely as others to develop the condition. Divorced men are at even greater risk than divorced women.

Hui Liu, PhD, professor of sociology, Michigan State University, East Lansing, and leader of an analysis of more than 15,000 people, published in *Journals of Gerontology: Series B*.

A New Early Symptom of Alzheimer's Disease?

Daniel Z. Press, MD, associate professor of neurology at Harvard Medical School, and a specialist in cognitive neurology at Beth Israel Deaconess Medical Center, both in Boston. His research has been published in *Neurology, Journal of Alzheimer's Disease* and other leading medical journals.

Even though a seizure can be caused by conditions ranging from drug or alcohol withdrawal to stroke, most people associate this surge of electrical activity in the brain with epilepsy.

Now: An increasing body of scientific evidence links seizure activity to Alzheimer's disease. This area of research is so important that it was a major focus of the 2019 Alzheimer's Association International Conference (AAIC) in Los Angeles.

With estimates showing that up to 16 million Americans will be diagnosed with Alzheimer's disease by 2050—and still no cure or effective therapy to slow it down—researchers hope that early treatment of seizure activity may offer a new way to stop the progression of this relentless disease.

What you need to know...

A DIFFERENT TYPE OF SEIZURE

Seizures occur in about 10% to 22% of people with Alzheimer's, according to research published in *JAMA Neurology.* These seizures are often less dramatic than commonly known seizures that involve erratic movements and loss of consciousness (see next page).

In Alzheimer's patients who have seizures, their symptoms, including the classic loss of memory and other mental abilities, known as cognitive impairment, are typically more severe.

Cognitive impairment also may occur about five to seven years earlier in these people than in those with Alzheimer's and no seizures. In individuals with early-onset Alzheimer's, for example, which can begin in one's 50s, the likelihood of having seizures is more than 25%.

At the AAIC, research was presented showing that seizures can occur even before other cognitive impairment symptoms are noticeable. For example, a study of close to 300,000 US veterans found that vets over age 55 who had a first seizure had twice the risk of developing Alzheimer's disease within nine years. This research had not been published at the time that it was presented at the AAIC.

Other studies presented at the conference found that...

•**Alzheimer's patients are over six times more likely to have seizures than older adults without Alzheimer's.**

•**Alzheimer's seizures are more likely to be recurrent.** Two-thirds of patients have a second seizure within eight months.

•**The longer a person has Alzheimer's disease, the higher the risk for seizures.**

A TRIGGER OR A SYMPTOM?

Even though the most recent research suggests that seizures can occur before Alzheimer's disease symptoms become apparent, it's not clear whether the seizure is a trigger, a symptom or a risk factor for a more accelerated form of Alzheimer's. It is known, however, that the accumulation of abnormal proteins called amyloid plaques and tau tangles in the brains of people with Alzheimer's destroy brain cells—and loss of brain cells can lead to abnormal brain activity and seizures.

Interestingly, even before seizures develop, 42% of people with Alzheimer's disease (some of whom did not have apparent memory problems) had abnormal brain waves detectable on an electroencephalogram (EEG), known as subclinical epileptic activity, versus 10% of study participants without Alzheimer's, according to research published in *Annals of Neurology*.

As scientists try to sort out the role that seizures play in people with Alzheimer's, the best explanation for now is that the abnormal brain waves of preclinical epilepsy are an early result of Alzheimer's disease. These changes can lead to seizures that cause more damage and speed up the progression of Alzheimer's. As Alzheimer's worsens, it can lead to more seizures…and more damage—in short, a vicious cycle.

WHAT SHOULD YOU DO?

If you or a loved one has early-stage Alzheimer's—or a diagnosis of mild cognitive impairment (which may become Alzheimer's)—be on the lookout for any seizure activity. These seizures, especially the early ones, may not be the classic grand mal type of epileptic seizure, usually marked by a fall, loss of consciousness and uncontrollable muscle jerking.

Instead, it may be a type of seizure called a partial seizure, which is easy to miss. This type of seizure may be just a brief period (a few minutes) of staring off into space…being confused or unresponsive…fumbling…stumbling…or losing the ability to speak.

Any such behavior should be reported to your primary care physician. An EEG may show abnormal brain waves that indicate seizure activity. If this is the case, a neurologist can be consulted, and antiseizure medication may be prescribed.

Important: Because there are many causes of seizures, any type of seizure activity in an older adult (with or without Alzheimer's) needs to be evaluated. Don't assume that a seizure in an older person means a future diagnosis of Alzheimer's disease.

Currently, there is no evidence that treating a new seizure in a person without Alzheimer's will stop the disease from developing. However, researchers say that any patient with Alzheimer's who has a seizure should be treated, since seizures may make the disease worse.

Promising treatment: A study led by researchers at Beth Israel Deaconess Medical Center (BIDMC) in Boston and published in *Journal of Alzheimer's Disease* found that brain wave activity returned to a more normal pattern in early-stage Alzheimer's patients with subclinical epileptic activity who received a single dose of the antiseizure drug *levetiracetam* (Keppra). Their cognitive function did not improve, but this was not expected after a single treatment.

The BIDMC researchers have received funding from the National Institutes of Health to conduct a larger and longer study in which they hope to find that treating preclinical epilepsy will not only restore normal brain waves but improve or delay cognitive decline. In past studies, levetiracetam and another antiseizure drug, *lamotrigine* (Lamictal), were found to be more effective at controlling Alzheimer's seizures than *phenytoin* (Dilantin) and other older antiepileptic drugs.

Bottom line: Any seizure in a person with Alzheimer's disease should be recognized and treated. Future studies should tell us if treating seizure activity can alter the course of Alzheimer's—something that would be a big breakthrough for this baffling disease. Levetiracetam is currently the best established therapy for seizures in people with Alzheimer's disease.

Another Early Sign of Alzheimer's…

Patricia A. Boyle, PhD, neuropsychologist, is associate professor of behavioral sciences at the Rush Alzheimer's Disease Center, Rush University Medical Center, Chicago, and lead author of a study published in *Annals of Internal Medicine*.

Susceptibility to scams may be an early sign of Alzheimer's disease and cognitive impairment. Scam awareness taps into a number of complex behaviors such as the ability to detect fraud, evaluate an offer and manage emotions under pressure. Seniors who have difficulty detecting scams should consider a clinical assessment for Alzheimer's and cognitive impairment, particularly if other changes, such as difficulty managing finances, are present.

Tests Rule Out Alzheimer's

D.P. Devanand, MD, professor of psychiatry and neurology, Columbia University Vagelos College of Physicians and Surgeons, New York City.

When 749 men and women, ages 70 to 83, with mild cognitive impairment (MCI) took a test that measures cognition and a test that assesses the ability to identify odors, nearly all (96.5%) who performed well on both tests did not develop dementia over the next four years.

Implication: These assessments, typically used to predict dementia risk, could help older adults with MCI avoid further invasive and expensive diagnostic tests.

Surprising Headache Link to Alzheimer's

Suzanne Tyas, PhD, associate professor, School of Public Health and Health Systems, University of Waterloo, Ontario, Canada. She is coauthor of the study titled "Migraine and the risk of all-cause dementia, Alzheimer's disease, and vascular dementia: A prospective cohort study in community-dwelling older adults," published in *International Journal of Geriatric Psychiatry.*

We know a lot more than we used to about dementia, which currently affects about 5.8 million Americans. But we still do not have a way to accurately predict who will get it. Now, a new study has found that having a certain type of headache may be a clue to increased risk—especially for Alzheimer's disease. *Here's what you need to know...and what you should do if you get these headaches.*

Dementia is the most common neurological condition in older adults...while headaches are the most common neurological condition in people of all ages. Considering how common both conditions are, researchers from University of Waterloo in Ontario, Canada, wanted to see if there was a link.

Study: The researchers looked at a severe form of headache, migraines, and dementia among 679 men and women (62% of them were women) age 65 and older who had participated in a long-term study on healthy aging. The data included history of migraine, as well as other factors associated with dementia risk. The participants had no memory problems at the start of the study. The researchers then followed the participants for five years, checking for various forms of dementia, including vascular dementia (dementia that occurs as vessels that supply blood to the brain become blocked, such as following a stroke) and Alzheimer's disease.

Results: 51 participants were diagnosed with dementia over the study period. Those who had reported a history of migraines were three times more likely to be diagnosed with any type of dementia...and four times more likely to have Alzheimer's disease, after considering the effects of age, education, gender, depression, diabetes and cardiovascular conditions such as high blood pressure, stroke and heart attack. However, the association was found only among women, because no men in the study had both migraines and dementia. Migraines and dementia are more common in women. The study authors say larger studies are thus needed to further examine the migraine/ dementia association among men.

The researchers also had expected to find a strong association between vascular dementia and migraines, which is considered a vascular condition—blood vessel swelling in the brain is thought to drive the pain. However, no association was found, suggesting that another pathway may be involved in the development of dementia.

WHAT THIS MEANS

If further research confirms that migraine history is a risk factor for Alzheimer's disease, it may pave the way toward earlier diagnosis and enhanced prevention efforts, the researchers hope. For instance, doctors may want to screen earlier for signs of cognitive decline in people with a history of migraines in order to treat other risk factors for Alzheimer's disease more aggressively.

Meanwhile, if you have a history of migraines, it might be worth mentioning this research to your doctor. And whether or not you have migraines, it doesn't hurt to keep up healthy, brain-protecting activities, such as staying physically and mentally active and socially engaged…eating a healthy diet…and managing health conditions such as high blood pressure and diabetes that put your brain at risk. If it's good for your heart, it's also good for your brain!

Age-Related Memory Decline Reversed

Robert Reinhart, PhD, assistant professor, department of psychological and brain sciences, is director of Visual Cognitive Neuroscience Laboratory, Boston University.

Age-related memory decline can be temporarily reversed through electrical stimulation.

Preliminary study: People in their 60s and 70s given 25 minutes of extremely low-powered electrical current through a skullcap performed as well on tests of working memory as people in their 20s. The current temporarily resynchronizes parts of the aging brain that no longer communicate well. Preliminary data suggest it can boost long-term memory. This therapy is not yet available.

To Improve Your Memory, Declutter Your Brain

Maureen K. O'Connor, PsyD, assistant professor of neurology at Boston University and director of neuropsychology at Bedford Veterans Affairs Medical Center. She is coauthor, with Andrew E. Budson, MD, of *Seven Steps to Managing Your Memory: What's Normal, What's Not, and What to Do About It.*

If you have always prided yourself on having an excellent memory, chances are you don't make a shopping list or put that weekend dinner with a friend on a calendar. You simply point to your forehead and say, "It's all in here."

Even though this might feel like a good way to continually test your memory, you're likely missing out on more than just an occasional forgotten quart of milk.

People who don't use simple memory aids—everything from handwritten lists to new-fangled phone apps—forgo a key strategy that's embraced by most highly accomplished people. You also are "cluttering" that wonderful brain of yours with a lot of stuff that could be kept elsewhere.

Some people are reluctant to use lists, schedules, alarms and other aids because they think it will make their brains lazy. But that's not true! Using memory aids can, in fact, help reduce the stress and annoyance that inevitably come from age-related memory errors.

Memory aids also can help you establish lifelong habits that will make a big difference when you experience those normal age-related memory lapses, such as losing things from time to time or sometimes forgetting which word to use.

These changes happen to everyone—including people who never develop Alzheimer's disease or other serious memory disorders. What's interesting, though, is that people who use memory aids handle those little memory glitches more easily.

6 TOP MEMORY AIDS

Memory aids to choose from…

•**Keep a notebook.** Get a small notebook that you can slip into a pocket or carry in a handbag to jot down grocery lists…questions for your doctor or accountant…and information you get at an appointment or meeting.

Smart strategy: Use a note-taking app on your smartphone.

•**Rely on technology.** In addition to apps, smartphones have built-in features that are easy to use and do wonders to support your memory.

Smart strategy: If you're out running errands and remember something you need to do the minute you get home, call your landline from your cell phone and leave yourself a message. If you use the calendar on your smartphone, ask for alerts a day, an hour or a few minutes before an appointment or phone call.

You can use your phone's alarm feature or timer to remind you to check the cookies in the oven or the wet laundry in the washer. You can even label the alarms you set as "meeting" or customize them for specific tasks (such as "take out neighbor's garbage can").

Also helpful: Your phone's camera is a memory aid, too—use it to take a picture of the street sign near your parking space before walking away from your car.

•**Create a memory table (or bowl or basket).** This is where you toss your keys when you walk in the door—and find them when you go out again. It's also a good spot for the bills you want to mail in the morning and the book you want to return to your neighbor.

Smart strategy: Put a memory table, bowl or basket near the door you use to leave and enter the house. Some people like to pair it with a hook for their keys and a wastebasket for incoming promotional mail.

Important: It will defeat the purpose if you allow this area to become cluttered—it should be a temporary landing spot for a few small essential items.

Also helpful: If you have room, the space above your memory table or basket is ideal for a whiteboard or chalkboard, where you can leave messages for other household members—or for yourself. ("Take out the trash today!")

•**Use a "workhorse calendar."** Some people love an old-fashioned wall calendar with big squares for writing details. Others never use anything but the calendar on their phones. Still others like to blend paper and portability with a planner they tote everywhere. Any of these choices is fine, though a digital calendar has some advantages, including the ability to share your schedule with others and get pop-up reminders before events.

Smart strategy: Use a calendar of your choice—but make sure it's kept in a place you can easily access every day. Wherever your calendar is, make it a workhorse. When you add an appointment, be sure to include When, Who and Where (including, if needed, an address), along with What—what is the appointment for and what do you need to bring? And add a phone number—you will thank yourself if you end up running late or have to cancel at the last minute. Check your calendar every morning and evening.

•**Get a pillbox.** People have all sorts of systems for keeping track of medications, but nothing beats a pillbox. The basic version has a compartment for each day's medications (and/or supplements) and holds enough for one to four weeks. You also can get compartments for morning and evening meds or meds taken three times a day. These are all available online or at your local drugstore, often for less than $10.

Fancier versions have built-in alarms to remind you that it's time to take pills and sensors that link to apps you can set to communicate with others—if, for instance, you want a family member to know you are on track with your pills. You can even get boxes with vibrating alarms or braille lettering for people with hearing problems or vision challenges.

Smart strategy: Once you have a pillbox, pick a regular refilling day and time (add it to your calendar!)…and put your box where you will see it at medication time.

•**Use sticky notes.** The beauty of these little slips of paper is that you can put them anywhere and move them as needed.

Smart strategy: Whenever you have an errand to run or a task that needs to be done on a certain day, place a sticky note in a visible spot as a reminder. If the sticky note doesn't attach to the surface you're using, tape it to the door (or the handle of your bag) so that you'll see it when you're leaving your house.

THE GOLDEN RULES

To get the greatest benefit from memory aids, follow these rules…

RULE #1: **Don't delay.** When you make an appointment, write or type it into your calendar immediately. When the alarm goes off, go get the laundry, take your pill or make your call.

RULE #2: **Keep it simple.** Have one calendar, not four.

RULE #3: **Make it routine.** When you use your memory aids all the time, they become automatic and easier to use—even when you get tired, distracted or rushed.

How to Remember Names...

Cynthia R. Green, PhD, a psychologist and assistant clinical professor in the department of psychiatry at Icahn School of Medicine at Mount Sinai in New York City. Dr. Green is president and founder of Total Brain Health and CEO of TBH Brands LLC. She also is author or coauthor of six books on memory and brain health, including *Your Best Brain Ever*. TotalBrainHealth.com

You met Beth minutes ago but already you can't remember her name. Forgetting names is one of the top memory complaints of adults. *Here's how to get your brain in gear for better name recall...*

•**Prime your brain to pay attention.** If you know in advance that you will be meeting a lot of new people, make sure you're well rested. Your memory doesn't work as well when you lack sleep.

Also: Limit your intake of alcohol. Alcohol has been shown to impair our ability to learn new information. Too much caffeine or sugar can be overstimulating and make it harder to concentrate on what you're learning.

•**Repetition.** When you are introduced to Tom, say, "Hi, Tom. It's nice to meet you." Continue to repeat his name in the course of the conversation. Say, "Tom, where do you live?" Repetition is a simple and straightforward way to help you remember something.

•**Use a simple association strategy.** Find a connection to something familiar. If you meet a Barbara, think of Barbara Bush, Barbra Streisand or your cousin Barbara. Making a connection between something that you know and something that you're learning is a powerful way to remember.

•**Create a visual association.** If you meet someone named Robin, you might picture a red "robin" bird. By creating a snapshot in your mind, you are less likely to forget.

•**Tell yourself a story.** Make up a silly little one-liner to go with the name. Think, "Kristen kissed Kris Kringle." When you see her again, this line will come back to you. "Oh right, Kristen kissed Kris Kringle." Storytelling is a great way to amplify your memory.

•**Make a mental movie.** If you meet someone named Frank Hill, you might imagine frankfurters marching over a hill. The more absurd and bizarre the image, the more memorable it's going to be.

WHEN YOU FORGET

In spite of all your best efforts, sometimes you are going to forget someone's name.

•**Make a deal with your significant other or someone from work**—"If I am talking to someone you don't know and I don't introduce you within 15 seconds, stick out your hand and introduce yourself."

•**Admit that you don't know.** Say, "I'm sorry, I don't remember your name." The person might turn around and say, "Gee, I'm sorry, I don't remember your name either." Everyone forgets sometimes.

Just Thinking About Coffee Can Boost the Brain

Sam Maglio, PhD, associate professor of management, University of Toronto, Canada, and coauthor of a study published in *Consciousness and Cognition*.

People who regularly drink coffee get some of the same effects of being alert, awake and attentive when they simply think about drinking it.

Have Fun and Keep Your Memory Sharp

Cynthia R. Green, PhD, a psychologist and assistant clinical professor in the department of psychiatry at Icahn School of Medicine at Mount Sinai in New York City. Dr. Green is president and founder of Total Brain Health and CEO of TBH Brands LLC. She also is author or coauthor of six books on memory and brain health, including *Your Best Brain Ever*. TotalBrainHealth.com

Solitary pursuits such as crossword puzzles, Sudoku or even online and app-based games can help you stay mentally sharp, but there's something special about joining friends or family for a fun board, card or tile game.

These real-time, in-person gatherings ratchet up the brain-boosting effects. And regularly engaging in such games and other intellectually stimulating pursuits has been linked to lower rates of dementia. Chess, checkers, bridge and Scrabble are all good contenders—there's no strong research showing that one nonsolitary game is better than another. *But to try something different, consider…*

MAHJONG

The game that originated centuries ago in China and caught on in the US in the 1920s is enjoying a new wave of popularity here. This four-person game is played with domino-style tiles. Rules can vary, but the most common American version is played much like the card game rummy.

What you do: Players are dealt a set of tiles—including "suits" decorated with dots, bamboo and Chinese characters—and have chances to discard and pick up tiles, with the aim of collecting sets and pairs. The first player to collect a winning hand calls out "Mahjong" and wins the game. A game typically consists of four rounds of about 45 minutes each. A mahjong set can cost less than $50 to more than $100. *When you play mahjong, the mental muscles you exercise include…*

•**Attention skills.** You need to keep track of your own tiles (typically, 13 to 14) and what the other players are doing.

•**Short-term memory.** As you play, you must keep in mind not only the tiles you have in front of you but also the ones you need.

•**Planning and strategizing.** Each time you hold or discard a tile, you weigh its future value in creating sets and pairs.

•**Mental flexibility.** You need to adjust your strategy as the game progresses.

•**Long-term memory.** If you are a veteran player, you draw on strategies that worked for you in the past.

SET

The card game SET, which was designed by a research scientist, isn't widely known, but it will give your brain a good workout. You can buy this game online for less than $10.

SET consists of a deck of 81 cards, each of which displays four features—a color, number, pattern and shape. Each feature comes in three variations. So, a card can be red, green or purple…with one, two or three objects…with shaded, unshaded or striped patterns…and with diamond, oval or squiggle shapes.

What you do: You lay out 12 cards at a time and race other players to find groups of three cards that make a "set." A set consists of three cards, each having one feature (color, number, pattern or shape) that's either all the same or all different. At the end, the player with the most sets wins.

The concept can be tricky to grasp, but you will get better with practice—a sign that your brain is carving out new neural pathways. *SET works your…*

•**Attention skills.** To identify "sets," you must be attentive to the distinguishing features and variations on each card.

•**Flexible thinking.** Because there are multiple features (color, number, pattern and shape) and variations on each card, your thinking must be nimble enough to move back and forth from one feature and variation to the next.

•**Visual perception skills.** These skills help you identify the features and variations on each card.

•**Processing speed.** The time pressure involved in this game helps build faster mental-processing capacities.

Bonus: SET is a great game to play with kids and groups of varying sizes. You can play solo, too, but the biggest brain boost occurs when you play against others!

Can You Still Do Basic Math in Your Head?

Dharma Singh Khalsa, MD, founder, Alzheimer's Research & Prevention Foundation, Tucson, Arizona, and author of *Brain Longevity*.

As we age, the brain naturally takes a bit longer to make decisions or complete basic calculations. However, other factors can contribute to mental slowdown as well.

For example, some chronic health conditions, such as high blood pressure and diabetes, slow blood flow to the brain. Anticholinergic drugs, commonly used to treat allergies and many other conditions, slow brain activity as well—as can proton pump inhibitors (PPIs), used to treat heartburn. If you take one of these drugs, your doctor may be able to change your treatment.

Note: Never stop taking a prescribed drug without consulting with your doctor.

In some people, slowed thinking can signal the very early stages of memory loss that may lead to mild cognitive impairment (MCI) and then possibly dementia. But living a brain-healthy lifestyle may reduce risk for progression.

My advice: Visit your doctor, and start to incorporate the Four Pillars of Alzheimer's Prevention into your life…

#1. Healthy Diet. Cut down on saturated fats, such as those in red meat, and instead eat foods high in omega-3s, like salmon and nuts. Also, eat lots of vegetables and fruit.

#2. Exercise. A brisk 30-minute walk on most days of the week increases blood flow to the brain. Strength training has also been shown to enhance cognition.

#3. Yoga and Meditation. Research shows that a daily, 12-minute yoga/meditation technique called Kirtan Kriya (KK) offers significant brain-boosting benefits. Learn how to do KK at AlzheimersPrevention.org/research/kirtan-kriya-yoga-exercise.

#4. Spiritual Fitness. Staying connected to your spiritual side is also important for brain health. Volunteering, being close to loved

Two Simple Practices May Reduce Memory Loss

Memory and cognitive performance improved in 60 men and women with subjective cognitive decline (a strong predictor of Alzheimer's disease) after they practiced a beginner chanting meditation or listened to classical music for 12 minutes a day for 12 weeks, and then as often as they wanted for an additional three months. The gains remained or even increased at six months.

Theory: These practices promote memory and cognition by reducing stress and improving sleep.

Kim Innes, PhD, professor of epidemiology, West Virginia University School of Public Health, Morgantown.

ones and/or prayer all help develop spiritual fitness.

Noninvasive Treatment Stops Parkinson's Tremors

Gordon Baltuch, MD, PhD, professor of neurosurgery at University of Pennsylvania Perelman School of Medicine and a neurosurgeon at Pennsylvania Hospital, both in Philadelphia.

Magnetic resonance-guided focused ultrasound, or MRgFUS, uses ultrasound-wave technology in combination with magnetic resonance equipment to destroy targeted brain tissue and stop or reduce tremors. Now available at more than 100 medical centers, it can be used at an early stage, when medication isn't effective and as an alternative to brain-stimulation surgery.

Inflammation Makes the Brain Less Alert

Ali Mazaheri, PhD, principal investigator, Centre for Human Brain Health, University of Birmingham, UK, and senior coauthor of a study published in *NeuroImage*.

Inflammation—the body's response to illness—affects the part of the brain responsible for reaching and maintaining a state of alertness. This is the sluggishness or brain fog that many people report when they are ill or dealing with a chronic condition. Inflammation also may have an impact on other brain areas, such as those responsible for memory. More study could show that it is possible for anti-inflammatory drugs to improve or preserve cognitive function in some people with chronic conditions such as obesity, kidney disease and Alzheimer's.

Hip Fracture Alert

Esther S. Oh, MD, associate professor of geriatric medicine and gerontology, Johns Hopkins University School of Medicine, Baltimore.

Most patients hospitalized to repair broken hips with no signs of cognitive decline had abnormal levels of at least one biomarker for Alzheimer's disease, according to a study of 168 people ages 65 to 102.

Implication: Brain changes that can occur years before Alzheimer's symptoms surface may contribute to loss of balance, falls and fractures.

Self-defense: While not everyone who suffers a hip fracture will develop dementia, help hospital patients stay oriented by reminding them of dates and times, and to wear their glasses and hearing aids. Alert medical staff if they appear confused.

Air Pollution Linked to Depression and Suicide

Study of research data from 16 countries by researchers at University College London, UK, published in *Environmental Health Perspectives*.

Very fine particulates from dirty air can reach the brain and potentially cause inflammation, nerve-cell damage and changes in stress-hormone production, which can lead to poor mental health. People exposed to an increase of 10 micrograms per cubic meter ($\mu g/m3$) in the level of small particulates for a year or more had a 10% higher risk for depression than people not exposed to that extent. Researchers estimate that cutting pollution worldwide to the European Union's legal limit could prevent about 15% of the instances of depression and reduce cases of suicide. The World Health Organization estimates that 90% of the world lives with air pollution above recommended levels.

Nightmares May Help Us Face Real-World Fears

Study by researchers at Sleep and Cognition Laboratory, University of Geneva, Switzerland, published in *Human Brain Mapping*.

When people wake up after having nightmares, the brain areas responsible for emotion control respond more effectively to fear-inducing situations. Researchers believe this means that bad dreams may help prepare people to react better to real-world frights.

Drugs Linked to Dementia

The Anticholinergic Cognitive Burden (ACB) Scale, which was developed by scientists at the Aging Brain Program of the Indiana University Center for Aging Research, ranks both prescription and over-the-counter drugs with a score of 1 to 3, according to their anticholinergic effect.
To use the scale, look to see if a medication you are taking is listed in one of the three categories…

Possible anticholinergics include those listed with a score of 1…**definite anticholinergics** include those listed with a score of 2 or 3.
To determine your risk…

- Each definite anticholinergic may increase the risk for cognitive impairment by 46% over six years.
- For each one-point increase in the total ACB score, a decline in the Mini Mental State Examination (MMSE) score of 0.33 points over two years has been suggested.
- Additionally, each one-point increase in the ACB total score has been correlated with a 26% increase in the risk for early death.

If you are taking a medication that appears on the ACB Scale, ask your physician whether there is a suitable alternative medication or treatment approach available.

Drugs with ACB Score of 1

GENERIC NAME	BRAND NAME
Alimemazine	Theralen™
Alverine	Spasmonal™
Alprazolam	Xanax™
Aripiprazole	Abilify™
Asenapine	Saphris™
Atenolol	Tenormin™
Bupropion	Wellbutrin™, Zyban™
Captopril	Capoten™
Cetirizine	Zyrtec™
Chlorthalidone	Diuril™, Hygroton™
Cimetidine	Tagamet™
Clidinium	Librax™
Clorazepate	Tranxene™
Codeine	Contin™
Colchicine	Colcrys™
Desloratadine	Clarinex™
Diazepam	Valium™
Digoxin	Lanoxin™
Dipyridamole	Persantine™
Disopyramide	Norpace™
Fentanyl	Duragesic™, Actiq™
Furosemide	Lasix™
Fluvoxamine	Luvox™
Haloperidol	Haldol™
Hydralazine	Apresoline™
Hydrocortisone	Cortef™, Cortaid™
Iloperidone	Fanapt™
Isosorbide	Isordil™, Ismo™
Levocetirizine	Xyzal™
Loperamide	Immodium™, others
Loratadine	Claritin™
Metoprolol	Lopressor™, Toprol™
Morphine	MS Contin™, Avinza™
Nifedipine	Procardia™, Adalat™
Paliperidone	Invega™
Prednisone	Deltasone™, Sterapred™
Quinidine	Quinaglute™
Ranitidine	Zantac™
Risperidone	Risperdal™
Theophylline	Theodur™, Uniphyl™
Trazodone	Desyrel™
Triamterene	Dyrenium™
Venlafaxine	Effexor™
Warfarin	Coumadin™

Drugs with ACB Score of 2

GENERIC NAME	BRAND NAME
Amantadine	Symmetrel™
Belladonna	Multiple
Carbamazepine	Tegretol™
Cyclobenzaprine	Flexeril™
Cyproheptadine	Periactin™
Loxapine	Loxitane™
Meperidine	Demerol™
Methotrimeprazine	Levoprome™
Molindone	Moban™
Nefopam	Nefogesic™
Oxcarbazepine	Trileptal™
Pimozide	Orap™

Source: Regenstrief Institute, Inc., Regenstrief.org, copyright © 2008, 2012, all rights reserved.

Drugs with ACB Score of 3

GENERIC NAME	BRAND NAME
Amitriptyline	Elavil™
Amoxapine	Asendin™
Atropine	Sal-Tropine™
Benztropine	Cogentin™
Brompheniramine	Dimetapp™
Carbinoxamine	Histex™, Carbihist™
Chlorpheniramine	Chlor-Trimeton™
Chlorpromazine	Thorazine™
Clemastine	Tavist™
Clomipramine	Anafranil™
Clozapine	Clozaril™
Darifenacin	Enablex™
Desipramine	Norpramin™
Dicyclomine	Bentyl™
Dimenhydrinate	Dramamine™, others
Diphenhydramine	Benadryl™, others
Doxepin	Sinequan™
Doxylamine	Unisom™, others
Fesoterodine	Toviaz™
Flavoxate	Urispas™
Hydroxyzine	Atarax™, Vistaril™
Hyoscyamine	Anaspaz™, Levsin™
Imipramine	Tofranil™
Meclizine	Antivert™
Methocarbamol	Robaxin™
Nortriptyline	Pamelor™
Olanzapine	Zyprexa™
Orphenadrine	Norflex™
Oxybutynin	Ditropan™
Paroxetine	Paxil™
Perphenazine	Trilafon™
Promethazine	Phenergan™
Propantheline	Pro-Banthine™
Propiverine	Detrunorm™
Quetiapine	Seroquel™
Scopolamine	Transderm Scop™
Solifenacin	Vesicare™
Thioridazine	Mellaril™
Tolterodine	Detrol™
Trifluoperazine	Stelazine™
Trihexyphenidyl	Artane™
Trimipramine	Surmontil™
Trospium	Sanctura™

CHAPTER 3

Cancer Breakthroughs and Care

Beware This Hidden Cause of Lung Cancer

When most people hear lung cancer, they think cigarettes. But that can be a mistake. While cigarette smoking is hands down the number-one risk factor for lung cancer, radon is a very real danger that doesn't get the attention it deserves.

Radon is the leading cause of lung cancer in nonsmokers—and accounts for about 21,000 deaths from the disease each year, according to the Environmental Protection Agency (EPA). Many of these deaths occur in people who never smoked. If you do smoke—and your home has high radon levels—this one-two punch makes your risk for lung cancer especially high. *Facts to know about this silent killer…*

A WIDESPREAD INDOOR THREAT

Radon occurs naturally when uranium, an element found in rocks and soil, decays. As the element breaks down, it releases radon gas. Even though radon can be found outdoors in harmless amounts, it can accumulate in homes and buildings that are constructed on soil with natural uranium deposits, as the air is trapped inside the building.

Radon is an insidious threat because it cannot be seen, tasted or smelled. When radon is inhaled, it causes no symptoms even though invisible particles are attacking the body's cells with cancer-causing radiation.

Thousands of lung cancer deaths would be avoided each year if home and building owners tested and fixed high levels of radon, according to the American Lung Association.

So why are there still so many deaths linked to radon? Over the years, several myths have emerged, undermining efforts to eradicate this pervasive health threat. *For example…*

Gary G. Schwartz, PhD, chair of the department of population health in the School of Medicine & Health Sciences at University of North Dakota in Grand Forks. Dr. Schwartz is coauthor of "Radon and Lung Cancer: What Does the Public Really Know?" recently published in *Journal of Environmental Radioactivity.*

DON'T BE FOOLED BY THESE MYTHS

***MYTH #1:* Radon is a concern only in certain parts of the country.**

Fact: It's true that radon exists in higher concentrations near uranium-dense rock deposits, but radon can be found everywhere. In total, nearly one in every 15 homes in the US is estimated to have radon levels that exceed the EPA's recommendation. The EPA has mapped the country into three zones. While the highest levels are generally found in northern states, moderate-risk counties exist in every state except Louisiana. And even in low-risk areas, a single neighborhood might be sitting on a pocket of uranium. For a US map that indicates average radon levels by state and zone, check the EPA Map of Radon Zones (at EPA.gov/radon, search "map of radon zones").

***MYTH #2:* I've lived in my home for decades, so there's no point in testing now.**

Fact: Regardless of whether your home was tested for radon when you purchased it, testing should be repeated every five to 10 years. Radon levels can change over the years as your home settles, the ground shifts and new cracks form. And if a test you conduct now indicates that radon levels in your home are high, that doesn't necessarily mean you've had long-term exposure. But because the harmful effects of radon are cumulative, the sooner you address the problem, the lower your risk.

***MYTH #3:* I have a brand-new home, so there's nothing to worry about.**

Fact: Some states do require new homes to be radon-resistant, but most don't. Because new homes are built to be more energy-efficient,

This Simple Test Could Save Your Life

Radon testing is simple—and takes only minutes to set up. Stop by your local hardware store or go online to pick up a test kit…place the cannister in the lowest level of your home that you spend time in…give it time (typically 48 hours) to collect an air sample…and mail the cannister to the lab. That's all you have to do! Results are typically mailed and/or e-mailed to you within a week or so.

Here's how to evaluate your test results, based on recommendations from the EPA…

•**Below 2 pCi/L.** Relax, but remember to retest every five or 10 years.

•**Borderline levels (2 pCi/L to 4 pCi/L).** Do a second test. If the second test confirms the first, you have a choice—either begin remediation now or monitor levels by retesting.

•**High levels (4 pCi/L or above).** There are literally no "safe" levels of radon exposure, but the EPA says that you should take action if radon is this high in your home. If DIY sealing doesn't bring down the levels—and a repeat test confirms that they are high—find a radon mitigation contractor. Consult your state's radon office for advice on licenses, registration or certification that may be required for mitigation experts.

Until you can arrange for remediation, keep the windows open. Fresh air will help to dilute the radon concentration indoors. Also, try not to spend significant amounts of time in the basement. Radon levels there are typically two to three times higher than on the first floor.

Important: For the most accurate results, be sure to follow instructions on the test kit carefully. For example, do not move the test device or open doors and windows in the testing area while the air sample is being collected. Weather patterns, such as high winds or storms, can make your results lower or higher than normal.

For more information, read the EPA's "Consumer's Guide to Radon Reduction." It'll walk you through the process and guide your decision-making.

For renters: Get more information about radon testing and remediation in rental properties from the EPA's report "Radon Guide for Tenants." Both reports can be found at EPA.gov/radon.

—Gary G. Schwartz, PhD

they're more efficiently sealed. That means new homes can trap whatever radon might emerge from the soil under the house—so they may become even more prone to higher radon levels than older homes.

Myth #4: **Testing is too expensive and time-consuming.**

Fact: You can buy a basic home test for under $15 at many hardware stores, and some states even provide them for free.

With most tests, you set it up, leave it in place for a minimum of 48 hours and then mail it to a lab for evaluation. Long-term tests may remain in a home for 90 days or more—these tests are used when home owners want a more stable, average level. However, when researchers at University of Calgary recently compared a five-day radon test against a 90-day test, the longer-term testing was significantly more precise. If you can, use long-term testing.

MYTH #5: **If I test my home and the levels are too high, I won't be able to sell it later on.**

Fact: Radon testing is a routine part of home inspections in many states, so if you have a problem, it could hold things up when you do decide to sell your home. Plus, remediation may be easier than you think. If you have obvious cracks in your basement floor, for example, DIY sealing can be easy and inexpensive—hardware stores sell products made for this purpose. Just retest after performing this type of sealing to ensure that radon levels were adequately reduced.

If the levels are still dangerously high, you may need a remediation system that uses a vent pipe and fan to pull radon to the outside. Such systems cost about $800 to $2,000, depending on your home and location.

Smoked Fish May Raise Cancer Risk

The New York Times.

The American Institute for Cancer Research places smoked and cured fish in the same category as processed meats, which are asso-

Cell-Phone Radiation Danger

Cell-phone radiation can cause tumors. Research from the National Toxicology Program has connected radiofrequency radiation with malignant brain and heart tumors in rats exposed to nine hours a day of 2G and 3G radiation.

Best: Don't hold your cell phone against your body…and use headphones. For every millimeter you move the phone away from your body, exposure is reduced by 10% to 15%.

John Bucher, PhD, is senior scientist of the National Toxicology Program at National Institute of Environmental Health Sciences, Durham, North Carolina.

---

ciated with higher cancer risk—and, in some scientists' view, actually can cause cancer when eaten regularly in large amounts.

Yogurt and Fiber Linked to Lower Lung Cancer Risk

Xiao-Ou Shu, MD, PhD, MPH, Ingram professor of cancer research, Vanderbilt Ingram Cancer Center, Nashville.

People who ate the most fiber (about 30 g daily) and yogurt (three to four ounces daily) had a 33% lower risk for lung cancer compared with those who ate the least, according to a study that followed up to 1.4 million men and women for nine years.

Theory: High-fiber foods and probiotic-rich yogurt reduce lung cancer–promoting inflammation.

Faster Lung Cancer Test

Vassiliki A. Papadimitrakopoulou, MD, professor of medicine, University of Texas MD Anderson Cancer Center, Houston.

Compared with a traditional surgical tissue biopsy, a new liquid (blood-based) biopsy called Guardant360 detected biomarkers that can lead to more effective treatments in those with non-small cell lung cancer as accurately and in nearly half the time (nine days versus 15 days). The test identifies patients with gene mutations that can be treated with targeted molecular therapies that result in up to two to three times higher response rates compared with chemotherapy or immunotherapy.

Good News for Melanoma Patients

NYU School of Medicine.

A blood test quickly gauges the effectiveness of drug treatments in melanoma patients. The test, in development, tracks the circulating DNA (ctDNA) that's released by cancer cells— ctDNA won't be detected after successful drug treatments, and a positive test might indicate that a drug change is needed.

The Ultimate Guide to Skin Checks

National Institutes of Health, medlineplus.gov/ lab-tests/skin-cancer-screening/

Frequent head-to-toe self-exams are one of the best ways to detect skin cancer early, when it is most treatable. Be sure to check the areas that are often overlooked, which are indicated in the following graphic. A skin-cancer screening performed by a doctor (see adjacent page) should also include these areas.

To perform a self-check: You'll need to fully undress and do the exam in a well-lit room in front of a full-length mirror (and have a hand mirror available).

To ensure that you are checking your skin correctly, follow these steps...

1. Stand in front of the mirror and look at your face, neck and stomach. (Women should look under their breasts.)

2. Raise your arms and look at your left and right sides.

3. Look at the front and back of your forearms.

4. Look at your hands, including between your fingers and under your fingernails. (Be sure to remove any nail polish from fingers and toes.)

5. Look at the front, back and sides of your legs.

6. Sit down and examine your feet, checking the soles and the spaces between the toes. Also, check the nail beds of each toe.

7. Check your back, buttocks and genitals with a hand mirror.

8. Part your hair and examine your scalp. Use a comb or a hair dryer along with a hand mirror to help you see better. (Have a friend or loved one help with this if needed.)

Signs to watch for: If you find signs of skin cancer, see your health-care provider for a more thorough screening. *Signs vary depending on the type of skin cancer, but they may include...*

•**Change in an existing mole or spot.**

•**Mole or other skin mark that oozes, bleeds or becomes crusty.**

•**Mole that is painful to the touch.**

•**Sore that doesn't heal within two weeks.**

•**Shiny pink, red, pearly white or translucent bump.**

•**Mole or sore with irregular borders that may bleed easily.**

Remember ABCDE: During a self-exam, be alert for signs of melanoma, the most serious type of skin cancer. *An easy way to remember the signs of melanoma is to think of "ABCDE," which stands for...*

•**Asymmetry.** The mole has an odd shape, with half of it not matching the other half.

•**Border.** The border of the mole is ragged or irregular.

Often-Overlooked Areas in Skin Checks

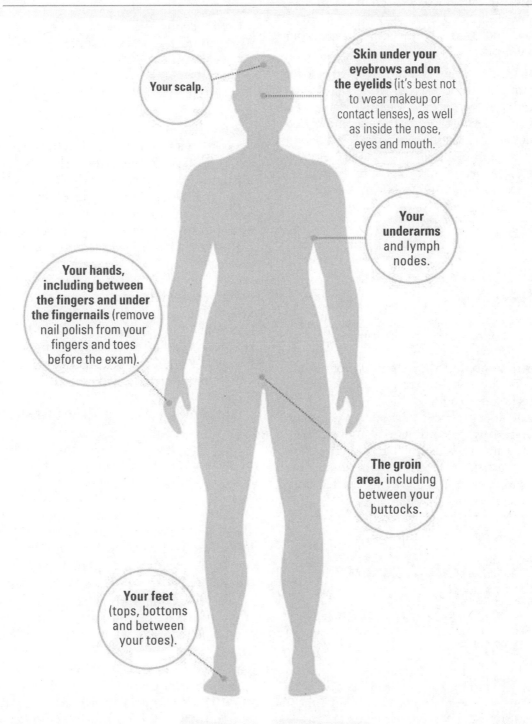

Your scalp.

Skin under your eyebrows and on the eyelids (it's best not to wear makeup or contact lenses), as well as inside the nose, eyes and mouth.

Your underarms and lymph nodes.

Your hands, including between the fingers and under the fingernails (remove nail polish from your fingers and toes before the exam).

The groin area, including between your buttocks.

Your feet (tops, bottoms and between your toes).

© 2019 Bottom Line Inc. BottomLineInc.com

•**Color.** The color of the mole is uneven.

•**Diameter.** The mole is bigger than the size of a pea or a pencil eraser.

•**Evolving.** The mole has changed in size, shape or color.

If you find signs of melanoma, see your health-care provider as soon as possible.

Also: Talk to your health-care provider for advice on the frequency of your self-checks and regular skin-cancer screening exams performed by a dermatologist. The recommended frequency of skin exams performed by a doctor is based on your personal risk factors, including skin type, history of sun exposure and family history, according to the American Academy of Dermatology.

Sore Throat Linked to Cancer

Elizabeth Shephard, PhD, research fellow, University of Exeter College of Medicine and Health, UK.

When combined with shortness of breath, difficulty swallowing or earache, throat pain was linked to a 5% to 7% increased risk for laryngeal cancer (cancer of the larynx, known as the voice box), according to a study of more than 800 patients with this cancer. This compares with a risk of 2.7% for hoarseness alone, the symptom most commonly associated with laryngeal cancer.

When Cancer Spreads to the Brain

Nduka Amankulor, MD, a neurosurgeon and neuro-oncologist at UPMC Hillman Cancer Center and assistant professor of neurological surgery at University of Pittsburgh School of Medicine.

An astounding 20% to 30% of people with cancer develop metastatic brain cancer (MBC)—cancer that has spread from another organ to the brain.

Breast cancer, lung cancer, kidney cancer and melanoma are the main types of cancer that invade the brain. But almost any cancer can produce brain metastases, with an estimated 170,000 new cases every year.

Until recently, the prognosis for people with MBC was grim—only 8% of patients were alive two years after diagnosis, and 2% after five years. But those sad statistics are changing.

Now: The treatment of MBC is being revolutionized by targeted drug therapies that attack genetic mutations driving cancer…immunotherapies that stimulate the body's own immune system to fight cancer…and precisely focused radiation.

Immunotherapy more than doubled the average survival time of melanoma patients with MBC—from 5.2 months to 12.4 months, according to a study published in *Cancer Immunology Research*. The effects are even better for melanoma patients with MBC but no other metastases—research found that those who received immunotherapy had an average survival rate of 56 months, compared with 7.7 months for those receiving standard treatment, such as chemotherapy. In other words, MBC patients treated with immunotherapy lived about seven times longer!

What cancer patients and their families need to know…

Many oncologists don't recommend screening for brain metastases, except for certain tumor types that have a significant predilection for spreading to the brain. Of course, if the patient develops neurological symptoms, such as headaches, numbness, blurred vision, balance difficulties, cognitive decline and/or seizures, then brain screening for a brain tumor is recommended, regardless of the type of cancer.

New thinking: Early detection can extend survival time in patients without neurological symptoms who are at high risk of developing MBC.

My advice for who should get screened…

•**Any patient with a new diagnosis of stage II to stage IV lung cancer,** whether it's non-small cell (the most common type) or small cell.

•**A melanoma patient with metastatic disease elsewhere in the body**—because two out of three of these patients will also develop MBC.

•**A breast cancer patient who is positive for HER2** (a gene that plays a role in the development of breast cancer)…or whose tumor lacks hormone receptors (estrogen and progesterone receptors)…or lacks any markers at all (triple-negative breast cancer). The rate of MBC is significantly higher (10% to 15%) in all these breast cancer patients.

The gold standard for early detection is a brain MRI with contrast dye, which can detect brain tumors as small as 2 millimeters in diameter (less than one-tenth of an inch). Especially in patients who are at high risk of developing MBC, insurance may cover the MRI even if there are no neurological symptoms, but be sure to check first. Once MBC is diagnosed, MRIs are obtained roughly every two to four months.

•**Targeted therapies** are drugs (oral or IV) that block or alter specific genes and/or proteins that drive cancer. There have been dozens of clinical trials of targeted therapy in patients with brain metastases—with some remarkable results. *For example…*

Researchers from the MD Anderson Cancer Center at University of Texas studied melanoma patients with MBC who had the BRAF mutation, which occurs in about half of patients with this disease. The patients received two drugs—*dabrafenib* (Tafinlar), which targets BRAF…and *trametinib* (Mekinist), which targets MEK, a mutation similar to BRAF. In a group of 76 patients with BRAF who had never been treated for MBC and whose neurological symptoms were under control, 58% had significant shrinking of their brain tumors—and in four patients the tumors vanished, according to the research, which was published in *The Lancet Oncology*. The response lasted, on average, six to seven months.

•**Immunotherapy drugs** are a class of drugs that stimulate a patient's immune system, essentially calling it into action. The most widely used immunotherapies are drugs that block checkpoint proteins, such as PD-1 or PD-L1, which suppress inflammatory responses in the immune system.

Scientific evidence: Impressive results with combined drug therapy—*ipilimumab* (Yervoy) and *nivolumab* (Opdivo)—were cited in a study published in *The New England Journal of Medicine*. In that research, when 94 melanoma patients with MBC took both drugs, 81% were alive after one year and 70% after two years—a dramatic increase over the typical survival rate of four to five months before the introduction of immunotherapy.

•**Focused radiation** in the past, the standard radiation treatment for MBC was whole-brain radiation—multiple treatments of the entire brain with low-dose radiation.

However, whole-brain radiation has significant side effects, such as a marked decrease in memory and other cognitive abilities. Doctors are now using highly focused radiation therapies called stereotactic radiosurgery. Employing a flexible robotic arm to deliver radiation (CyberKnife), or using a helmet with built-in radiation sources (Gamma Knife), this treatment delivers less total radiation…faster…and more accurately. And its cancer-killing efficacy is as good as whole-brain radiation—with less severe side effects.

To take advantage of the breakthrough treatments for MBC, you need a plan of action. *Here are four steps to follow…*

STEP #1: **Treat the primary cancer.** The key in treating cancer is always minimizing your overall cancer burden using the full range of treatments available—such as chemotherapy, radiation, surgery, targeted therapies and immunotherapy. Controlling the primary malignancy reduces the risk of the cancer spreading to the brain.

STEP #2: **Ask your oncologist, "Has my tumor been sufficiently molecularly characterized?"** Sophisticated genetic tests will show if you're a candidate for targeted therapy or immunotherapy.

For example, if such testing shows that you have the ALK mutation, treatments for the primary tumor may include targeted therapies such as *alectinib* (Alecensa), *brigatinib* (Alunbrig) or *lorlatinib* (Lorbrena)—all of which also help prevent and/or treat brain metastases.

If a tumor biopsy shows that you have high levels of PD-1 or PD-L1, then you may be a candidate for an immunotherapy drug such as *pembrolizumab* (Keytruda), *nivolumab* (Opdivo) or *atezolizumab* (Tecentriq).

STEP #3: Ask your oncologist, "Are there effective therapies that treat the molecular pathways affecting my cancer—and should we use those therapies to treat my brain cancer?" Once your tumor has been tested for molecular mutations, talk with your oncologist about the targeted and immunological therapies available to treat those problems. You and your doctor should develop a complete list of the targeted therapies and immunotherapies (see examples above) that may be right for you—and then decide which to use.

STEP #4: Demand a multidisciplinary team approach. The best treatment for primary cancer and for MBC is a team approach, typically involving a medical oncologist, a radiation oncologist and a cancer surgeon. The best treatment decisions are made when the entire team talks to one another, face-to-face. This type of multidisciplinary approach is typical of cancer centers that are designated by the National Cancer Institute for offering cutting-edge treatments.

To find such an NCI-designated cancer center near you, go to: Cancer.gov/research/nci-role/cancer-centers/find.

Cancers Linked to Bad Behavior Get the Least Research

Journal of the National Comprehensive Cancer Network.

Cancers linked to "stigmatized behavior," such as smoking (lung cancer) or excessive drinking (liver cancer), are among those receiving the least research funding relative to how common they are and how many deaths they cause. The best-funded cancers include breast cancer and leukemia.

Takeaway: Well-funded cancers deserve continued support, but underfunded cancers need more dollars to pay for research and drug development.

Psoriasis and Cancer Risk

Alex M. Trafford, MSc, is a PhD candidate in the department of biology, medicine and health at University of Manchester in the UK and lead author of a study published in *JAMA Dermatology*.

Psoriasis increases risk for many types of cancer by an average of 18%. Esophageal, liver, pancreatic and squamous cell skin cancers were among the highest risks. The exact link is unclear but could be related to inflammation, a hallmark of both psoriasis and cancer. Keeping up with recommended cancer screenings can help with early detection and diagnosis.

Psoriasis Drugs for Cancer

Cancer Discovery

Psoriasis drugs could help patients with osteosarcoma, a rare bone cancer that often affects young men. The drugs target an inflammatory immune molecule that can trigger the formation/progression of cancer.

Catch Pancreatic Cancer Early for the Best Care

Diane M. Simeone, MD, an internationally recognized surgeon and scientist, the associate director for translational research at Perlmutter Cancer Center at NYU Langone Health and director of its Pancreatic Cancer Center in New York City. Her research has been widely published in leading medical journals including *Cancer Cell, Journal of Clinical Oncology* and *Cancer Discovery*.

When a pancreatic cancer is found via a screening program, there is an 80% to 90% chance that the tumor can be removed, and up to 30% to 35% of those individuals will live for five or more years.

However, when a pancreatic cancer is found in a person who has not been regularly screened and he/she has already developed symptoms (such as abdominal or back pain, weight loss, nausea and/or jaundice), there is only a 15% chance that it can be removed. This lack of early detection, along with the need for improved therapies, has resulted in a persistently low overall survival rate of 9% for pancreatic cancer patients.

Here's how to spot pancreatic cancer before it's too late…

KNOW YOUR RISK FACTORS

The first step to staying ahead of pancreatic cancer is knowing how to assess your risk factors. *Your risk is higher if you have any of the following…*

•**Two or more relatives with pancreatic cancer,** including one first-degree relative (parent, sibling or child).

•**A first-degree relative who developed pancreatic cancer before age 50.**

•**An inherited genetic syndrome linked to pancreatic cancer such as Lynch syndrome,** which is also associated with colorectal cancer…or BRCA mutations, which predispose a person to breast, ovarian and prostate cancers.

Note: People of Ashkenazi Jewish (Central and Eastern Europe) descent aren't the only ones who can have BRCA mutations. Though less common, individuals of Norwegian, Swedish, Italian and other ethnic groups have been found to also carry certain BRCA mutations.

Other factors that increase your risk for pancreatic cancer…

•**Long-standing type 2 diabetes (more than five years),** which increases pancreatic cancer risk by twofold.

Note: New-onset diabetes—especially when weight loss instead of weight gain appears—may be an early sign of pancreatic cancer.

•**Chronic pancreatitis,** which can be caused by heavy use of alcohol (usually four or more drinks a day), increases risk for pancreatic cancer by about threefold.

•**Personal history of another type of cancer,** such as breast or colon cancer or melanoma.

•**Smoking.** About 25% of all pancreatic cancer cases are associated with smoking.

•**Age.** Most people with pancreatic cancer are diagnosed after age 45.

•**Gender.** Men are slightly more at risk than women.

•**Obesity.** People with a body mass index (BMI) of 30 or more are 20% more likely to develop pancreatic cancer.

•**Workplace exposure to certain chemicals.** Research has found significant links between workplace exposure to chemicals, such as pesticides, asbestos, benzene and chlorinated hydrocarbons, and increased risk for pancreatic cancer.

•**Diet.** Eating a diet high in processed meats and/or red meat has been linked to increased risk for pancreatic cancer. For every 50 g of processed meat consumed daily (roughly the equivalent of one hot dog or four strips of bacon), risk for pancreatic cancer increases by 19%. The increased risk linked to red meat consumption is less significant but also present—especially in men.

Important: An easy-to-use online Pancreatic Cancer Risk Assessment tool (Find-PanCancer-Early.org) can help determine your risk level based on your answers to a few brief questions about your personal and family medical history. You also can work with your own physician to do a thorough family history if you're more comfortable with that approach.

NEXT STEPS

If you have any risk factors for pancreatic cancer that are controllable, take immediate action. For example, stop smoking…reduce or eliminate alcohol if you are a heavy drinker…lose weight if you're overweight…and avoid diabetes or treat it if you've already been diagnosed with this condition.

Meanwhile, if you have a family history of pancreatic cancer, talk to your doctor about getting your DNA examined through germline genetic testing, a blood test that looks for specific hereditary mutations in your cells and can help determine your risk. The cost of germline testing has plummeted in recent years, and there are validated tests that check a panel of gene mutations that can be performed for as little as $250. In individuals with a family history of pancreatic cancer, germline testing is typically covered by insurance.

Guidelines published in 2018 in *Journal of Clinical Oncology* recommend that all patients with pancreatic cancer consider having germline testing. Individuals with a strong family history of pancreatic cancer also are advised to undergo testing and screening.

At the multidisciplinary Pancreatic Cancer Center at the NYU Perlmutter Cancer Center, we found that 15% of pancreatic cancer patients have a germline mutation (also known as a "hereditary mutation") that increased the patient's risk of developing the disease, even if a strong family history wasn't present.

Knowing whether such a hereditary, or germline, mutation is present in a pancreatic cancer patient may change the treatment strategy…and have implications for testing siblings and children who might also be at higher risk.

Genetic counseling will help you understand the test results and decide whether it's appropriate to consider enrolling in a screening program run by specialists in pancreatic cancer. To locate a certified genetics counselor, consult the National Society of Genetic Counselors at NSGC.org.

If an individual is deemed to be high risk, annual imaging of the pancreas is recommended. Two types of tests are used—a pancreatic MRI/MRCP (a special type of MRI)…and an endoscopic ultrasound (EUS).

We usually start with the MRI/MRCP and then check with an EUS the next year, alternating the exams each year. The two tests are complementary and examine the pancreas in slightly different ways. Insurance should cover these tests.

The MRI is noninvasive. With EUS, an upper endoscopy is performed, passing a thin scope down the esophagus into the stomach and the first part of the small intestine after sedation is given (much like a colonoscopy, but no prep is needed). The scope has an ultrasound probe at the end, and the pancreas can be readily visualized, as it is next to the stomach.

Both tests have only very minor risks, but it's important that the screening be done in a multidisciplinary clinic where there's collaboration among various health-care providers, such as genetic counselors, gastroenterologists, pancreatic surgeons, radiologists and social workers as well as a tumor board, where this team of experts, along with oncologists, meets to discuss each patient's unique situation. Pancreatic cancer is a complicated disease, and decision-making in high-risk individuals is best done with an experienced team guiding your care.

Important: Even with a genetic mutation linked to pancreatic cancer, most people will not get the disease. But with an increased risk, it is crucial to know that screening can be an effective strategy to combat pancreatic cancer. I tell my patients, knowledge is power. As we do a better job in identifying individuals at risk, we will be much better positioned to shift the disease from the advanced state to one in which many more patients have easier-to-treat, surgically resectable disease.

With a concerted effort in early detection (and prevention), along with the development of more effective therapies and clinical trial strategies, it is likely that we will see a change in survival in pancreatic cancer patients in the coming years—and it's about time.

This is a rapidly moving field, so ask questions and seek information from doctors who are at the forefront of the research.

GETTING THE BEST CARE

The Pancreatic Cancer Action Network (Pan Can.org) is a patient-advocacy group that serves as a resource for finding a high-quality pancreatic cancer center. It's the driving force behind Precision Promise, a multicenter "adaptive" clinical trial initiative that allows multiple novel therapies to be evaluated alongside standard-of-care approaches to speed the development of new treatments.

Other excellent resources: Rolfe Pancreatic Cancer Foundation (RolfeFoundation.org), a nonprofit dedicated to early diagnosis of pancreatic cancer, research that aims to cure the disease and resources for patients and their families…and Project Purple (ProjectPurple.org), another nonprofit group that funds research to defeat pancreatic cancer and supports patients and their families.

Pancreatic Inflammation Increases Cancer Risk

Science

Pancreatic inflammation, a common cause of hospitalization, can greatly increase cancer risk.

New finding: Patients with both pancreatitis and pancreatic cancer have high levels of a dangerous sugar structure known as CA19-9. Blocking the sugar could prevent pancreatitis from progressing to cancer.

Hair Dyes and Straighteners Linked to Cancer

Dale Sadler, PhD, chief, epidemiology branch, US National Institute of Environmental Health Sciences, Research Triangle Park, North Carolina, and leader of a study published online in *International Journal of Cancer.*

African-American women had a 60% increased risk of developing breast cancer if they used hair dye every five to eight weeks or more often, and white women had an 8% increased risk. Women using chemical straighteners with the same frequency were 30% more likely to develop breast cancer than those who did not use them. The study did not prove cause and effect—and all the women studied had a sister who had been diagnosed with breast cancer, even though they did not have the disease themselves when the study began. Further research is necessary.

Easing Fears for Cancer Survivors

Fear of cancer recurrence is associated with significant distress for more than one-third of survivors. Survivors might view any physical change or oddity as a sign that the cancer is coming back, leading to anxiety or even suicidal thoughts. Medical appointments and other people's cancers also trigger fears. There will be about 19 million cancer survivors in the US by 2024. Relaxation training and mindfulness meditation are some ways to ease fears and potentially strengthen the immune system, too.

Daniel L. Hall, PhD, is an integrative medicine research fellow, Harvard Medical School, and clinical fellow in psychology, Massachusetts General Hospital, both in Boston. Health.Harvard.edu

Common Mouth Bacteria Make Colon Cancer More Dangerous

Study titled "Fusobacterium nucleatum promotes colorectal cancer by inducing Wnt/b-catenin modulator Annexin A1" by researchers at Columbia University College of Dental Medicine, New York City, published in *EMBO Reports.*

Colon cancer, a disease that affects one out of 23 adults, has recently been linked to gum disease. But how the one might be driving the other has not been known—until now. A new study has discovered what it is in our mouths that causes colon cancer to become most deadly...and may lead to better tests and new treatments.

Fusobacterium nucleatum is a common bacterium found in the mouth that plays a role in forming dental plaque, which can lead to tooth decay, gingivitis and periodontitis. The bacterium also has been implicated in diseases outside the mouth, including colorectal cancer, atherosclerosis, rheumatoid arthritis and Alzheimer's disease. In fact, research has found that about one-third of colorectal cancer patients test positive for F. nucleatum bacteria—and those patients usually have more aggressive tumors.

Researchers at Columbia University College of Dental Medicine had previously discovered that F. nucleatum produces a molecule called FadA adhesin. They also observed that FadA adhesin interacted with cancerous colon cells but not with healthy colon cells. To learn more, the researchers reviewed cellular data from more than 450 patients with colorectal cancer.

Results: The researchers found that FadA adhesin molecules bind to a protein called Annexin A1 that is produced only in the cancerous cells, not in the noncancerous cells. Annexin A1 stimulates cancer growth and leads to a more aggressive and deadly prognosis. In fact, the patients in the study with the highest levels of Annexin A1 in their cancer cells had the fastest-growing cancers.

Vicious cycle: FadA adhesin molecules bind to the Annexin A1 protein, triggering the cells to produce more Annexin A1. This in turn causes more binding and more cancer growth—a sequence called a "positive feedback loop" in scientific terms.

The researchers hope that the results of their study might lead to development of a test for Annexin A1 levels to identify which cancers are more likely to become aggressive, as well as new treatments for colorectal cancer.

While the researchers were able to show in cell cultures and mouse studies that blocking Annexin A1 prevented F. nucleatum from binding to cancer cells, no research has yet shown that reducing oral F. nucleatum will protect people with colorectal cancer from more aggressive disease. However, it is known that F. nucleatum increases with the severity of gum disease and is also higher in smokers. So, if you have been diagnosed with colorectal cancer it makes sense to be especially persistent about maintaining good oral hygiene. And if you smoke, here's one more good reason to quit.

Obesity-Related Cancers On the Rise

Hyuna Sung, PhD, cancer epidemiologist, American Cancer Society, Atlanta, and leader of a study published in *The Lancet Public Health*.

Obesity-related cancers are on the rise among millennials and other young adults. Rates for six of 12 cancers linked to obesity—colorectal, endometrial, gallbladder, kidney,

multiple myeloma and pancreatic—rose from 1995 to 2014. For some of the cancers, people born between 1980 and 1989 had twice the risk of people born from 1945 to 1954.

My Secret for a More Effective and Gentler Colonoscopy Prep

Jamison Starbuck, ND, naturopathic physician in family practice in Missoula, Montana, and producer of *Dr. Starbuck's Health Tips for Kids*, a weekly program on Montana Public Radio, MTPR.org. She is a past president of the American Association of Naturopathic Physicians and a contributing editor to *The Alternative Advisor: The Complete Guide to Natural Therapies and Alternative Treatments.* DrJamisonStarbuck.com.

It's not news that colonoscopy is a wonderful screening and diagnostic tool.

What you may not know: According to the American College of Gastroenterology, bowel preparation is inadequate in up to 20% to 25% of colonoscopies. This means you may get inaccurate results, including missed abnormalities, or you may be asked to reschedule the test involving another round of the dreaded prep!

In the typical colonoscopy prep, patients need to drink a laxative solution anywhere from 12 to 24 hours before the procedure in order to empty the bowels completely. Unfortunately, many patients do not accomplish this goal—sometimes they don't finish the solution due to a strong reaction such as nausea, vomiting and/or painful elimination, they start the prep too late or they don't follow other instructions.

I've developed a plan for my patients that makes typical colonoscopy prep more successful and gentler on the system. The object is to gradually reduce stool volume for a few days before you even begin drinking the prep solution. This helps ensure that the bowels will be well prepared for the test. *What I suggest…*

Four days before your colonoscopy, make your diet simple and clean. Your goal is to have one or two good-sized, complete stools each day during the days prior to drinking the colonoscopy prep solution. *To help achieve this…*

•**Avoid fried and high-fat foods.** Use olive oil and mashed avocado for fats.

•**Become a vegetarian or limit protein to fish or a small amount of turkey.** Eat lots of baked or steamed vegetables. Avoid salads and limit raw vegetables to one or two small servings per day.

•**Avoid corn, nuts, berries and legumes as they can sometimes linger in the bowel.** Whole grains, such as brown rice, are OK.

•**Limit fruit to apples and pears.** Applesauce and baked apples and pears are excellent—delicious and high in fiber.

•**Avoid dairy because it's often not easy to digest.**

Also, cut out any foods with dyes as well as beets, which can discolor your bowel wall. And avoid preservatives and sugar substitutes and alcohols, which can irritate your colon. These ingredients may affect your test results.

Thirty-six hours before your colonoscopy, switch to an all-liquid, low-protein, low-fiber diet. Drink only clear or lightly colored fruit juices, such as apple or pear…miso…broth…preservative- and color-free, unsweetened electrolyte solutions…and lots of water. Black coffee or tea is OK. Do not drink milk or nondairy milk (soy, almond, etc.).

After using my plan, begin your colonoscopy prep as directed by your doctor. Hydrate with water up until the time your doctor has told you to stop drinking.

•**After a colonoscopy.** Load up on probiotics. I advise an acidophilus/bifidus supplement, 20 billion colony-forming units (CFUs), for 14 days.

Caution: If you have a severe illness or a significantly compromised immune system, talk to your doctor before using probiotics—they can increase risk for infection in these individuals. For three days after, rehydrate with lots of water and eat a simple diet of whole foods.

Aspirin for Colon Cancer

Charles H. Hennekens, MD, DrPH, senior academic advisor, Schmidt College of Medicine, Florida Atlantic University, Boca Raton.

The US Preventive Services Task Force has recommended that aspirin be considered to reduce risk for colorectal cancer in people with advanced colon polyps, after an analysis found that it reduces the risk by 40%.

However: In a study of 84 patients ages 40 to 91, only 42.9% of patients with advanced colon polyps, determined by biopsy, were taking aspirin.

Note: Even if you have been diagnosed with colon polyps, daily aspirin increases bleeding risk. Ask your doctor for advice.

Battling Cancer at 65 or Over? This Can Make Chemo More Bearable

Arti Hurria, MD, former director of the Center for Cancer and Aging. Dr. Hurria, who died in 2018, was coauthor of the report titled "Practical Assessment and Management of Vulnerabilities in Older Patients Receiving Chemotherapy: ASCO Guideline for Geriatric Oncology," published in *Journal of Clinical Oncology.*

The American Society of Clinical Oncology (ASCO) now recommends every cancer patient 65 and older get a geriatric assessment—a questionnaire either done by the patient's own regular doctor and then shared with the oncologist or done by the oncologist him/herself—before beginning chemotherapy.

How it will help improve patients' quality of life during cancer treatment…

Weighing the risks and benefits of therapy involves more than its effect on your cancer. For example, if you have a separate chronic condition, such as high blood pressure, diabetes or even a balance issue, how chemo affects it also needs to be considered. In addition to your medical conditions, a geriatric assessment includes questions about your activity level, diet, social support, depression and anxiety, memory issues and other information about your daily life.

Having the results of your geriatric assessment enables your cancer doctor to know you better, more precisely tailor your treatment plan to you, help predict how severe the side effects of chemotherapy will be, and determine what additional help you might need to get through cancer therapy with the best outcome.

For instance, research has shown that people who suffer from depression can have increased trouble functioning while on chemotherapy. Or, your balance may be worsened by chemo. So, part of your treatment plan may include working with a physical therapist to improve your balance and an occupational therapist to help make your home safer. If you don't have social support, a social worker may be the additional resource you need.

The assessment will help your doctor give you a more accurate prognosis and life expectancy by taking into account not only your cancer, but also your other medical conditions. This, too, may influence your choice of treatment.

TAKING THE INITIATIVE

You don't have to wait for your doctor to get the process started. You can take the geriatric assessment at the Cancer and Aging Research Group website (MyCARG.org), then print out the results to bring to your oncologist.

Suicide Risk with Cancer Patients

Katherine E. Henson, MSc, DPhil, a senior analyst in Public Health England's National Cancer Registration and Analysis Service, London, and author of a study on cancer and suicide risk published in *JAMA Psychiatry*.

Suicide risk is highest in the first six months after cancer diagnosis, contrary to the common belief that risk is highest in the palliative-treatment stages. These new findings suggest that mental health care should be integrated into cancer care early on to help patients with anxiety and hopelessness. Talk to your doctor about counseling or support groups at the start of treatment.

Promising Treatment for Mouth Ulcers

Supportive Care in Cancer

Painful mouth ulcers (oral mucositis) are among the worst side effects of cancer treatment.

Promising research: Photobiomodulation (low-dose light therapy) is one of the most effective ways to relieve pain and promote healing in patients who receive radiation (with or without chemotherapy) for head and neck cancers.

CHAPTER 4

Cardiovascular Disease and Stroke

Little-Known Heart Attack and Stroke Triggers

Cardiovascular disease causes one out of every three deaths in the US—and it has three main henchmen...

•**Heart attack,** when a blocked cardiac artery cuts off blood flow to the heart muscle, affecting about 735,000 people each year.

•**Sudden cardiac death (SCD),** commonly known as cardiac arrest, when chaotic activity in the heart's electrical system causes it to stop functioning—a condition that strikes 325,000 people yearly.

•**Ischemic stroke,** when blood flow is blocked to the brain, occurring in nearly 800,000 people every year.

If you ask most cardiologists what leads to these "acute cardiovascular events," they'll talk about conventional risk factors, such as elevated cholesterol, high blood pressure, a sedentary lifestyle, diabetes and smoking.

There's more to the story: Roughly half of all acute cardiovascular events are precipitated by little-known physical, emotional and chemical stressors, according to research. Exposure to these stressors can trigger a sudden, potentially harmful increase in the activity of the sympathetic nervous system, the "fight-or-flight" mechanism that prepares the body to respond to stress by temporarily accelerating heart rate, raising blood pressure and increasing blood clotting.

Because an estimated 85% of adults over age 50 have some degree of atherosclerotic cardiovascular disease, largely due to the risk factors listed above, the already-compromised arteries

Barry A. Franklin, PhD, director of Preventive Cardiology/Cardiac Rehabilitation at Beaumont Health in Royal Oak, Michigan. He is past president of the American Association of Cardiovascular and Pulmonary Rehabilitation and the American College of Sports Medicine, as well as a former editor in chief of *Journal of Cardiopulmonary Rehabilitation and Prevention.*

of the heart muscle or brain may not be able to handle these abrupt physiological changes... and you can end up suffering a heart attack, SCD or stroke. *What you need to know...*

PHYSICAL TRIGGERS

Major surgery is the leading little-known physical trigger. Surprisingly, it's not just heart surgery, but any invasive surgery that requires general anesthesia.

Important finding: Among more than 10 million adults (age 45 and older) who underwent a major noncardiac operation (such as orthopedic, gynecologic, vascular and neurosurgery), 3% of patients (or one in 33), on average, had either a heart attack or stroke while hospitalized, according to a nine-year study published in *JAMA Cardiology.*

The risks were especially high for certain types of operations—nearly 8% of patients undergoing vascular surgery suffered a heart attack or stroke while hospitalized...and more than 6% undergoing chest (thoracic) surgery. Patients who were at greatest risk were older, obese, smoked and/or had chronic conditions such as diabetes, kidney disease or high blood pressure.

What can happen: The surgery may cause arterial plaque to rupture and form a blood clot, triggering a heart attack or stroke.

And the risk for an acute cardiovascular event remains elevated for some time. One in 20 patients (5%) who had major noncardiac surgery had a heart attack within 30 days of the surgery, according to a study published in *Annals of Internal Medicine.*

Self-defense: To protect yourself against an acute cardiovascular event during or after major surgery, improve your aerobic fitness—which is associated with lower resting heart rates—before surgery. For example, in the study mentioned above, every 10 beat-per-minute increase in resting heart rate before surgery (for example, 80 versus 70 beats per minute) was linked to about a 30% relative increase in the odds of a heart attack during hospitalization after surgery.

You can achieve a good level of fitness simply by walking briskly (where you can have a conversation, but you'll be breathing harder than usual) for at least 30 minutes, five or more times a week.

EMOTIONAL TRIGGERS

Intense negative emotions—such as grief and anger—also stimulate the sympathetic nervous system, raising the risk for an acute cardiovascular event.

Compelling study: When researchers at Harvard Medical School tracked nearly 2,000 people (mean age of 62) over a five-year period, the risk for heart attack increased by 21-fold the day after the death of a "significant person," such as a spouse, and declined on each subsequent day, according to research published in *Circulation.* The risk was greatest among those who already had heart disease.

When researchers reviewed nine studies on anger and acute cardiovascular events, they found that rates of heart attack, stroke and arrhythmia (a risk factor for SCD) all increased—some by nearly eight-fold—in the two hours after outbursts of anger compared with other times, according to research published in *European Heart Journal.*

Women with diagnosed heart disease are particularly vulnerable to negative emotions. Those who had the highest levels of "psychological distress"—depression, post-traumatic stress, anxiety, anger, hostility and perceived stress—were 44% more likely to have a heart attack or stroke than those not experiencing those negative emotions, noted a study published in *Journal of the American Heart Association.*

How to protect yourself: If you have cardiovascular disease, stay fit (as described earlier) and take your prescribed medications, whether it's a beta-blocker, statin or low-dose aspirin. These drugs may reduce one's vulnerability to an acute cardiovascular event when an emotional trigger occurs.

To reduce, or even prevent, the adverse consequences of negative emotions, complementary approaches include meditation, deep breathing, yoga, tai chi, mental stress-reducing exercises and anger-management interventions.

CHEMICAL TRIGGERS

Air pollution and secondhand smoke are the two main chemical triggers of acute cardiovascular events.

Startling new findings: When levels of air pollution—from traffic and non-traffic emissions—in urban areas in New York state were tested and correlated with levels of hospitalization for acute cardiovascular events the next day, the higher pollution levels were linked to a more than doubled rate of hospitalization for arrhythmia and a nearly quadrupled rate of hospitalization for stroke, according to research published in *Environment International*.

Two years after smoke-free legislation was implemented in Uruguay—prohibiting people from smoking indoors in the workplace or in public places—hospitalizations for heart attack decreased by 22%, according to research published in *Tobacco Control*.

How to protect yourself: Limit your outdoor activities when pollution is high…and steer clear of people who are smoking. To monitor air quality in your local area, check the website AirNow.gov. As mentioned earlier, it's also crucial to get (and stay) fit and take your cardioprotective medications, as prescribed.

Other strategies to protect yourself against triggered cardiovascular events include avoiding unaccustomed heavy physical exertion (such as snow removal) and prolonged periods of sleep deprivation. It also helps to strive for strict enforcement of environmental regulations regarding air pollution.

Your Heart Needs Sleep

Céline Vetter, PhD, is assistant professor of integrative physiology and director of the Circadian and Sleep Epidemiology Lab at University of Colorado, Boulder, and senior author of a study published in *Journal of the American College of Cardiology*.

Getting less than six hours of sleep in 24 hours can up your heart attack risk by 20%. Ten or 11 hours can also increase heart attack risk by 34%, although we don't know the reasons for this yet. Staying in the healthy zone and sleeping six to nine hours per night can offset other risks for heart disease—even if those risks are genetic.

Heart Attacks That Start Slowly Could Be More Deadly

Study titled "The Association Between Symptom Onset Characteristics and Prehospital Delay in Women and Men with Acute Coronary Syndrome" led by researchers at University of Illinois at Chicago, published in *European Journal of Cardiovascular Nursing*.

Sudden chest pain or discomfort is a classic red flag for heart attack, but sometimes the symptoms start out mild and develop gradually. How do slower symptoms affect treatment and survival?

To find out, researchers recently looked at the time that elapsed between the first symptoms that occurred in 474 heart attack patients (average age 62) and their arrival at emergency departments (EDs) at various locations across the US.

The study, which was published in *European Journal of Cardiovascular Nursing,* found that people who experienced gradual symptoms, which tend to start with mild discomfort that slowly worsens, took eight hours, on average, to get to an ED versus 2.6 hours for those with abrupt symptoms that were characterized by sudden and severe pain from the beginning.

"Both are a medical emergency and require urgent help," explained Sahereh Mirzaei, PhD, RN, study author and a clinical practitioner in the open-heart intensive care unit at the University of Illinois at Chicago. "But our study shows that gradual symptoms are not taken seriously."

Other study findings…

•**Slow-to-develop symptoms are common.** Even though 56% of the study participants experienced abrupt symptoms, including sudden chest pain, 44% suffered gradual symptoms, such as mild and slowly progressive chest discomfort or pain.

•**Abrupt symptoms are linked to physical activity.** Sudden heart attack symptoms were more likely to occur after some type of exertion such as shoveling snow, climbing stairs, heavy gardening or jogging. This can signal a serious type of heart attack that requires prompt restoration of blood flow to blocked arteries.

•**Driving to the ED is a mistake.** A major cause of delay for all patients was driving to the ED instead of calling for an ambulance. Only 45% of the study participants called for emergency medical services. Differences in delay time between men and women were not significant.

•**The uninsured are at greater risk.** Being uninsured was linked with a longer delay.

Key takeaways…

•**Don't delay.** When medical care for heart attack symptoms is not sought promptly, there can be dire consequences. For example, the American Heart Association has set a goal of two hours for getting a patient with heart attack symptoms to the ED. Research has shown that every 30-minute delay reduces life expectancy by one year. After six hours, standard treatment with angioplasty, in which a catheter is inserted and the blocked artery is opened by inflating a tiny balloon, does little to reduce the rate of heart attack deaths.

•**Call 911.** Driving to the hospital was linked to slower arrival times at the ED. Despite repeated warnings that driving is not safe and delays treatment, studies consistently show that most people with heart attacks arrive at the ED by car. Calling 911 has several advantages, according to the National Heart, Lung, and Blood Institute. For one, it allows the 911 operator to give you advice (such as taking an aspirin if you're not allergic). Once emergency medical services (EMS) personnel arrive, they can assess your condition and start lifesaving medicines and other treatments right away. In addition, people who arrive by ambulance often receive faster treatment at the hospital.

Heart attack symptoms—either sudden or slow—are a medical emergency. *They include…*

•**Chest pain, discomfort or pressure**

•**Pain or pressure in the throat, neck, shoulder, arms or back**

•**Shortness of breath**

•**Pain may include nausea, vomiting or cold sweats.**

Heart Drug Alert

Hanno Tan, MD, PhD, cardiologist and project leader of European Sudden Cardiac Arrest network (ESCAPE-NET), University of Amsterdam, the Netherlands.

Patients taking high doses (60 mg or more daily) of *nifedipine,* such as Procardia, typically prescribed to treat angina and high blood pressure, had up to twice the risk for cardiac arrest, a potentially fatal stoppage of the heart, according to a review of more than 60,000 people.

Possible explanation: Nifedipine may disturb the heart's electrical properties.

Important: Consult your doctor about medication options. Do not stop this—or any drug—on your own.

New A-Fib Guidelines: What You Need to Know

Ijeoma A. Ekeruo, MD, assistant professor, department of internal medicine, division of cardiology, McGovern Medical School at UTHealth, Houston.

For more than 50 years, the gold standard drug to prevent stroke for patients with atrial fibrillation (A-fib) has been *warfarin* (Coumadin). Now new guidelines for treating A-fib bump that drug out of first place in favor of newer anticoagulants. If your doctor prescribed warfarin for your A-fib, should you change medications? *Facts to consider…*

Warfarin works by blocking the effect of vitamin K, which is involved in the cascade of proteins called "clotting factors" that help blood to clot. Vitamin K levels fluctuate naturally, and consuming dietary sources—including leafy greens—also influences levels of the vitamin in the body. Since the effectiveness of warfarin depends on how much vitamin K is in the body, dosage of the drug has to be carefully monitored—too much can lead to bleeding, while too little doesn't protect against stroke. So patients need to have their blood levels of warfarin checked often and, if necessary, the

Food for a Healthy Heart

Spicy Stop to Fatal Heart Attacks

People who ate chili peppers at least four times a week were 44% less likely to die from a heart attack over an eight-year period, compared with people who did not eat the hot peppers. Chili peppers also were associated with a big reduction in the risk for death from cerebrovascular disease—61%—in people who ate them at least four times every week. It is possible that the ingredient that gives the peppers their heat—capsaicin—may have protective effects. Animal studies have found it is associated with lower cholesterol and with blocking expression of a gene that causes blood vessels to tighten.

Marialaura Bonaccio, PhD, epidemiologist, IRCCS Neuromed Mediterranean Neurological Institute, Pozzilli, Italy, and leader of a study of 22,811 people, published in *Journal of the American College of Cardiology.*

Blueberries for Heart Health

Overweight adults with high blood pressure, elevated blood sugar and/or other cardiovascular risk factors ate a cup or a half-cup of blueberries, or a placebo, daily for six months.

Result: The one-cup group reduced their risk for cardiovascular disease by nearly 15%, while the half-cup and placebo groups showed no improvement.

Theory: One cup of blueberries daily provided adequate levels of heart-healthy anthocyanins.

Aedín Cassidy, PhD, professor of nutrition, Norwich Medical School, University of East Anglia, Norwich, England.

Red...White...or No Meat?

Red...white...or no meat?

Recent study: Healthy adults, ages 21 to 65, ate a diet rich in red-meat protein (such as beef)...a white-meat diet (chicken)...and then a no-meat diet, for four weeks each, with a "washout" period of two to seven weeks in between.

Result: LDL cholesterol levels were similarly higher (6% to 7%) after eating the red or white meat, versus the nonmeat diet.

For cholesterol control: Aim for a diet limited in meats and rich in plant-based proteins, such as nuts, beans, lentils, quinoa and tofu.

Ronald M. Krauss, MD, director of atherosclerosis research, Children's Hospital Oakland Research Institute, California.

---

dosage adjusted. And they need to keep dietary sources of vitamin K at a steady level.

NONVITAMIN K ANTICOAGULANTS

Alternative anticoagulants known as direct oral anticoagulants (DOACs) block clotting factors without depending on vitamin K. There's no need for blood tests or dietary restrictions.

It would seem like a no-brainer to just switch patients over to these new medications. But without years of clinical trials attesting that they are safer and more effective than warfarin, doctors have been holding off. Now the American Heart Association has published updated guidelines for treating A-fib that strongly recommend DOACs over warfarin, with some important qualifications. *According to the available research, all four DOACs are about equally effective for A-fib, but with some differences to consider...*

•*Dabigatran* (Pradaxa). FDA-approved in 2010, the drug showed lower rates of stroke and systemic embolism compared with warfarin but had similar risks of bleeding. It can cause nausea or heartburn and is not recommended for patients with kidney problems. It is taken twice a day.

•*Rivaroxaban* (Xarelto). Approved in 2011, it's taken only once a day. Another plus is that there are established dosing recommendations for patients with compromised kidney function, although it's not advised for patients on dialysis or with severe renal dysfunction.

•*Apixaban* (Eliquis). Approved in 2012, it was shown to be superior to warfarin with regard to stroke and systemic embolism...and also caused less bleeding and resulted in lower mortality. While it, too, is not recommended for patients with severe kidney dysfunction, apixaban is the only DOAC recommended for patients with Afib on dialysis. It is taken twice a day.

•**Edoxaban** (Savaysa). Approved in 2015, edoxaban is unique among DOACs in that it can be used by patients who have some kidney damage and at a reduced dose by patients with more severe decreased kidney function. It is taken once daily and not recommended for patients on dialysis.

Important: The guidelines advise that patients with a heart valve problem stick with warfarin. There's not enough evidence to say that DOACs are safer or more effective for this condition.

SIDE EFFECTS

When first introduced, there was concern about life-threatening bleeding from DOACs because there was no reversal drug as there is for warfarin. However, research finds the risk of bleeding from DOACs to be lower than with warfarin. Also, *idarucizumab* (Praxbind) is now an approved antidote for dabigatran...Andexxa is approved for rivaroxaban and apixaban...and other reversal drugs are being developed. Still, bleeding is a serious concern when taking any anticoagulant. *Signs to watch for include...*

•**Unexpected bleeding,** such as from the gums, bladder/urine...or sudden swelling of the joints

•**Unexplained bruising**

•**Bloody or black and tarry stool.**

DOACs are very expensive, so check with your insurer regarding coverage before talking to your doctor about changing your prescription.

Heart Attacks Are On the Decline

Analysis of the health records of 4.3 million Medicare beneficiaries by researchers at Harvard University, Boston, and Yale University, New Haven, Connecticut, published in *JAMA Network Open*.

And when they do occur, they are less likely to be fatal. Between 1995 and 2014 (latest data available), the rate of heart attacks fell by 38% among people age 65 and older. And the death rate within 30 days of an attack dropped by about one-third to 12%.

Reasons: Increased use of statins and other cholesterol-lowering drugs...use of coronary angioplasty to open arteries...lifestyle changes such as quitting smoking, eating a balanced diet, exercising regularly and reducing stress.

E-Cigarettes May Harm the Heart More Than Regular Cigarettes

Study titled "Chronic E-Cigarette Users Demonstrate More Consistent Coronary Endothelial Dysfunction Than Chronic Combustible Cigarettes," by researchers at Smidt Heart Institute at Cedars-Sinai Medical Center in Los Angeles and presented at the 2019 American Heart Association Scientific Sessions in Philadelphia.

If you're a cigarette smoker looking to quit, e-cigarettes, also known as vape pens, may seem like a good alternative.

Battery-operated or rechargeable e-cigarettes do not contain any tobacco. Instead, a cartridge of liquid nicotine, flavorings and other chemicals is heated to make a vapor, which is then inhaled by the user. The ease of use, lack of ash and smoky odor and variety of flavors make these electronic nicotine delivery systems appealing to many people, including teenagers.

But a study presented at the 2019 American Heart Association Scientific Sessions concludes that using e-cigarettes may carry as much risk for heart disease—and maybe even more—as traditional tobacco cigarettes.

This finding comes at a time when, despite increased reports of lung-related e-cigarette injuries, manufacturers continue to claim that these electronic systems are safe and can help cigarette smokers to quit.

Recent study: Researchers at the Smidt Heart Institute at Cedars-Sinai Medical Center in Los Angeles measured blood flow to the heart—a marker of how well the heart is functioning—of regular smokers ages 18 to 38 before and after smoking either e-cigarettes or traditional cigarettes. The measurements were taken while the participants were at rest and after they performed a handgrip exercise. The tobacco cigarettes caused blood flow to decrease after physical stress, but not while at rest. The e-cigarettes, however, caused impaired blood flow both after physical stress and while at rest. Decreased coronary blood flow increases the risk for heart disease.

"It's not just the nicotine that makes e-cigarettes harmful to the heart and lungs. It's the completely unknown bucket of manufactured products used to form vapors that is likely causing the most harm," said senior study author Florian Rader, MD, MSc, medical director of the Human Physiology Laboratory at the Smidt Heart Institute.

Note: The Centers for Disease Control and Prevention recently identified vitamin E acetate as a "very strong culprit" in lung injuries related to vaping.

And because e-cigarettes are associated with blood flow dysfunction not just during physical stress but at rest as well, they may be even more harmful than traditional cigarettes, despite what their distributors would like you to believe, the study reports.

The researchers add that because the practice of vaping is still relatively new, scientists may not yet know all of the ways it can damage hearts and lungs. Dr. Rader advises, "The use of any electronic nicotine delivery system should be considered with a high degree of caution until more data can be gathered."

Bottom line: At this point, we need to assume that cigarettes of any kind may hurt your health. If you don't smoke or vape, don't start. If you need help quitting, you can find useful tools and tips at SmokeFree.gov.

Aspirin for Heart Health

Christina C. Wee, MD, MPH, associate professor of medicine at Harvard Medical School and director of the Obesity Research Program in the Division of General Medicine at Beth Israel Deaconess Medical Center (BIDMC), both in Boston. She is also associate program director for the Internal Medicine Program at BIDMC and deputy editor of *Annals of Internal Medicine.*

Taking a daily low-dose (81-mg) aspirin has long been considered a bedrock therapy for people striving to prevent cardiovascular disease (including heart attack

and stroke). The reasoning was simple. Aspirin interferes with the formation of blood clots that develop inside blood vessels and can lead to a heart attack or stroke.

Here's the rub: Interfering with blood clotting also can lead to harmful bleeding—especially from the stomach. So it's been a balancing act to identify the people who are most likely to get more help than harm from aspirin therapy.

Until recently, most studies found that the benefit of low-dose aspirin therapy outweighed the risk of bleeding for people with a history of cardiovascular disease (a past heart attack or stroke) and for those with risk factors such as elevated cholesterol, diabetes, high blood pressure or a strong family history of heart attack or stroke.

New thinking: As researchers have continued to investigate this widely used therapy, a more nuanced view of the individuals who can benefit from daily aspirin—and who is at risk of experiencing more harm than good—has emerged.

What you need to know about a more customized use of aspirin therapy...

HOW WE GOT HERE

While aspirin therapy has been recommended for decades, the backdrop for its use in preventing cardiovascular disease has changed during that time. The risk of bleeding from aspirin has stayed about the same, but the risk for cardiovascular disease has been going down due to better treatment of key risk factors. Statin drugs have lowered cholesterol, and doctors have been doing a better job of treating diabetes and high blood pressure. Many people have stopped smoking, eliminating another major risk factor.

This means that the risk-benefit balance has shifted for people taking a daily low-dose aspirin to prevent a first heart attack or stroke (primary prevention). However, the therapy should still be used by those who have already had a heart attack or stroke.

This more customized view resulted from three landmark studies that came out in 2018, looking at primary prevention in adults with diabetes...adults at average risk for cardiovascular disease...and older adults. Taken together, these studies found few benefits compared with a consistent risk of bleeding.

Note: These studies do not apply to those with preexisting heart disease or stroke. The new studies prompted the American Heart Association (AHA) and the American College of Cardiology (ACC) to update their 2019 guidelines for aspirin therapy in primary prevention.

Why is the bleeding risk so concerning? With daily aspirin therapy, the main risk for internal bleeding is from a peptic ulcer. These ulcers, which are more common as people age, occur in about one out of 10 people. Bleeding can lead to anemia and the need for hospitalization and blood transfusion if it's acute.

Back in 2015, AHA guidelines said it was reasonable to use aspirin for primary prevention in anyone with an increased risk for cardiovascular disease and without an increased risk of bleeding. The AHA and ACC now say that people ages 40 to 70 should take it only if they are at significant risk for a first heart attack or stroke, and they are not at increased risk of bleeding, due to such factors as use of blood-thinning medication and a history of peptic ulcer or kidney disease, which also increase bleeding risk. And people over age 70 are strongly discouraged against routine aspirin use for primary prevention.

The big takeaway is that you should not start daily aspirin therapy to prevent heart disease on your own. Unless your primary care doctor has ruled out bleeding after taking your medical history and has calculated that you are at high enough risk for cardiovascular disease, the risk of using aspirin therapy is greater than the reward.

WHAT ABOUT PEOPLE ALREADY TAKING ASPIRIN?

As the landscape for recommended aspirin use has changed, it's worth noting that a lot of Americans are now taking it outside the guidelines. A recent study by researchers at Beth Israel Deaconess Medical Center and Harvard Medical School analyzed health data from 2017 for more than 14,000 adults over age 40 to determine how many people in the US were taking a daily aspirin for primary prevention—and estimated the total number of aspirin users from this representative survey.

Based on the study's findings, published in *Annals of Internal Medicine,* an estimated 30 million Americans over age 40 with no history of heart disease or stroke were taking a daily aspirin. This included close to 10 million people over age 70. More than six million Americans were taking aspirin without a doctor's approval. Researchers also found that Americans with a history of peptic ulcer—putting them at increased risk of bleeding—were not significantly more likely to report reduced use of aspirin.

This research, along with the new guidelines, is a warning that millions of Americans are probably using daily aspirin contrary to the new guidelines and are subjecting themselves to more risk than benefit by doing so. The researchers urge doctors to ask their patients about aspirin use and counsel them about the risks and benefits.

WHAT SHOULD YOU DO?

If your doctor has told you to take a daily aspirin because you have cardiovascular disease (that is, you've had a heart attack or stroke or undergone bypass surgery or received a heart stent), the warning above does not apply to you. To be safe, have another discussion with your doctor to make sure his/her recommendation has not changed based on the new guidelines.

If you do not have cardiovascular disease and you have been taking a daily aspirin, here's what you need to do…

•**If you are over age 70,** talk to your doctor. You probably do not need to be on aspirin if you don't have preexisting heart disease or stroke.

•**If you are any age and you are taking aspirin for heart health without your doctor's approval,** talk to your doctor to find out if your risk outweighs your benefit.

•**If you are age 40 to 70 and have any bleeding risk, but no cardiovascular disease,** talk to your doctor. You probably need to stop aspirin.

Doctors are doing a better job of reducing heart attack and stroke risk factors. To help reduce your own risk factors, don't smoke…eat a heart-healthy diet…and get regular exercise. If you are at low-to-moderate risk for cardiovascular disease, adding a daily aspirin may no longer be worth the risk. Risk assessment is complex but typically includes your doctor's clinical evaluation based on a risk calculator such as the tool provided on the ACC's website. Go to ACC.org and search "risk estimator."

Note: These guidelines do not include recommendations for aspirin use to treat other conditions such as headache and fever and to help reduce risk for colon cancer in people who are at increased risk. Consult your doctor for advice on these uses.

Glucosamine May Reduce Heart-Disease Risk

Lu Qi, MD, PhD professor of epidemiology at Tulane University, New Orleans, and coauthor of a study published in *The BMJ*. SPH.Tulane.edu

Glucosamine is a dietary supplement known to lessen joint pain, but a large study found that regular users were 15% less likely to experience cardiovascular events. Earlier research suggests that these benefits might be related to glucosamine's ability to reduce inflammation or its ability to mimic a low-carbohydrate diet that is related to lower risk for heart disease.

Mouthwash/Blood Pressure Alert

Nathan Bryan, PhD, adjunct professor of molecular and human genetics, Baylor College of Medicine, Houston.

Recent finding: After one week of using an oral rinse containing the antiseptic chlorhexidine, which is used to fight plaque and gingivitis, participants' tongues had a decrease in "friendly" bacteria that produce nitric oxide (NO), a substance that helps maintain normal blood pressure. In addition, their systolic (top number) blood pressure increased significantly—by 5 mmHg to 26 mmHg. Once the mouthwash was stopped, NO-producing bacteria in the mouth were replenished and blood pressure returned to normal after seven days.

Fiber for Your Heart

Give Your Heart a Fiber Boost

Heart failure patients often have less diversity in their gut microbiota.

Recent finding: Reduced gut bacteria was linked to lower dietary fiber intake, according to stool samples taken from more than 300 participants with and without heart failure.

Self-defense: Choose fruits, vegetables, cereals and other high-fiber foods to stimulate healthy gut flora.

Cristiane Mayerhofer, MD, cardiologist, Oslo University Hospital, Rikshospitalet, Norway.

Fiber Supplement Controls Cholesterol

The popular fiber supplement psyllium has been shown to help reduce LDL ("bad") cholesterol and two other lipids that are associated with heart disease. Those benefits are in addition to psyllium's treatment of constipation, the purpose for which it usually is used.

Analysis of the findings of 28 studies of people with normal and high cholesterol, led by researchers at St. Michael's Hospital, Toronto, Canada, published in *American Journal of Clinical Nutrition*.

Breathing Technique Can Lower Blood Pressure

Daniel Craighead, PhD, postdoctoral researcher, integrative physiology department, University of Colorado at Boulder and leader of a study of 50 people, presented at the recent Experimental Biology conference in Orlando, Florida.

Inspiratory Muscle Strength Training (IMST) involves breathing in vigorously through a special handheld device originally developed to help critically ill people breathe without ventilators. This technique also has been shown effective in helping develop the weak breathing muscles of people with obstructive sleep apnea. Now early results of a new study show that regular use of IMST can lower systolic blood pressure (the top number) nearly twice as much as aerobic exercise does. IMST users also had better large-artery function and lower heart rate and oxygen consumption during exercise than study subjects not using the technique. Inspiratory muscle trainers already are commercially available—ask your doctor if you should consider IMST.

Timing Your Blood Pressure Medication

Compared with people who took their blood pressure medication in the morning, those who took one or more blood pressure–lowering drugs at bedtime had 34% lower risk for heart attack…and 49% lower risk for stroke, according to a six-year study of nearly 20,000 men and women with hypertension.

Reason: Sleep-time blood pressure is the most significant marker for cardiovascular risk.

Important: Talk to your doctor before changing the time of day you take your medication.

Ramón C. Hermida, PhD, director, Bioengineering and Chronobiology Labs, University of Vigo, Spain.

No Fasting Needed Before Cholesterol Test

Samia Mora, MD, director, Center for Lipid Metabolomics, Brigham and Women's Hospital, Boston.

Prior to a cholesterol blood test, fasting has traditionally been advised for nine to 12 hours beforehand.

Recent finding: Nonfasting cholesterol levels were similar to fasting levels measured four weeks apart in the same participants, according to a study of more than 8,000 people with cardiovascular risk factors. This research supports the recent guideline change from the American College of Cardiology/American Heart Association that no longer requires fasting before a cholesterol test.

Statins Increase Risk for Staphylococcal Skin Infections

Humphrey Ko, BSc (Pharm) (Hons), doctoral candidate at School of Pharmacy and Biomedical Sciences at Curtin University in Perth, Australia and lead author of the study published in *British Journal of Clinical Pharmacology.*

Statins increase the relative risk for staphylococcal skin infections by 40%. The risk was statistically significant and similar over three, six and 12 months of taking these drugs, which previously had been linked to diabetes risk. This study shows increased risk for skin infections, whether or not patients had diabetes.

Cutting Back on Salt May Harm You

Michael Alderman, MD, emeritus professor at Albert Einstein College of Medicine, New York City, and former president of the American Society of Hypertension. He has studied extensively the effects of sodium on hypertension.

Salt has a reputation for being bad for your health. The main cause for alarm is sodium, which at very high levels can throw the body's fluid balance out of whack, causing high blood pressure, heart disease and even death. Government organizations say that we consume too much salt and recommend cutbacks. But in fact, sodium is a nutrient that's essential for myriad physiological processes in our bodies, and getting too little salt is also harmful to our health. The truth is, most of us are fairly conservative with the salt shaker.

Although it's true that cutting back on sodium can lower blood pressure in people who have hypertension, no studies have shown that doing so will help reduce heart attacks or death. What's more, cutting back too much also is likely to have some unexpected side effects—higher cholesterol, triglyceride and blood sugar levels.

Recent research summarizing six decades of studies that included more than one million people worldwide suggests an optimal range for sodium intake that's associated with the lowest risk for disease and death from all causes. That sodium "sweet spot" is roughly 3,500 mg to 4,500 mg a day. (Most people consume 3,600 mg to 3,700 mg daily.) That's a lot higher than the 1,500 mg to 2,300 mg a day recommended by the American Heart Association (AHA), the World Health Organization and numerous other health bodies.

Instead of trying to lower your sodium, it may make more sense to increase your intake of potassium, which helps control blood pressure by upping your ability to process sodium out of your body and by relaxing blood vessel walls. (Fruits and vegetables such as bananas, oranges, spinach and cucumbers are good sources.) Research has shown that higher levels of potassium are linked to fewer cardiovascular events and deaths across the globe.

Stents Don't Help Most Patients

Suzanne Steinbaum, DO, cardiologist in private practice in New York City and a national spokesperson for the Go Red for Women campaign. She is author of *Dr. Suzanne Steinbaum's Heart Book.* DrSuzanneSteinbaum.com

Yes, inserting a stent to open a blockage that's causing a heart attack can be life-saving for a patient having a heart attack—but there is growing controversy about how much it can help if used preemptively.

Stenting, an invasive and potentially risky procedure, has become standard practice for more than 1.8 million people a year in the US, even though multiple studies have questioned its effectiveness.

In the latest trial of more than 5,000 participants, researchers found that placing stents in arteries of people with stable and mild coronary artery disease as a preemptive measure doesn't prevent heart attacks or extend life for most patients and is no more effective than medication and lifestyle changes. Worse, risks include blood clots, strokes, heart attack and infection.

Why doesn't stenting help? Heart disease is a disease of the endothelium—the tissue that lines blood vessels and organs—and the stent fixes just one damaged spot. For a system-wide problem, you need a whole-body approach that includes managing blood pressure, cholesterol, blood sugar and your weight.

If your doctor suggests a stent, ask about both the risks and benefits for your particular circumstances. For example, a stent may be the answer when symptoms such as the pain of angina make it too challenging to exercise—a stent might allow you to adopt a healthier lifestyle.

If you already have a stent, remember that it didn't fix your heart disease. It only added support.

Best advice: Exercise and eat a primarily plant-based diet to avoid developing more blockages.

Dogs Help You Heal

Tove Fall, VMD, PhD, professor of epidemiology, Uppsala University, Sweden.

Dog owners live longer after a heart attack or stroke. Compared with people who did not own a dog, dog owners had a 21% lower risk of dying after a heart attack and an 18% lower risk of dying after a stroke in an 11-year study.

Bonus: Dog owners living alone fared even better. They were about 30% less likely to die after a heart attack or stroke than non–dog owners living alone.

Heart Patients: Block Out the Nighttime Light

Laura K. Fonken, PhD, assistant professor in the division of pharmacology and toxicology at University of Texas at Austin and lead author of the study published in *Experimental Neurology.*

Exposure to hospital light at night could harm recovering cardiac patients. Mice subjected to seven nights of even dim light after cardiac arrest had increases in mortality, compared with those that had no light disruption.

Theory: Nighttime light disruption upends our circadian rhythms, which in turn negatively impacts our immune systems and can lead to inflammation.

Self-defense: Since patients can't control hospital lighting, they should wear a sleep mask while there to block nighttime light.

Get Prompt Help for DVT

Arina ten Cate-Hoek, MD, clinical epidemiologist, Maastricht University, Maastricht, the Netherlands.

Patients with deep vein thrombosis (DVT)—blood clotting that often occurs in the legs—had a 20% lower risk for continued clotting when compression therapy was started, along with medication, within 24 hours of diagnosis, according to a new study of 600 DVT patients.

How it works: Compression therapy, which involves bandaging the legs or wearing compression stockings, reduces swelling and pain and prevents residual clots by improving blood flow in the legs.

Infections Linked to Stroke Risk

The study "Infection as a Stroke Trigger: Associations Between Different Organ System Infection Admissions and Stroke Subtypes," led by researchers at Icahn School of Medicine at Mount Sinai in New York City and published in *Stroke*.

If you are an older adult with diabetes, high blood pressure, atrial fibrillation, high cholesterol or migraine, you likely know that you are at higher risk for stroke. But did you know that an infection also may boost your odds of having a stroke?

While it's been known by scientists that a nasty urinary tract infection or respiratory infection may increase one's vulnerability to a life-threatening stroke, questions have remained around the specific types of stroke that may be triggered by different infections.

Now: To find out exactly which infections most often preceded three types of strokes, researchers at the Icahn School of Medicine at Mount Sinai in New York City delved further into the data.

Study details: For their study, researchers searched databases at New York state hospitals and analyzed admissions for three types of stroke along with hospital or emergency room admissions for five types of infection.

Ischemic stroke, the most common type of stroke, which is typically caused by a blood clot that blocks blood supply to the brain…intracerebral hemorrhage, due to bleeding into the brain…and subarachnoid hemorrhage, resulting from bleeding in the inner lining of the brain, were the types of stroke studied.

In addition, the researchers looked at five types of infection—skin…urinary tract…sepsis (a life-threatening infection of the bloodstream)…abdominal…and respiratory (including pneumonia and other lung infections). The odds of an infection triggering a stroke seven to 120 days after infection were then calculated.

Study results: Every type of infection included in the study increased the odds of an ischemic stroke. Urinary tract infection had the strongest association, increasing the risk by threefold within 30 days after infection.

For intracerebral hemorrhage, urinary tract and respiratory infections and sepsis increased risk. This time, the strongest association was found with sepsis, which tripled the risk within 60 days after infection.

Only a respiratory infection increased the risk for subarachnoid hemorrhage. This infection tripled the risk in the shortest period of time—within 14 days.

The good news is, with all types of infection studied, the risk for any stroke decreased over time.

The researchers theorized that various factors could be at play. People who develop infections may be more likely to suffer a stroke because the infection leads to inflammation that damages blood vessels…and increased numbers of white blood cells and platelets may contribute to the formation of blood clots. Infections also tend to make people less active, which also may increase the risk of blood clotting.

What this research could mean for you: The study did not analyze whether avoiding infection helps protect people from stroke. However, it's always wise to guard against infection—regardless of one's stroke risk.

During cold and flu season, for example, this includes avoiding illness-causing germs by washing your hands frequently, staying away from sick people and crowds whenever possible—and getting a flu shot and pneumonia vaccine. Warning signs of a urinary tract infection include chills, fever and burning pain when passing urine.

Prevent Stroke with Good Oral Hygiene

Pekka J. Karhunen, MD, PhD, professor of forensic medicine, Tampere University, Finland.

Nearly 80% of blood clots removed from 75 stroke patients contained DNA from mouth bacteria.

Theory: The bacterium *Streptococcus mitis* is harmless to the mouth, but when it enters the circulation from infected gums or a tooth extraction, it can bind to platelet receptors, making a person more prone to blood clots.

Important: Brush, floss and see a dentist at least twice a year for cleanings and oral exams.

A Severe Stroke Didn't Stop Him

Ted W. Baxter, a stroke survivor who now volunteers at hospitals and universities, providing his firsthand expertise in recovery from communication deficits. He is also active in philanthropic organizations and is author of *Relentless: How a Massive Stroke Changed My Life for the Better.*

Ted Baxter had what many people would consider a charmed life. He had an MBA from a prestigious school and traveled the world for his job at a top hedge-fund company.

Then, in 2005, at age 41, Ted's life collapsed when he had a massive ischemic stroke (due to a blood clot)—a life-threatening and often disabling condition that strikes nearly 700,000 people in the US each year.

Extensive damage on the left side of Ted's brain resulted in limited muscle control over the right side of his body. Worse, Ted was left with global aphasia—he couldn't speak, write or read.

Remarkably, Ted is now thriving. We spoke with him about his relentless drive to recover—and why he believes that the stroke changed his life for the better.

What did you think when you were told that your stroke had caused global aphasia?

I was terribly frightened. Global aphasia means that all communication is broken. It was difficult for me to understand what people were saying unless they spoke slowly and clearly. Because of the aphasia, I couldn't speak—the words weren't there—nor could I read or write.

What steps have you taken to recover?

Like most stroke survivors, my recovery involved physical therapy, occupational therapy and speech therapy. Working to regain my words has been much harder than regaining the use of my body. I've had to focus and practice constantly.

In the beginning, I had to start with kindergarten-level worksheets that paired simple nouns like "house" or "banana" with pictures. I moved on to exercises that had me work through various parts of a sentence—subject, verb, etc. I practiced for at least an hour every morning and an hour every night.

What role did acceptance play in your recovery?

It took months for me to finally understand and accept my new reality, but that's when my recovery took off. What I learned is that accepting reality doesn't have to mean losing hope.

How did you get through your down days?

The thing that saved me from disappearing into darkness and depression was getting a dog, a pug named Sullivan. I was never a dog person, but Sullivan saved me. A dog doesn't care if you can't remember his/her name or read a book. When Sullivan passed away, I got my dog Zorro.

It's also important to talk about your feelings and experiences. If you can't talk, find other ways to keep from growing apart from family and friends. Let them know that you'd like someone to come read to you or just watch TV with you.

You say your life is better now. In what ways?

I approach everything with a fresh appreciation, and I'm doing things that I never had the chance to do before.

I volunteer at hospitals and universities where they focus on strokes, traumatic brain injuries and aphasia. I run and attend group sessions with people who are experiencing the stages of trauma and tell them what helped me.

In my old life, I didn't make time for things like art, but now I'm visiting galleries and museums regularly. I have discovered that I love modern art!

Do you have any advice for caregivers?

The most important thing a caregiver can bring is patience. As stressful as it was for me to hunt for words, it was a crucial part of my recovery to let my brain do the work instead of loved ones filling in the blanks for me.

Also, do research so you can understand what is happening to your loved one, and locate your own support groups. Knowledge makes you more confident, and your loved one needs to feel that strength within you.

Where are you at today in your recovery?

I continue to work on my recovery every day—even 15 years later. My speech is not always smooth, but that doesn't stop me from giving public talks.

I still do physical therapy four times a week. I will never get back everything I lost, but I discovered that I have different facets of me that make my life fuller.

Any words of advice for people after stroke?

Hope and positive attitude come first. Determination is second. Doctors told me I had a two-year window for improvement in speech. After that, I would be stuck with whatever disability lingered. But I wanted to defy expectations. I continued to practice and continued to improve. For anyone who has had a stroke, just keep challenging yourself. When you get stronger, set new goals and keep doing more!

New Approaches for Aphasia

Susan Wortman-Jutt, MS, CCC-SLP, a certified speech-language pathologist in the outpatient speech department at the Burke Rehabilitation Hospital in White Plains, New York. She is involved in both patient care and research, with a special interest in rehabilitative speech and language therapies for adults.

Cutting-edge treatments can help stroke victims and others get their words back… About one million people in the US have aphasia. Some people with this condition have just a little trouble finding the right words. But others lose virtually all of their ability to speak, read, write and understand language. Most cases fall somewhere in between.

The cause of aphasia is most often a stroke or head injury. But brain tumors and other neurological disorders such as frontotemporal dementia also can lead to aphasia.

Latest news: Exciting new treatment approaches are being developed. *Best options now…*

INTENSIVE PROGRAMS

In traditional speech-language therapy for aphasia, patients typically have 30-to-60-minute appointments two or three days a week for a limited period of time. In contrast, with a new

The 15-Minute Stroke Alert

Getting treated for stroke just 15 minutes earlier could save your life.

Recent finding: For every 1,000 stroke patients whose time from hospital arrival to start of treatment was 15 minutes sooner, 15 fewer died…and 17 more walked out of the hospital without assistance, compared with the average stroke patient undergoing treatment, according to a study of more than 6,500 hospital patients with ischemic stroke (caused by a blood clot). The average time from arrival to treatment was one hour and 27 minutes.

Reza Jahan, MD, professor of neurosurgery, David Geffen School of Medicine, University of California, Los Angeles.

type of treatment program called an Intensive Comprehensive Aphasia Program (ICAP), many types of therapy for aphasia, including individual, group, computer-based and sometimes cutting-edge or experimental therapies, are provided for at least three hours a day, four to five days a week for two to six weeks.

Scientific results increasingly support the role of intensive therapy programs for boosting aphasia recovery.

There are currently only a handful of ICAPs in the US, mostly at universities or hospitals, but the number is growing. Ask your speech-language pathologist for locations and if an ICAP would be appropriate for you.

OTHER TREATMENT ADVANCES

Even if you can't participate in an ICAP, some of the latest treatments are available in traditional therapy programs. *Breakthrough and experimental approaches…*

•**Constraint-induced aphasia therapy (CIAT).** With this treatment, the patient is urged to use only spoken words—with no compensatory strategies such as gestures or writing—during therapy sessions that might last for two or more hours per day. Scientific results on its effectiveness are encouraging.

•**Computer software programs and apps** can allow patients to work on speech skills independently—whether at a speech clinic or at home.

Examples: In one software program called AphasiaScripts from Shirley Ryan AbilityLab in Chicago, a virtual therapist gives patients scripts for handling a variety of common situations, such as ordering a cup of coffee. Practice can give patients the confidence to use these words outside of therapy. And Constant Therapy is an app that provides speech, language and cognitive exercises that change as you make progress. The company can send progress reports directly to a patient's therapist. Aphasia.org lists other recommended apps for aphasia.

Important: Check with your therapist to find out which apps and programs might work for you and how best to use them.

Noninvasive brain stimulation. This involves using a painless electrical current to stimulate or inhibit certain areas of the brain,

with the hope of enhancing speech recovery. This is currently available only through clinical trials (see below).

On the horizon: Hybrid therapies. Combining aphasia treatment and movement therapy for stroke survivors and others who struggle with both kinds of impairments is in the early stages of investigation but holds promise for poststroke speech and movement recovery.

HANDLING THE COSTS OF THERAPY

Insurance typically covers only a specific number of sessions and may not cover newer or experimental treatments. However, you may be able to get free or reduced-cost therapy at a university clinic staffed by students supervised by licensed therapists…or be eligible for a clinical trial that explores innovative treatments—costs are often covered. Check ClinicalTrials.gov.

VITAL FOR IMPROVEMENT

Patients see more improvement if they practice their skills at home and in their communities and have the support of family and friends who encourage them to communicate.

To find aphasia therapy programs and speech-language pathologists near you, go to Aphasia.org or ASHA.org.

Women: Don't Hesitate to Call an Ambulance

Marek Gierlotka, MD, PhD, research coordinator and associate professor of cardiology, University of Opole, Poland.

Women: Don't wait to call an ambulance for yourself. In a study of 7,582 men and women who suffered a heart attack, significantly fewer women (41%) were treated within the recommended 90-minute window than men (47%).

Possible reasons: Women hesitate to call an ambulance for themselves and fail to recognize that their heart attack symptoms may include jaw, back, shoulder or stomach pain, instead of the classic chest pain and left-arm pain.

Eat Breakfast to Help Recovery

Marcos Minicucci, MD, professor of medicine, São Paulo State University, Brazil.

Skipping breakfast and eating a late dinner hinders heart attack recovery. Heart attack sufferers with these eating habits were four to five times more likely to die, have another heart attack or suffer from angina within 30 days of hospital discharge. Each habit alone was also linked to these outcomes.

Get Up and Move for Your Heart's Sake

Study of 150,000 people in Australia by researchers at University of Sydney, Australia, published in *Journal of the American College of Cardiology*.

Risks from prolonged sitting can be offset by about 20 to 40 minutes of exercise a day. If you regularly sit for six hours or more per day, you need 150 to 300 minutes of moderate-intensity exercise per week to offset the negative effects on your cardiovascular system.

Stronger Body = Stronger Heart

Stefanos Tyrovolas, PhD, principal investigator, Frailty, Sarcopenia and Nutrition Group, Parc Sanitari Saint Joan de Déu, Barcelona, Spain.

Men and women with the highest muscle volume were 81% less likely to suffer heart attack or stroke compared with those who have the lowest, according to a 10-year study of 2,020 adults, ages 45 and older.

Theory: Muscle mass helps maintain normal inflammatory, endocrine and metabolic function, which can stave off cardiovascular disease.

Takeaway: Include resistance training in your exercise routine.

CHAPTER 5

Consumer Health Alerts

The Truth About Skyrocketing Drug Prices

Here's the real story behind those astronomical costs—and what you can do to fight back... Many modern drugs are lifesavers. With their help, countless Americans are now living longer and better. Remarkably, new drugs can even allow some people with otherwise lethal cancers to survive for years.

But make no mistake. Pharmaceutical breakthroughs come at a price—and it's a high one. Headlines regularly announce stratospheric costs such as a hemophilia drug with a tab of $1.5 million. Everyday drugs are also taking an ever-heftier chunk of the average paycheck.

What's driving these runaway drug costs? For the real story, we spoke with Robin Feldman, JD, a renowned legal scholar who specializes in pharmacy and patent law.

Have drug prices really gone up as much as people think?

Yes! Even after accounting for rebates, Medicare spending for brand-name drugs rose 62% between 2011 and 2015. And while the cost of new drugs and those for rare conditions contributes to the sticker shock, drug companies have raised prices most sharply for commonly used drugs such as those prescribed for chronic conditions, including diabetes, elevated cholesterol, high blood pressure, asthma and the like.

But doesn't health insurance generally pick up the tab?

Not everyone has health insurance, and not all insurance covers drugs. Many people who are insured through their jobs pay a deductible before drug coverage kicks in. Many Medicare

---

Robin Feldman, JD, Arthur J. Goldberg Professor of Law and director of the Institute for Innovation Law at University of California Hastings College of the Law, San Francisco. She is author of *Drug Wars* and, most recently, *Drugs, Money, and Secret Handshakes.*

participants pay coinsurance—a proportion of the drug cost—and then there's the "donut hole," a gap in coverage when the insured pays a percentage of the cost (25% of the list price) up to $6,350 out-of-pocket for 2020. Though many people assume that it's the insurance companies that are swallowing these higher drug prices, the fact is, health insurers pass them on in higher premiums.

Sadly, the human cost can be extraordinarily high when people are forced to choose between medication and other basic bills like food and heating…or they halve the dose or only take their meds on alternating days.

What about the pharmaceutical companies' contention that they need high prices to finance the development of lifesaving drugs?

Research and development (R&D) is indeed expensive, and a pharmaceutical company that makes an important discovery should get a handsome reward. But the billion-dollar R&D costs that drug manufacturers commonly cite are "one of the great myths of the industry," according to Andrew Witty, former CEO of Glaxo-SmithKline, one of the biggest pharmaceutical companies.

Patent protection allows the company to sell the product it developed without competition for a decade or more. But companies constantly play the system, extending patents by slightly tweaking a drug with "me-too" drugs… adding new dosages…putting it in a pill instead of a capsule…or repurposing it for a new disease.

When patents do expire, companies may find it worth their while to pay generic manufacturers to actually keep cheaper versions off the market. But the real reason for ever-rising drug costs has to do with how they're sold.

How so—isn't it a free market?

It's complicated. Few people realize that private and government health plans don't deal directly with drug companies. These insurers hire middlemen, known as "pharmacy benefit managers" (PBMs), to help choose what drugs they'll cover, negotiate prices and set consumer costs, such as co-pays and coinsurance. PBMs initially operated mainly as claims processors,

but when Medicare added drug coverage in 2006, their roles expanded so that they now help establish formularies (the lists of drugs that insurers cover) and are the ones to negotiate drug costs directly with the pharmaceutical companies.

This is where it gets tricky. PBMs should be bargaining with the drug companies to get the best deals, but pharmaceutical companies usually put a high price on their drugs and then offer discounts or rebates to the PBM. (It's like Macy's jacking up the "list price" for a suit and then lowering it by 60% for a doorbuster sale.)

To sweeten the pot further, manufacturers offer volume discounts to PBMs whose health-plan clients buy more of their drugs. In return, the PBM gives preferential treatment to the company's drug by denying coverage for a competitor's products or tacking a higher co-pay on them. This is why you may be asked to pay more for a generic medication than for the brand-name drug. Or why cheaper drugs aren't covered by your insurance.

The trouble is, the rebate or discount may go to the PBM, but no further. The insurer—and you—pay the rising list price. The shocking part is that the deals struck between PBMs and drug companies are considered "trade secrets"—they are hidden from the consumer, the insurer, the employer and even the government.

Is this why drugs are so much cheaper elsewhere?

It's true that the systems in other countries are quite different from those in the US. To an extent, we subsidize the pharmaceutical manufacturers' profits—drug companies know they can cut prices in Europe and Canada and make it up in the free-for-all American market. This is why you pay $200 for a prescription that your cousin in Toronto fills for $10.

Short of moving to Canada, what can we do to keep our drug costs down?

First, be an intelligent consumer. If you're paying out of pocket, shop around for lower prices. For example, on the website GoodRx. com, you can compare costs at local pharmacies. The website also offers coupons to reduce the purchase price for certain drugs.

In addition…

•**Don't assume that health insurance will reduce your cost.** If a drug covered by your policy carries a hefty co-pay, it's sometimes cheaper to buy it yourself.

•**Ask your doctor if there's a generic or less costly alternative with the same therapeutic effect.** And don't be fooled by advertising. Manufacturers of brand-name drugs advertise, but companies don't do the same for their generic medications.

•**If you're prescribed a combination drug, price its components separately.** For example, Treximet, a brand-name migraine drug, costs just over $900 for nine tablets (a typical 30-day supply). It's a combination of the drug sumatriptan, an older, off-patent medication now available as a generic, and naproxen, a generic pain reliever that's available over the counter. Buying the drugs separately would cost about $36.

Note: You may not be able to find the exact dosages that are in a combo drug by purchasing the drugs separately. Discuss with your doctor how to adjust the drugs if taking them separately to still meet your needs.

•**Review every medication that you take with your doctor,** and make sure you still need them all.

•**Talk to your doctor about nondrug therapies.**

•**Buy a pill splitter ($5 to $10 at most drugstores).** Many drugs cost the same regardless of dosage. If you're prescribed a 5-mg daily dose of an expensive medication, ask your doctor to write a script for 10 mg—you'll get a two-month supply for the price of one. Just be sure to ask your pharmacist if the pill can be split.

•**Consider using a pharmacy discount card.** Organizations such as AARP and AAA offer these cards to members, but don't forget to comparison shop to make sure the card is offering you the best price.

Cancer Genetic Testing: Is It Right for You?

Scott M. Weissman, MS, CGC, a board-certified genetic counselor and a clinical faculty member at the Northwestern University Graduate Program in Genetic Counseling in Chicago. He also is the founder of Chicago Genetic Consultants, a personalized genetic-counseling service based in Northbrook, Illinois.

As cancer treatments become increasingly sophisticated, so too has the testing for this disease. Genetic tests that can determine one's risk for cancer—or help guide treatment in those who've already been diagnosed—are now becoming the standard of care.

Latest development: For certain patients, Medicare will now cover cancer genetic tests that have been approved by the FDA—tests that detect whether your DNA has a genetic mutation that increases your risk of developing cancer or underlies a diagnosed cancer. Many private health insurers also are picking up the tab.

Whether you're a woman or a man, the testing might show, for example, that you have a mutation (or variant) in the BRCA1 or BRCA2 gene, which increases risk for breast cancer by up to 85% or ovarian cancer by up to 60%…and risk for prostate cancer by up to 30% to 40%.

For insights about the new world of cancer genetic testing, we spoke with genetic counselor Scott M. Weissman, MS, CGC, a leading authority on this topic.

WHAT'S AVAILABLE

There are two main types of cancer genetic tests…

•**Germline.** A saliva or blood test is used to detect specific, heredity-based genetic mutations that may predispose you to cancer. If you already have cancer or you're a cancer survivor, the test can detect whether it was tied to a hereditary cause—this will tell you if you're at increased risk for a second occurrence of the same cancer or perhaps another type of cancer…or whether family members should also consider testing. Medicare typically covers this test only if you currently have cancer or are a cancer survivor. Most private insurers also cover people who have not had cancer.

Germline tests can be obtained in three different ways...

•Health-care provider–ordered. Following a risk assessment conducted by a doctor or genetic counselor who documents your personal and family history risk factors, a doctor may order the test. This type of test is 90% to 95% accurate.

•Direct-to-consumer. In this case, you order the test yourself. You receive a kit, provide a saliva sample and send it back to the company. The DNA in the saliva is analyzed, and results are delivered directly to you. For example, 23andMe is the only company offering FDA-cleared direct-to-consumer cancer genetic testing—for BRCA1 and BRCA2 mutations in breast and ovarian cancer...and for MUTYH mutations, which raise the risk for colon cancer. Direct-to-consumer testing is not covered by insurance.

Caution: The 23andMe BRCA test is only for the three genetic variants of the BRCA gene that are prevalent among Ashkenazi Jews—and misses the roughly 90% of people who have other types of BRCA mutations.

•Consumer-initiated, doctor-ordered. With this approach, you order the test from one of several laboratories (see below)—but the lab that conducts the test works with an independent network of genetic counselors and physicians to review the request, with a physician approving the test...or deciding that the test isn't warranted.

This type of testing (typically saliva) can detect dozens of genetic mutations that indicate an increased risk of developing certain cancers (such as breast, ovarian, uterine, colon, pancreatic, prostate, thyroid and brain). Many laboratories across the US now provide this service, but the three most reliable are Color Genomics...Invitae...and Helix/PerkinElmer.

Helpful: The best laboratories are accredited by the College of American Pathologists, CAP. org, as well as Clinical Laboratory Improvement Amendments, CDC.gov/CLIA. To see if a lab that you are considering using is accredited, check the above websites or the lab websites...or call the lab and ask.

Watch out: Some unscrupulous laboratories are "cold calling" seniors and offering cancer genetic testing—whether the individual needs it or not. Before ordering, talk to your doctor about the benefits of the test.

•**Somatic.** This test uses cancer tissue or blood to see if there is a genetic mutation fueling the cancer. This type of mutation spontaneously develops over the course of a lifetime and cannot be passed on to your children. If a mutation is found, the oncologist can prescribe one of the many "targeted" therapies now available to inhibit the action of the mutated genes.

Examples: The EGFR mutation in lung cancer is targeted by the drug *erlotinib* (Tarceva)...and the BRAF mutation in melanoma is targeted by the drug *vemurafenib* (Zelboraf). Insurance almost always covers a somatic cancer genetic test, which must be ordered by a doctor.

SHOULD YOU GET TESTED?

If you're interested in preventing cancer, it's important to realize that only 5% to 10% of all cancers have a genetic component. When does genetic testing make sense if you have *not* had cancer? *Some criteria...*

•**When a close relative (a parent, sibling or child)** has been diagnosed with cancer before the age of 50...or a cancer genetic test in a close relative shows a germline cancer mutation...or you have three or more close relatives with the same cancer regardless of age.

•**For a woman,** when there are both breast and ovarian cancers in close relatives...when there is breast cancer in two or more relatives on the same side of the family...when there is a close relative with cancer in both breasts.

•**For colon cancer,** if a colonoscopy detects more than 10 precancerous colorectal polyps regardless of family history.

If you have cancer, you should get a cancer genetic test.

Why this is important: Finding a genetic mutation can determine the best treatment options.

Or if you had cancer years ago, before germline testing was common, and the cancer recurs, that could be a good time to do a risk assessment to see if a germline test is indicated.

POST-TESTING STRATEGY

If your screening test results are positive—meaning that you have a genetic risk for cancer—take action.

Your test results may indicate that you need earlier or more frequent screenings, such as colonoscopies. If you have a genetic risk for breast cancer, for example, along with earlier screening, you might also consider taking an estrogen-blocking drug or getting a preventive mastectomy.

And if you find out that you have a hereditary risk, you should also tell your close relatives (parents, siblings and children), as well as aunts/uncles, cousins and grandparents, that they should consider testing, too.

Important: Even if your tests results are negative, if you have a strong family history of cancer, you may need increased monitoring. Ask your doctor for advice.

HOW GENETIC COUNSELING HELPS

It's a complex process to decide whether or not to take a genetic cancer test…choose which test to take and which laboratory to use…understand the results…act on the results…and cope emotionally with positive results. That's why there are genetic counselors—health professionals specially trained in genetics and psychology to help people in the process of genetic testing.

To find a genetic counselor near you: Go to the website of the National Society of Genetic Counselors, FindAGeneticCounselor.com, and enter your zip code. Some insurers will cover the cost of genetic counseling.

Beware New Genetic Testing Scam

Shimon Richmond is assistant inspector general for investigations at US Department of Health and Human Services, Washington, DC. HHS.gov

By mail, telemarketing or at health fairs, seniors are offered "free" genetic screenings. Scammers ask for a cheek swab and Medicare number, which may be used for identity theft. Also, the scammers bill Medicare $6,000 to $11,000. Medicare pays only for medically necessary, doctor-approved tests. If Medicare balks, the senior may have to pay the entire cost.

Beware At-Home DNA Tests. False Positives. False Negatives

Marwan Sabbagh, MD, director of the Cleveland Clinic's Lou Ruvo Center for Brain Health in Las Vegas. He is coauthor of *Fighting for My Life: How to Thrive in the Shadow of Alzheimer's.* ClevelandClinic.org

It sounds easy. For less than $200 you can buy a DNA testing kit that provides information about your ancestry and identifies health risks in your genes. But while the ancestral information can be interesting, that health component can be troubling.

Unlike genetic tests through your doctor, direct-to-consumer genetic health tests are unreliable. A 2018 report published in *Genetics in Medicine* uncovered a 40% false-positive rate—for every 10 people given the life-altering news that they have a potentially serious genetic variant, four are being misinformed. Additionally, at-home genetic tests don't check the full spectrum of risk markers for many conditions—they check only the most common and omit others.

Inaccurate results have significant consequences—unnecessary visits with specialists, wasted money, emotional distress. And for those with false-negatives, there is a risk that other symptoms of a problem will go ignored because they think they're "safe." At-home tests usually don't provide access to genetic counselors to help people deal with the results, either, increasing the odds of misunderstandings. What's more, insurance companies could withhold life, disability or long-term-care insurance based on the results, although health insurers are prohibited from considering genetic test results.

Your privacy is at risk, too. At-home genetic-testing companies sell customers' data to pharmaceutical companies, and their databases could be vulnerable to hackers.

73

If you have already taken one of these tests, review the results—positive or negative—with your doctor and ask what he/she recommends as a next step. Do not make important decisions based on the test alone.

If you're concerned about your risk profile, opt for FDA-approved genetic testing that's arranged through your doctor and, often, covered by health insurance or Medicare. There is the "CGx" test, which screens those at high risk for cancer for a broad spectrum of genes believed to play a role in 5% to 10% of cancers—and the "PGx" test for genetic reactions to prescription drugs.

Emergency Room Finder

Emergency Medicine Network. EMNet-USA.org

The nationwide app, EMNet findERNow, quickly determines your location…finds the ERs that are closest in terms of distance and time…and provides directions and other information. Listings are researched by Boston's Massachusetts General Hospital.

The "New" Rx We Should All Be Getting

Rebecca Shannonhouse, editor-in-chief, health content, Bottom Line Inc.

Plenty of research shows that our food choices dramatically affect our risk for chronic diseases, such as heart disease, high blood pressure (hypertension), cancer and diabetes. Not surprisingly, the majority of health-care costs involve the very same chronic diseases. So what would happen if our doctors sent us home with prescriptions for food instead of drugs? Until recently, food prescriptions were little more than a novel idea.

Now: A recent study by researchers at Tufts University has calculated some of the real-world benefits that would result from food prescriptions.

In one scenario, Medicare/Medicaid would cover 30% of the cost of "prescribed" fruits and vegetables. In another scenario, the same insurance coverage would extend not only to fruits and vegetables but also to whole grains, seafood, nuts and seeds, etc.

The projected benefits were stunning. Over the lifetime of a typical study participant, the fruit-and-vegetable plan was projected to reduce deaths due to cardiovascular disease (CVD) by 350,000. The more extensive healthy-food plan had even better results—620,000 fewer CVD deaths. Oh, and there was a whopping $100 billion reduction in health-care costs! According to Yujin Lee, PhD, a co-first author of the study, healthy-food prescriptions could be "as or more cost effective as other common interventions, such as preventative drug treatments for hypertension or high cholesterol."

Sobering fact: More than two-thirds of all doctor visits generate a prescription for one or more drugs, adding substantially to health-care costs. With today's tight budgets, an insurance-company-issued debit card for the grocery store might sound like an expensive indulgence. But the fact is, it could be one of the smartest moves of all.

Get Your Insurer to Cover a "Controversial" Diagnosis

Charles B. Inlander, consumer advocate and health-care consultant based in Fogelsville, Pennsylvania. He was the founding president of the nonprofit People's Medical Society, a consumer-advocacy organization credited with key improvements in the quality of US health care, and is author or coauthor of more than 20 consumer-health books.

As much as you hear and read about chronic Lyme disease, adrenal fatigue and chronic fatigue syndrome, most health insurers (and even some doctors) do not consider these conditions to be "real." The problem is, there is no single diagnostic test that proves any of those conditions is the cause of symptoms you are experiencing—even if your doctor and experts who specialize in treating those conditions conclude that you do have the disease. Some of these conditions have diagnostic codes that are required to file an insurance claim, but many insurers deny the treatment protocol being prescribed, such as long-term antibiotic therapy for chronic Lyme disease.

As foreboding as this sounds, there are ways to improve your chances of getting the health insurance and disability insurance coverage you need. *Here's my four-step plan for overcoming the controversial diagnosis barrier…*

•**Check the fine print.** A number of health insurers exclude certain conditions, many of which are controversial diseases. Carefully review your policy for these exclusions or call customer service and ask for a list of excluded conditions. Make sure to also check under specific categories—such as alternative treatment for chronic fatigue—for exclusions that may not be on the main list.

Insider tip: If you're shopping for your own coverage, try to purchase policies with as few exclusions as possible. If your employer provides your health and/or disability insurance, see if there are options with fewer exclusions.

•**Get it in writing.** When you're diagnosed with a controversial condition, it is crucial that your doctor give you his/her diagnosis in writing along with copies of all test results that led him to make that diagnosis. If a claim or course of treatment is denied, it's your doctor's written treatment plan justifying the recommended course of treatment that you'll need to give to the insurer.

Insider tip: Emphasize to your doctor the importance of a detailed explanation supporting his treatment program.

•**Seek a top-notch expert's opinion.** If an insurer denies your claim, get a second opinion from an expert in the field. You may have to go outside your local area to find such expertise. Second opinions are typically covered by insurance, but even if you must pay for it up front, it will be money well spent if it helps get your claim approved. Start your search by contact-

ing a major teaching hospital in your region to locate a specialist. If you strike out there, extend your search to one of the nationally known medical centers such as Mayo Clinic or Cleveland Clinic.

Insider tip: Because some experts can base their second opinions on a review of your test results and treatment plan, you may not need to be physically present.

•**See how others have fought—and won—insurance denials.** Seeking help from others with your condition can be especially useful when it comes to dealing with insurance. There are self-help groups for just about every condition imaginable, and most have local or state chapters that offer support and suggestions based on the members' own experiences, including how they fought insurance denials. You can find these groups by doing an online search. Simply enter "support groups for (list the condition)."

Best Pharmacy Chain

"J.D. Power 11th Annual US Pharmacy Study," based on responses from 12,059 pharmacy customers, reported at JDPower.com.

Top-ranked pharmacy chain: Good Neighbor. It scored 914 points out of a possible 1,000 in a J.D. Power survey. Second place went to Health Mart, with a score of 893…followed by Rite Aid, with 865.

Among brick-and-mortar mass merchandiser pharmacies: Sam's Club scored highest, with 890…followed by Costco with 879 and CVS inside Target with 869.

Among supermarket pharmacies: Wegmans scored highest, with 915, followed by Publix with 897 and Winn-Dixie with 896.

Among mail-order pharmacies: Humana scored highest, with 900…followed by Kaiser Permanente with 886 and OptumRx with 869.

How to Be Heard in the Health-Care Debate

Charles B. Inlander, consumer advocate and health-care consultant based in Fogelsville, Pennsylvania. He was the founding president of the nonprofit People's Medical Society, a consumer-advocacy organization credited with key improvements in the quality of US health care, and is author or coauthor of more than 20 consumer-health books.

Health care is the number-one issue in state primaries and in the general election, according to most polls. And regardless of our political persuasions, access to quality, affordable health care is something all of us want for ourselves and our families.

That's why it is vital to let the candidate you support for president and those running for the US House or Senate know about the health-care issues that affect you. It's also important to be in touch with candidates for your state legislature, since states license and regulate doctors and hospitals as well as all the health insurance plans offered in your state. Your voice can make a difference. *To get your views heard…*

●**Know where to start.** First off, you've got to find the proper mailing address, e-mail and/or phone numbers. If you are contacting an incumbent member of the US House of Representatives, go to House.gov/representatives. You can search by state or zip code. For the US Senate, go to Senate.gov/senators/contact and search by name or state. To contact your state legislators, go to Congress.gov/state-legislature-websites and click on your state. You'll then see links to contact incumbent members. To contact a candidate for any office, search online by entering the candidate's name and the phrase "contact info." This will usually call up the candidate's website, where you can find contact information.

●**Put it in writing.** Write a succinct letter or e-mail to an incumbent legislator or a candidate. Keep it to one page, if you can. Limit each communication to one issue. For example, if you are unable to afford your medications, explain that. Name the drugs you cannot afford…and point out that, even with your insurance (if you have coverage), the co-pay or deductible is beyond

your means. If you have a recommendation to fix the problem, mention it. Make the message as personal as possible by telling your situation or a family member's situation.

●**Put it in your own words.** You may belong to an organization promoting a specific piece of legislation or issue. Often, these groups send out examples of letters you can use. Do not use these boilerplate letters. Incumbents and candidates get hundreds of these letters and e-mails, and Congressional staffers have told me that they usually end up in the trash. Instead, explain your view on the issue and why you either support or are against a given proposal—these messages are read.

●**Pick up the phone.** A direct telephone call to your elected official or to a candidate's campaign office is also very effective. Unless the matter is being voted on in a matter of days, the best office to call is the incumbent's district office—the one closest to you. In addition to offices in Washington, DC, all incumbents have district offices, which are staffed by knowledgeable personnel who handle constituent issues. For a nonincumbent candidate, contact the campaign office in your district. Ask to speak with the campaign director and explain your concerns. In most cases, that person will take your call. Briefly summarize your situation and state your opinion on pending legislation. Health care is an issue that's too important to sit back and let others decide for you.

Groupon Discounts for Health Services

Kaiser Health News. KHN.org

Groupon discounts for health services are available in some markets, including Atlanta and parts of Oklahoma and California. The discount site has made physical therapy and ultrasounds available at reduced prices.

Other sites offer discounts, too: MDsave has deals with 250 hospitals for reduced prices on everything from MRIs to back surgery. Deals of this sort have been around since about 2011 and actually were more popular earlier in the decade—but are generating renewed interest as debates on health-care costs heat up. The deals are intended to make services available to people who do not have health insurance.

Get the Best Deal on Gym Membership

Roundup of experts on gym memberships, reported at Grow.Acorns.com.

To get the best deal on a gym membership…

•**Do not sign up for auto-pay.** Pay manually for a few months, until you find out whether you are using the gym regularly and whether the price works for you—if it does not, you may want to switch to a different gym.

•**Ask about fees and freezing.** Avoid gyms that charge a fee for canceling membership, and confirm that you can freeze the account, taking a break from payments, if you cannot use the gym for a while.

•**Do not take the first offered price.** Gyms need your business and are always offering deep discounts, free months and similar inducements.

Example: One national gym recently offered a $1 charge for the first month instead of the usual $50.

•**Check out your insurance and employee benefits.** Some insurers and employers offer discounted gym memberships or reimbursements if you use designated facilities.

Save on Contact Lenses

Dallas Cox, researcher and writer with Clark Howard's Team Clark Consumer Action Center and lead author of its recent contact lens price study. Clark.com

The best contact lens deals are from Lens.com, ContactLensKing.com and Costco. The websites Lens.com and ContactLensKing.com feature prices well below other retailers for five popular lenses, according to a recent study—sometimes as much as 50% less. Costco's prices are the best among brick-and-mortar stores.

Easy Ways to Cut the Cost of Dental Care

MoneyTalksNews.com

Have work done at a dental school—students do the procedures under close supervision. For routine cleanings, try a dental-hygienist school. If these schools are not nearby and you have low income, look for a dental clinic associated with a federally funded community-health center—charges are based on income. If you need to use a regular local provider, ask in advance about pricing and payment policies—you might get a discount for immediate payment or a chance to pay the bill over time without interest. If you have dental insurance, your out-of-pocket costs should be lower—but only up to coverage limits. Know what they are and what procedures are excluded completely. Visit the dentist regularly for preventive services that can avert high-cost procedures in the future.

Lower the Cost of Dentures

Money.USNews.com

Dentures usually last just five to eight years before needing replacement, so consider alternatives such as bridges or implant crowns. Comparison shop with other nearby dentists—if you like your current provider but find a lower price elsewhere, ask whether your dentist will match it. Consider a payment plan—many dentists offer them, and some do not charge interest. If you have a local dental school, find out if it does denture fittings by students who are closely supervised by experienced clinical faculty. If quotes for your dentures are very high, consider medical tourism—you may be able to take a vacation and have dentures fitted at the same time.

Antibiotics for a Toothache?

Peter Lockhart, DDS, chair, American Dental Association expert panel that developed the guideline, and research professor, Carolinas Medical Center–Atrium Health, Charlotte, North Carolina.

Not so fast. Antibiotics are often prescribed to relieve pain and prevent worsening of a toothache.

Now: A new review found that treatment by a dentist and, if needed, over-the-counter pain relievers, such as *acetaminophen* (Tylenol) or *ibuprofen* (Advil), are more effective at reducing pain and swelling and avoid the side effects and overuse of antibiotics.

Exception: Antibiotics may be needed if you are unable to see a dentist right away and/or have fever, swollen lymph nodes or extreme tiredness, symptoms that suggest the infection has spread beyond the tooth.

Antibiotics and Pesticides in Milk

Jean A. Welsh, PhD, associate professor, department of pediatrics, Emory University, Atlanta, and leader of a study published in *Public Health Nutrition*.

A study of four brands of organic milk and four brands of conventional milk found no such residues in organic samples but some level of them in 26% to 60% of samples of conventional milk. Residue levels were above federal guidelines for *amoxicillin* in one sample and for *sulfamethazine* and *sulfathiazole*—two common antibacterial agents—in several samples.

Unknown: Whether residues at the levels found have any impact on human health.

Beef Raised with Antibiotics Still Served Here...

Chain Reaction Report 2019, issued by six consumer groups, reported at ConsumerReports.org.

Beef from animals raised with antibiotics is still served at most fast-food chains. Fifteen of the top 25 chains were given a grade of F for having no policy on using beef from antibiotic-treated animals and no plan to reduce use of antibiotics in their beef supply. Only two chains—Chipotle and Panera Bread—got a grade of A or A– for using beef raised without antibiotics. But 13 of the top 25 chains—such as Burger King, McDonald's, KFC and Taco Bell—have responsible antibiotic-use policies in place for chicken. For a list of the chains and grades, go to USPIRG.org and search for "Chain Reaction V."

"Grass-Fed" Beef Labeling Can Be Deceptive

Mark Hyman, MD, practicing family physician and founder and director of The UltraWellness Center, Lenox, Massachusetts. His most recent book is *Food Fix: How to Save Our Health, Our Economy, Our Communities, and Our Planet—One Bite at a Time*. DrHyman.com

You have probably heard that grass-fed beef is the healthier choice—if you are going to eat beef. As with other healthful products that swell in popularity, however, cheap imitators have snuck in behind the real deals, and they are lying on labels to give the impression that their animals were grass-fed. Identifying the real deal can be a challenge.

True: Grass-fed beef has assorted health benefits vs. its grain-fed and fattened cousins. It has higher levels of vitamins, antioxidants and other nutrients, including more anti-inflammatory omega-3s and conjugated linoleic acid and fewer pro-inflammatory omega-6s. Also, grazing helps restore natural pasture ecosystems, leading to less reliance on chemical pesticides and herbicides. And since antibiotics are not used, grass-fed beef is significantly less likely to harbor drug-resistant bacteria. A 2015 study found that 18% of conventional beef samples were contaminated with "superbug" bacteria resistant to several classes of antibiotics, compared with 9% of sustainably raised (including grass-fed) samples.

Problem: There are no federal government standards for grass-fed beef nor for grass-fed beef labeling—meat companies can label meat "grass-fed" even if grass was only a minor part of the animals' feed.

Potentially misleading label: "Grass fed, grain finished" typically means that the animal ate grass much of its life but was fed a grain-rich diet to boost its weight in its final months. This is less than ideal even if the animal truly was grass-fed for most of its life—altering diet in these final months leads to changes in the nutritional composition of its meat.

What to look for on the label: A label identifying beef as grass-fed can be trusted if it's certified by a reliable third-party verifier such as the American Grassfed Association (AmericanGrassfed.org) or the Food Alliance (FoodAlliance.org). In order to be certified grass-fed beef by these organizations, the animal must have lived on pasture and eaten an exclusively grass (and/or other "forage," such as hay) diet throughout its life. Whole Foods uses the term "pasture-raised," and its beef is third-party verified. Another option is to purchase beef from a local farm, perhaps at a local farmer's market.

Produce with the Most Pesticide Residue

Environmental Working Group, EWG.org

The advocacy organization Environmental Working Group says strawberries have more pesticide residue than any other fruit or vegetable, followed by spinach, kale, nectarines, apples, grapes, peaches, cherries, pears, tomatoes, celery and potatoes. The group says consumers should buy only organic versions of those items.

Produce with the least pesticide residue: Avocados, sweet corn, pineapple, onions, papaya, frozen sweet peas, eggplant, asparagus, kiwi, cabbage, cauliflower, cantaloupe, broccoli, mushrooms, cabbage, honeydew and kiwi. Growers' groups point out that the amount of pesticide residue, although detectable, is extremely low, and conventionally grown produce is much less expensive than organic.

Hidden Toxins Are Everywhere

Joseph Pizzorno, ND, a leading authority on science-based natural and integrative medicine. He founded and served 22 years as president of Bastyr University, the largest fully accredited university of natural medicine in the US, and is treasurer of the board of The Institute for Functional Medicine. He is author of *The Toxin Solution* and 11 other consumer books and textbooks for doctors.

Asbestos…pesticides…tobacco smoke. We do our best to steer clear of these well-known harmful substances.

But what about the toxins we haven't heard of—the ones that can be found in places we'd never suspect? The truth is, toxins are everywhere—in most rugs and paints…cleaning supplies…cosmetics and perfumes…and the fumes from a gas pump. Even most food cans and the ubiquitous pizza box, designed to hold heat and resist stains, pose risks because of chemicals that, in our bodies, alter our hormones and our immune systems.

Recent development: While most of these hidden toxins are feared for their potential to cause cancer, mounting research shows that these substances also increase risk for serious health problems, such as diabetes and asthma—and more mundane ills like fatigue, poor concentration and memory problems.

Only a few hundred of the more than 80,000 chemicals in use in the US have been adequately tested for safety. But if toxins are everywhere, how can you stay safe? The answer is to limit your "toxic load." *Here's how…*

STEP 1: Eat organic. A nutritious diet—lots of fruits, vegetables, whole grains, etc.—can prevent disease. But these foods aren't always as healthful as you would imagine.

Modern agriculture depends on synthetic brews of pesticides, fertilizers and herbicides. Many go-to healthy foods have been flagged by the Environmental Working Group for high pesticide levels.

My advice: I strongly advise patients to buy organic foods—both packaged foods and produce. They contain few (or none) of the most harmful chemicals.

If cost is an issue, be sure that you buy the following 12 foods identified by the Environmental Working Group as the most important to purchase as organic—strawberries, spinach, kale, nectarines, apples, grapes, peaches, cherries, pears, tomatoes, celery and potatoes. (For produce with the least pesticide residue, see page 79.)

STEP 2: Rid your body of toxins. Exposure to toxins increases levels of harmful bacteria in the intestines that overload the detoxifying capacity of the liver…decreases levels of beneficial probiotic organisms…and damages the intestinal lining, which allows harmful substances to pass from the gut into the bloodstream—a condition known as "leaky gut." *My advice…**

•**Take a fiber supplement** (such as Metamucil, one to two teaspoons) a half hour before or after meals. Fiber binds to toxins and harmful bacteria to accelerate their excretion in the stools.

•**Recolonize the intestine** with the probiotics *Lactobacillus* and *Bifidobacterium* to help heal the intestinal walls. Many brands contain both organisms. Take one capsule, at least one billion colony-forming units (CFUs), three times daily. I advise taking this supplement indefinitely.

STEP 3: Take a safer painkiller. People with arthritis or other painful conditions often take daily doses of nonsteroidal anti-inflammatory drugs (NSAIDs), such as *ibuprofen* (Motrin) or *naproxen* (Aleve)…or the pain reliever *acetaminophen* (Tylenol). But all of these drugs can impair the ability of your kidneys to remove toxins from the body.

*Before taking any supplement, check with your doctor if you have a chronic medical condition or take medication.

Other choices: Take a natural pain reliever, such as the herb butterbur. It reduces inflammation and can relieve pain from headaches and other conditions. Curcumin is another excellent anti-inflammatory. Follow label instructions.

STEP 4: Test your toxin levels. Your doctor may suggest "target testing" if he/she suspects that you've been exposed to a certain toxin, such as lead in your drinking water. But even if you don't have symptoms (or risk factors), I advise getting a general test for toxins and repeating it every year or two.

One such test is the urinary 8-OHdG, which looks at metabolites that are released when DNA is damaged—a potential sign of elevated toxins. If your results are abnormal, work with your doctor to identify which toxin levels are elevated and their source so you can decrease your exposure as much as possible.

Dangerous Table Salt?

Seung-Kyu Kim, PhD, marine-science professor, Incheon National University, South Korea, and leader of an analysis published in *Environmental Science & Technology*.

Table salt contains plastic. Of 39 salt brands tested, 36 contained microplastics. The salt samples analyzed came from 16 countries on six continents and included 28 sea salt brands. Brands from Asia had especially high levels of microplastics. The effect of human consumption of salt-containing microplastics is unknown.

What's in Your Cold Brew?

Consumer Reports. CR.org

Bottled cold-brew coffee may not be as innocent as it seems. It typically has more caffeine per ounce than is found in hot coffee. Some brands have twice as much caffeine per ounce as regular brewed coffee. Bottled cold brews often contain added sugars—as much as 16 grams per serving, which is around four teaspoons. And more than half of the brands contain ingredients such as baking soda (sodium bicarbonate), sodium phosphate and salt—up to 320 mg of sodium per serving, about as much as in 48 potato chips.

How to Get to the Bottom of Those Murky Hospital Charges

Charles B. Inlander, consumer advocate and health-care consultant based in Fogelsville, Pennsylvania. He was the founding president of the nonprofit People's Medical Society, a consumer-advocacy organization credited with key improvements in the quality of US health care, and is author or coauthor of more than 20 consumer-health books.

Let's say you're headed to the hospital for knee surgery...or perhaps a colonoscopy. It may end up costing you hundreds or thousands of dollars, yet you likely have no clue what the total will be—until you get the bill.

Latest development: Federal law now requires all hospitals in the US to post on their websites price lists of the medical services they provide. This new law, enacted at the start of 2019, is designed to make the cost of hospital care more transparent and is an extension of the Affordable Care Act (ACA), which already required hospitals to publicly release their prices if asked. In this era of high insurance deductibles, co-pays and, in some cases, limited coverage for certain procedures, knowing a hospital's charges can have a dramatic impact on your pocketbook.

Of course, this all sounds good—and maybe eventually it will be—but for now, what you find on most hospitals' sites is a hodgepodge of confusing codes, untranslatable medical abbreviations and disclaimers effectively stating that no one really pays the dollar figures listed! Making matters worse, there are no federal guidelines requiring hospitals to post these costs in any standard way.

If you do find a site with the information presented in a reasonably comprehensible manner, it is relatively useless for the average health-care consumer. That's because the fees listed are what the hospital claims as its cost for a procedure, pill or service—not what a private insurer, Medicare or Medicaid has negotiated to pay.

Fortunately, there are ways you can get a better idea of how much a hospital procedure is going to cost you. *Based on your insurance coverage, here's my advice...*

•**When to call the hospital.** If you do not have insurance, it's vital that you know what a hospital is going to charge.

Note: If you do have a health insurance policy but it has a very high deductible, call the hospital and the insurer (see below) to ensure that the service is covered. You'll also want to know the charges if you are using a hospital that is not part of your insurance company's network of providers. In that case, you may have to pay full hospital-claim charges, rather than get the discount an in-network provider gives your insurance company.

Be aware: Most hospital charges do not include physician fees, so doctors bill you separately. To protect yourself, check with your physician(s) about his/her fees for the services he might provide.

Instead of searching for the cost of a procedure online, call the hospital billing department and ask what the cost is for the procedure you are going to have. Remember, under the law, the hospital must disclose its prices. Ask the billing representative to also give you the cost for services typically associated with the procedure, such as medications, anesthesia, scans and lab tests.

Insider tip: If you cannot afford the procedure, ask about the hospital's charity-care programs, which provide free or reduced-cost services, or financial-assistance programs, where you pay out over time and/or charges are reduced. Eligibility requirements generally include limits on annual income, assets, debt and other expenses.

•**When to check with your insurance carrier.** If you have medical insurance, whether private or provided through the government, call the customer-service department or the number listed on your insurance card. Ask the insurance representative what your insurer typically pays for the in-network hospital procedure you are going to be having—in your area. Prices can vary greatly depending on your location.

Insider tip: Ask your insurer the maximum out-of-pocket costs you might be liable for with the anticipated procedure. This should include any deductible or co-pay.

Consider Seeing a Geriatrician

AARP.org

Consider seeing a geriatrician if you are over age 65 and/or have multiple chronic medical conditions that cause challenges with your day-to-day physical or mental functioning. Geriatricians are family doctors or internists who are specially trained to treat older adults. If you are taking multiple prescription drugs, feel unsteady on your feet or have trouble getting around or you have developed difficulties with your memory, a geriatrician can help you manage your everyday life and can assess issues such as cognitive impairment, balance, gait and the likelihood of falls—which are the leading cause of injuries and death from injuries among people over age 65.

Also: If you are hospitalized for a traumatic injury, a consultation with a geriatrician can help you do better after discharge.

How to Get Your Insurer to Pay for Home Health Care

Charles B. Inlander, consumer advocate and health-care consultant based in Fogelsville, Pennsylvania. He was the founding president of the nonprofit People's Medical Society, a consumer-advocacy organization credited with key improvements in the quality of US health care, and is author or coauthor of more than 20 consumer-health books.

Let's say you're recovering from an injury, major illness (such as a stroke or heart attack) or a surgery. If you're not yet well enough to take care of yourself—but do not need to be in a nursing home or hospital—the best solution is home health care. But home health care isn't cheap—and it can be tricky to figure out how to qualify for these services. *My advice on navigating home health services…*

• **Understand the lingo.** If you use certain health services and/or equipment in your home while you're "homebound," this is known as "home health services." The services may include nurse visits to monitor your vital signs… physical therapy to recover from surgery…and occupational therapy to help you regain skills needed to bathe or get dressed. It may also include medical equipment, such as a walker, hospital bed or portable commode, that you may need to assist in your recovery.

Be aware: Custodial services, such as assistance with shopping, cleaning the home or cooking, are often needed by people with Alzheimer's disease or cancer but are not covered by Medicare if this is the only care needed. These services typically must be purchased out-of-pocket from home-care agencies.

Note: Long-term-care insurance policies may cover some of these services.

• **Learn if you qualify.** Qualifying for home health-care services depends on the type of health insurance you have. Most people who use home health services are on Medicare or Medicaid. (Some private health insurance plans cover these services, but policies vary.) Before such services will be provided, strict qualifications must be met, and your doctor must certify the services. For example, you must be under the care of a doctor who will certify that you are homebound, meaning that you are unable to leave your home to obtain health services on a regular basis (other than for an occasional doctor's visit…or for church or other religious services). The doctor must sign off on a plan of care, and the care must be provided by a Medicare-approved home health-care agency.

For more on the requirements: Consult the Medicare website at Medicare.gov. Search "home health services." Or call 800-MEDICARE (633-4227) and ask the representative for information on home health-care qualification requirements.

•**See how much is covered.** For Medicare beneficiaries on traditional Medicare, 100% of approved services will be covered if they are provided by a Medicare-approved home health-care agency. (Ask the agency if it is Medicare-approved or check Medicare.gov.) Medicare will also pay for 80% of all Medicare-approved medical equipment. Home health-care agencies have nurses, therapists (such as physical, occupational or respiratory), social workers and other aides to provide the care in your home. If you are in a Medicare Advantage Plan, you may be limited to certain agencies that are contracted by the particular plan you hold. If you are on Medicaid, all approved costs are covered.

Bonus: In all 50 states and the District of Columbia, Medicaid has programs that will allow a family member to be paid to provide some care-giving services to the beneficiary after a caseworker has determined what home services are needed. For details on eligibility, contact your state Medicaid office at Medicaid.gov. Click on "About us" and then "Contact us."

Who Is Protecting Consumers Online?

Jeff Wilbur, technical director of the nonprofit Internet Society, Reston, Virginia, and leader of the annual Online Trust Audit. OTAlliance.org

Health-care industry ranks lowest in protecting consumers online. In an analysis of 1,200 entities, the federal government fared best—91% of its entities made the honor roll...followed by consumer services, 85%...news and media, 78%...banks, 73%...online retailers, 65%...and health care, 57%.

Self-defense: Avoid clicking on e-mail links, especially any seeking information for health-care accounts. And enable two-step authentication where available.

When You Do Travel... Don't Forget Travel Medical Insurance

Charles B. Inlander, consumer advocate and health-care consultant based in Fogelsville, Pennsylvania. He was the founding president of the nonprofit People's Medical Society, a consumer-advocacy organization credited with key improvements in the quality of US health care, and is author or coauthor of more than 20 consumer-health books.

Several years ago, a friend's college-age daughter became seriously ill while traveling on her own in China. The local health facilities were not equipped to meet her medical needs, so she had to be transported by helicopter to a hospital in a city 100 miles away. The cost for the medical transport was $5,000, and her hospital stay was another $2,000. As is typical, her health insurance plan from home covered none of those costs while abroad. Fortunately, she recovered. But the unexpected bills were a real burden on the family.

Her experience taught me a lesson. No matter how healthy you or a travel companion may be, regardless of your age, being prepared for an unexpected medical event if you are traveling—especially abroad—should be at the top of your pre-trip planning. The best protection is travel medical insurance that covers the services you may need at an affordable cost. (Your current health insurance plan will cover most medical emergencies occurring in the US.) *My advice...*

•**Don't count on Medicare or other health insurance.** While you are traveling abroad, Medicare provides no coverage. Some Medigap policies and some Medicare Advantage plans have limited benefits if a medical emergency occurs while you're out of the country. Check with your plan well in advance of departure. Employer-provided insurance usually does not provide overseas coverage but check with the carrier or your employer to be sure.

•**Know where to shop.** Depending on the type of policy you purchase, travel medical insurance will pay for most of your medical costs if you become ill or get injured while traveling outside the US. Policies can be purchased through airlines, travel agents or directly from the insurance companies themselves (an online search of "travel insurance companies" will give you many options). Prices vary by the scope of the coverage. So a policy that pays for air transport to the nearest hospital will be costlier than policies that cover only medical costs themselves. Not surprisingly, prices are higher the older you are. Plus, benefits may be limited or denied if you have a preexisting condition, such as diabetes, asthma or heart disease. Even though travel plans are not covered by the Affordable Care Act, which protects people with preexisting conditions, you can often get a waiver policy for a preexisting condition by paying extra.

•**Be sure to shop around.** Policy costs vary widely among insurers, even for the exact same coverage. For example, I priced policies that paid up to $1 million in medical coverage… $500,000 for medical evacuation costs…and trip-interruption costs of up to $5,000 for a one-week trip to Italy for a 70-year-old. Price quotes from travel insurers ranged from $80 to $220 per person. So you need to shop around.

•**Consider a "bundled" policy.** You may be better served by so-called "comprehensive travel insurance policies." These plans bundle health insurance policies with other travel insurance such as lost baggage coverage…trip-cancellation insurance (which allows you to recoup your prepaid travel expenses if you cancel for any reason, such as a health problem)…or coverage for tour or hotel operator bankruptcy. These policies generally run 10% to 15% of your total booking costs.

CHAPTER 6

Diabetes and Blood Sugar Breakthroughs

The Secret Food Fix That Stops Diabetes

If you want to avoid diabetes—and who doesn't?—then choosing foods that are low in sugar and fat is probably your mantra. But there's more to the diabetes story.

Exciting research: One of the most effective—but least talked about—ways to protect against diabetes is to load up on antioxidants, those ultra-healthy substances (think vitamins C and E, beta-carotene and others), according to a growing body of scientific evidence. *Why antioxidants are such heavy hitters in preventing this increasingly widespread disease...*

ATTACKING THE ROOT CAUSE

No doubt you have heard of antioxidants and their archenemy, free radicals. In healthy numbers, these volatile oxygen molecules roam our bodies performing useful functions such as fighting infection. But in excess numbers, these and other similar molecules can cause all kinds of damage to the body.

Enter antioxidants. These substances, which are found in the highest amounts in certain vegetables and fruits and are naturally produced by the body, keep the rogue oxygen molecules in check. When antioxidants run low, however, the result is oxidative stress, a condition widely known to hasten aging, heart disease and cancer.

What you may not realize: Oxidative stress has also been linked to insulin resistance, a major cause of type 2 diabetes. When insulin resistance develops, it means that the hormone insulin is not working effectively to get glucose (sugar) into the cells of your body to give them energy. This leads to too much sugar in the blood—with the result being diabetes or its precursor, known as prediabetes.

George L. King, MD, research director and chief scientific officer at Joslin Diabetes Center, and professor of medicine at Harvard Medical School, both in Boston. He is author, with Royce Flippin, of *Reverse Your Diabetes in 12 Weeks* and *The Diabetes Reset.*

THE ANTIOXIDANT FIX

If you are concerned about diabetes, you may think that the easiest solution is to take an antioxidant supplement, such as vitamin C. But the latest research shows that's not true.

In fact, research has shown that supplements are of limited or no use to most people struggling with blood sugar control—and may even cause harm. For example, vitamin C supplements were shown to interfere with the diabetes-fighting benefits of exercise—in part by blocking the body's production of its own natural antioxidants. The solution is as simple as choosing the right foods.

GETTING THE RIGHT FOODS

When choosing foods to help prevent diabetes, you want to load up on those that contain "phase 2 antioxidants," nutrients that stimulate the body's antioxidant defenses by activating a protein called nrf2 (short for nuclear factor erythroid 2-related factor 2). Nrf2 is a powerful switch that can turn on genes inside your cells, triggering the production of natural antioxidants. *Among the best nrf2 boosters…*

•**Cruciferous vegetables** such as broccoli, brussels sprouts, cauliflower and cabbage contain high levels of *sulforaphane*, a potent phase 2 antioxidant.

Goal: Two or more cups daily.

•**Blueberries** contain high levels of *pterostilbene*, an effective nrf2 activator.

Goal: One cup daily.

Filtered Coffee Helps Prevent Type 2 Diabetes

An analysis of specific blood metabolites showed that people who drank two to three cups of filtered coffee daily had 60% lower diabetes risk than those having less than one cup. The study did not test French press, espresso or pods.

Rikard Landberg, PhD, professor of food science at Chalmers University of Technology, Gothenburg, Sweden, and principal investigator of the study published in *Journal of Internal Medicine*.

•**Fatty fish.** Salmon, tuna, sardines, mackerel and herring contain omega-3 fatty acids that boost nrf2.

Goal: Eat fatty fish (3 to 4 ounces per serving) three times a week.

•**Green tea** contains a wide array of antioxidants and stimulates nrf2 activity. Replace soda and juice with green tea.

Goal: Two to three cups daily.

•**Curcumin.** The active ingredient in the Indian spice turmeric is a powerful nrf2 stimulator that also has anti-inflammatory effects.

Goal: Season with curcumin instead of salt.

A DIET THAT WORKS

What does an antidiabetes diet look like? One version of this eating style is the Rural Asian Diet, developed at the Joslin Diabetes Center. The overall mix calls for 70% complex carbs (such as vegetables and whole grains)…15% fat…and 15% protein, including at least 15 g of fiber for every 1,000 calories.

Important: When it comes to limiting oxidative stress, don't forget to also exercise regularly…reduce stress…stop smoking…and get plenty of sleep.

Diabetes and Depression

Vincent Chin-Hung Chen, PhD, professor of psychiatry, Chang Gung University, Taoyuan, Taiwan.

People with diabetes are up to three times more likely to have depression than those without the disease—and more than half go undiagnosed.

New finding: Taking an antidepressant reduced death rates by 35% in those with depression and diabetes, according to a 13-year study of more than 53,000 people.

Theory: Treating depression increases adherence to diabetes treatment.

Common Food Preservative May Trigger Diabetes

Amir Tirosh, MD, PhD, is director, division of endocrinology, at Israel's Sheba Medical Center, Tel-Aviv, and lead author of a study published in *Science Translational Medicine.*

Common food preservative may trigger metabolic changes linked to obesity and diabetes. In new mouse and human studies, *propionate*—an additive used widely in processed bread, baked goods and cheeses, among other foods—triggered complex hormonal changes that raised blood sugar and insulin levels. Mice fed regular doses for 20 weeks gained weight and became insulin-resistant—a characteristic of type 2 diabetes. Eating less cheese and processed food, including bread, will minimize exposure to propionate.

Got Diabetes? Here's How to Do a Better Job of Tracking Your Glucose

Marwan Hamaty, MD, MBA, a board-certified specialist in endocrinology, diabetes and metabolism. Dr. Hamaty practices at the Cleveland Clinic Diabetes Center. His research has been published in leading medical journals, including International *Journal of Experimental Diabetes Research.*

Continuous glucose monitoring is more precise than A1C and reduces finger sticks by at least 90%.

If you have diabetes, your blood sugar (glucose) levels tend to change throughout the day. Even when you monitor your glucose often enough (typically four to five times a day), you are getting only a small portion of the whole picture.

Fortunately, a recent technological advancement known as continuous glucose monitoring (CGM) is now changing that.

What's more, a growing body of evidence shows that this high-tech system is poised to eclipse standard hemoglobin A1C testing, com-

monly known as A1C, as the gold standard for managing glucose levels.

If you or someone you love uses insulin to treat diabetes and is not using CGM, it could be time to take the plunge.

WHAT IS CGM?

CGM relies on a tiny sensor that you insert yourself into the skin of your upper arm or belly and leave in place for several days. Because the sensor uses a tiny needle, the process is virtually painless.

The sensor continuously measures glucose in the thin layer of fluid that surrounds the cells beneath your skin—called interstitial fluid—and wirelessly sends the results to a monitor or a smartphone to record your glucose levels 24 hours a day. Results are displayed every few minutes. Retrospective data is also available to detect trends in your glucose levels.

A CGM device helps you and your doctor create a daily diabetes management plan. It could reduce the frequency (or take the place) of using a glucometer to measure your blood levels of glucose to determine your insulin needs.

CGM reduces the number of finger sticks typically needed to use a glucometer and test strips by 90%—or by close to 100% for some of the latest devices. The specifics vary among CGM devices, so be sure to discuss these details with your diabetes educator or medical provider.

An important feature of CGM devices is that they allow the information to be shared with others—for example, parents can monitor a child or adults can track how well elderly parents are controlling their diabetes.

Note: Your doctor may use a professional CGM device to see how well you're managing your diabetes. You might wear the monitor for days or weeks while trends in your glucose levels are stored in the sensor/device and can be downloaded to your doctor's computer. People with type 2 diabetes can benefit from this type of periodic monitoring even if they do not need insulin.

BEYOND THE A1C TEST

Since the 1980s, the A1C test has been uniformly used to monitor glucose levels. This simple and inexpensive blood test tells you and your doctor your average blood sugar over an eight- to 12-week period. The A1C test, which usually is performed in a doctor's office or lab, does this by measuring the percentage of your red blood cells carrying glucose.

For your glucose management to be effective in preventing complications, most diabetes guidelines recommend an A1C of 7% or less when possible. This goal needs to be personalized to each patient's circumstances, and it changes over time.

It helps to think of your A1C as a baseball batting average. It tells you how well you are hitting, but it does not tell you when you are getting lots of hits or when you are in a slump. These ups and downs are called glycemic variability.

That's where CGM shines. It shows your real-time highs and lows as well as your trends (and averages) over time. Studies show that people with diabetes who use CGM have improved A1C levels and less glycemic variability.

Why is that important? Research shows that the time you spend in hyperglycemia (glucose levels above 180 mg/dL two hours after eating) is directly related to your risk for diabetes complications, such as heart disease and stroke.

CGM also shows the time you spend in hypoglycemia (glucose below 70 mg/dL). That can be particularly useful if you have hypoglycemia at night or if you don't get warning signs of the condition, such as shakiness, dizziness and hunger.

Unrecognized hypoglycemia can progress to a dangerously low glucose level (below 50 mg/dL), which can cause confusion, heart-rhythm irregularities, blurred vision, accidents, loss of consciousness, seizures and even death.

A1C also has other weaknesses. Aiming for a reading of 7% or less does not fit everyone. This is especially true for older people who have a naturally higher A1C because they have fewer red blood cells. Forcing these individuals to lower their A1C to 7% or less can increase their risk for hypoglycemia. Additionally, when a person has anemia or other abnormalities of red blood cells, A1C may not accurately estimate the glucose average.

WHO BENEFITS MOST FROM CGM?

CGM, which is prescribed by a physician, is for people with type 1 diabetes or those with type 2 diabetes who use multiple daily injections of insulin. The device typically is best for those who require frequent finger sticks (at least four times daily) to control their glucose levels.

CGM can be especially beneficial for people who unknowingly experience hypoglycemia. Certain devices will warn you of a hypoglycemic trend, and some models will send you and family members a warning alarm if you dip into the danger zone.

If you use an insulin pump, you should consider a CGM device that is compatible with your insulin pump. Some CGM models and insulin pumps are integrated. Insulin delivery by the insulin pump could be automatically adjusted to prevent or reduce your chances of hypoglycemia.

When using a CGM device, you'll see in real time how your diet, activities and stress levels affect your glucose levels. With your doctor's help, you will learn how to anticipate these trends and tweak your insulin use to address them.

GETTING STARTED WITH CGM

If you're interested in trying a CGM device, talk to your doctor and your diabetes educator. If they think that you'd benefit, there are many different devices on the market.

Some have more bells and whistles, such as alarms for high and low glucose levels...graphs you can download onto your computer or smartphone...and some even are connected to an insulin pump that gives you a glucose reading to use for a programmed dose of insulin for your meal or to correct a high glucose level.

Not surprisingly, CGM can be pricey. Your doctor or diabetes educator can help you select the best model for your needs.* If you go with a basic CGM system and meet the required criteria, it often is covered by insurance. The out-of-pocket cost to use it may not be much more than what you would be paying for a glucometer and your test strips.

*To find a diabetes educator near you, go to the Certification Board for Diabetes Care and Educators at NCBDE.org/find-a-cde/.

Most CGM devices still require a few finger sticks to ensure that they are accurately reflecting your glucose levels. This is called calibration. Depending on the device you choose, you may need to calibrate occasionally or every day.

Important: There is about a 15-minute delay for glucose changes in your blood (as measured by a finger stick) to show up in interstitial fluid (as measured by CGM). In certain situations, you may need to do a finger stick before making any insulin dose changes based on just your CGM. (Your doctor or diabetes educator can advise you on managing special circumstances and what's best for you.)

Once you start using CGM, the data stored on your monitor will help your doctor recommend the timing and dose you should take of a longer-acting or shorter-acting insulin…or adjust the pump setting if you're using an insulin pump.

Your job will be to follow your doctor's insulin directions and to use your readings to make any necessary adjustments to your meals and activity levels.

Seniors with Diabetes May Be in the "Danger Zone" and Not Know It

Anders L. Carlson, MD, medical director, International Diabetes Center, director, HealthPartners diabetes program, and assistant professor, University of Minnesota Medical School, Minneapolis. Research presented at The Endocrine Society Annual Meeting 2019 by the International Diabetes Center in Minneapolis.

The constant high blood sugar of diabetes damages the body, harms your health and, in the long term, shortens lives. But blood sugar that's too low is also dangerous—and can cut life short more quickly. A new study now finds that seniors being treated for type 1 diabetes may be spending more than an hour daily with low blood sugar levels—and a significant part of that time with levels low enough to put them at risk for loss of consciousness, seizures…and even death.

Researchers from 22 sites across the US that are part of the T1D Exchange tracked glucose levels in 203 patients age 60 and older with type 1 diabetes for 21 days. The patients wore a continuous glucose monitor (CGM) to record their glucose levels around the clock.

Results: On average, patients were within a healthy blood glucose target range—defined as 70 md/dL to 180 mg/dL for at least 70% of the day—for only 57% of the day (about 13.4 hours). The rest of the time was spent in a state of hyperglycemia (high blood sugar) or hypoglycemia (low blood sugar). Of particular concern was that many spent about half an hour daily with blood sugar levels low enough to be dangerous. Worse, many of the patients in the study who experienced hypoglycemia did not recognize the warning signs.

Hypoglycemia can cause falls, loss of consciousness, seizures and even death if not treated. Warning signs to look for include blurred vision, confusion, slurred speech, numbness, sweating and shaking, poor coordination, dizziness or feeling light-headed, difficulty concentrating, feeling anxious or irritable, hunger or nausea and erratic changes in behavior. People with diabetes, especially those at risk for hypoglycemia, are educated about the symptoms. However, the symptoms can be mistaken for other health issues—which can mean that hypoglycemia does not get treated.

Most people with diabetes are able to recognize early symptoms and know that they need to eat a glucose snack—such as a sugar tablet or a glass of juice. If they experience severe hypoglycemia, they may need another person to inject them with the hormone glucagon, which raises blood sugar levels. However, many people with diabetes do not know that using insulin, especially for many years, and also having previous episodes of hypoglycemia can cause desensitization to hypoglycemia warning signs, a condition called hypoglycemia unawareness.

Hypoglycemia unawareness is most common among people with type 1 diabetes—an estimated 40% may have the condition. But it can also affect people with type 2 diabetes. Hypoglycemia unawareness increases the risk of slipping into the hypoglycemic danger zone, becoming too confused to eat a sugary snack by themselves…or passing out. In the current study, patients who spent the most time daily with low blood sugar were hypoglycemia unaware.

SELF-PROTECTION IF YOU HAVE DIABETES

If you are an older person with diabetes on insulin…

• **If you are aware of experiencing periods of hypoglycemia, don't ignore them…** and let your doctor know. You may be in the danger zone more often than you realize and may need to take additional steps to better control your blood sugar.

Likely periods of increased risk: At night while you're asleep…before lunch…after drinking alcohol…and after exercise.

• **If you find that you don't always realize when your blood sugar is low (hypoglycemic unawareness),** make family members and/or coworkers aware of the signs of hypoglycemia—and, if necessary, alert them that they may need to inject you with glucagon if you aren't able to. (It's a good idea to always carry a glucagon kit if you take insulin.)

Note: Avoiding hypoglycemia for up to four weeks can restore hypoglycemia awareness.

• **If blood sugar control continues to be problematic,** talk to your doctor about getting a continuous glucose monitoring system (CGM). A CGM sets off an alarm when glucose gets too low (or too high)…and also tracks periods of hypoglycemia and hyperglycemia so that you can tell how well you're doing.

Vinegar Can Do Wonders For Your Blood Sugar

Carol Johnston, RD, PhD, professor and assistant director of the School of Nutrition and Health Promotion at Arizona State University, Phoenix. Dr. Johnston has published various papers on the medical use of vinegar in leading medical journals.

Apple cider vinegar is a classic home remedy with traditional uses ranging from reducing age spots to easing arthritis. Only one use is scientifically proven—vinegar has a specific effect on blood sugar that is beneficial for anyone with diabetes or prediabetes. *Here's what you need to know…*

• **The scientific evidence of vinegar's blood sugar benefits is strong and consistent.** A recent statistical analysis of the 11 best studies concluded that consuming vinegar with a meal, compared with having the same meal without vinegar, reduced postmeal blood sugar spikes by an average of 40%.

Why this matters: Much of the metabolic damage caused by diabetes—and prediabetes—is caused by these spikes.

• **Any vinegar works.** Sorry, apple cider vinegar enthusiasts. It's the acetic acid—in every vinegar—that blocks absorption of carbohydrates and helps clear blood sugar from the bloodstream.

• **Raw vinegar is best.** Cooking can break down acetic acid.

• **You don't need much.** Studies suggest that two tablespoons of vinegar is a good "dose." Less isn't as effective—and more doesn't add any benefit.

• **Timing matters.** For the best effect on blood sugar, consume vinegar at or near the start of a meal.

• **Consider a premeal drink.** For the most reliable effect, dilute two tablespoons of vinegar in a glass of water and drink it with the first bites of the meal. You can sweeten it with a non-nutritive sweetener such as stevia. Or try a commercial flavored apple-cider-vinegar drink made by Bragg.

• **Make your own vinaigrette** if you'd rather incorporate vinegar into a salad or vegetable dish (after the vegetables are cooked). Why? Store-bought vinaigrettes often have more oil than vinegar. Mix your own using two parts vinegar to one part oil. Try red wine vinegar—it delivers acetic acid plus a healthy dose of cell-protecting polyphenols. Mustard counts, too—most mustards are rich in vinegar.

• **Start your next meal with a dish dressed with vinegar.** And while you don't want to be eating a lot of bread, if you do have a slice, instead of slathering it in butter, dip it in vinaigrette.

How to Tame a Sugar Addiction

Kathleen DesMaisons, PhD, an expert in addictive nutrition and author of an updated edition of *Potatoes Not Prozac: Simple Solutions for Sugar Addiction*. She is based in Albuquerque, New Mexico, and is founder of Radiant Recovery, RadiantRecovery.com, an online community for people dealing with sugar sensitivity.

Here's a little test: Imagine that you have just had a big lunch. You are not remotely hungry but when you come home, you find a plate of warm chocolate chip cookies, smelling delicious, on the kitchen counter. No one else is around. Do you dive into those cookies?

If you answer yes, and can't imagine why anyone would say no, you may be a sugar addict—a biochemical problem that can set the stage not only for unhealthy weight gain, but also for depression, mood swings and impulsive behavior.

To learn more, we spoke with Kathleen DesMaisons, PhD, who has spent several decades helping people with out-of-control sugar cravings.

THE ROOTS OF SUGAR ADDICTION

There's a growing scientific consensus that too much sugar is a leading cause of America's biggest health problems, from obesity to heart disease and diabetes. But not everyone appears to have the same risk. Why?

According to theories of "addictive nutrition," some people are more sensitive than others to the brain-altering effects of sugar. People who are affected by "sugar sensitivity" are believed to have a genetic makeup that makes them especially vulnerable to the blood sugar swings that can happen after eating sweets, white bread, white pasta and other highly processed carbohydrates. The roller coaster is both emotional and physical.

But that's not all. According to this theory, you also may have chronically low levels of two key brain chemicals—serotonin and beta-endorphin. Serotonin helps regulate mood and self-control. Beta-endorphin is the body's natural opioid, capable of blunting both physical and mental pain.

Low levels of these two brain chemicals can leave you reeling, living from one soda or bowl of ice cream to the next to get your feel-good boost—and then crashing with feelings of sadness, anger and self-loathing. When you do resist your cravings, you are consumed with thoughts of your next sweet fix.

There's no blood test or formal diagnostic process to identify sugar sensitivity—and it's not the same as diabetes, which is a disease marked by high blood sugar (glucose) levels.

But if you have an insatiable sweet tooth…a history of depression…and/or past or current abuse of alcohol or drugs, sugar sensitivity may be a contributing factor.

TO TAME SUGAR ADDICTION

To help you get off this roller coaster, here's Dr. DesMaisons' seven-step plan…

STEP #1: **Eat breakfast.** You've heard it before…breakfast is important—but what you eat is the key. You want to avoid starting the day with a blood sugar crash, followed by a donut rescue. Even if you think you hate breakfast or don't have time, eat within one hour of getting up.

To help keep your blood sugar levels stable, don't eat just anything—build your breakfast around protein (eggs are fine, but so are beans, cottage cheese, tofu, nut butters or last night's turkey breast). You should also eat some complex carbohydrates (such as oatmeal, whole-grain toast or brown rice).

Key advice: Get one-third of your daily protein at breakfast. Aim for one-half gram of protein for each pound you weigh. For example, a 150-pound person would aim for 75 g a day with 25 g being consumed at breakfast. That's roughly the amount in two eggs, two tablespoons of peanut butter and a cup of oatmeal.

Caution: If you have chronic kidney disease, speak to your doctor about your protein intake—too much can be hard on your kidneys.

Important: Be sure to master this step before moving on—even if it takes months. Take the same step-by-step approach as you go.

STEP #2: **Start a food journal.** Write down everything you eat, with dates and times. Also, your food journal should include how you are feeling physically and emotionally at any time of the day that you notice a shift. For example, you may note that you get tired every day around 2 pm when you eat a heavy lunch. The idea is to notice patterns, not beat yourself up. Use the food diary as an ongoing tool.

***STEP #3:* Get enough protein at each meal.** Once you've mastered breakfast, do the same with lunch and dinner. At each meal, get one-third of the daily amount of protein you need.

Why the focus on protein? Protein not only helps stabilize blood sugar, it's also a key source of tryptophan, an amino acid your body uses to make serotonin—as mentioned earlier, the brain chemical that increases impulse control and feelings of well-being. You probably know that turkey is a good source of tryptophan, but tuna, tofu, salmon and kidney beans are as well.

Also important: To avoid blood sugar crashes, space your meals no more than six hours apart, except overnight. Ideally, you will only eat at mealtime—because that teaches you how to start and stop eating—instead of grazing all day. But some people, including pregnant women and those with physically demanding jobs, need snacks.

Good choices: An apple and some cheese… or a handful of almonds and a pear.

And if you feel you need a sweet dessert, eat it right after your meal to temper the effects of the sugar. Be reasonable with dessert and don't obsess about it. Focusing on your meals rather than sweets will naturally help quiet your cravings.

***STEP #4:* Try vitamins and…a nightly potato.** You should get most of your nutrients from food, but vitamin C, B-complex and zinc supplements may help balance your brain and body chemistry. Discuss this with your healthcare provider.

The most surprising part of the plan—a nightly potato with the skin—has a specific purpose. The idea is to end your day with a complex carbohydrate that will raise your serotonin levels. Complex carbohydrates do this by triggering the gradual release of insulin, which, in turn, enables tryptophan to travel from the bloodstream to the brain and produce serotonin.

A potato (with a little butter, if you like) fits the bill. It can be a small red potato, a medium Yukon Gold or even a sweet potato, roasted, boiled or baked. The skin has fiber which helps curb the potato's effect on your glucose levels. Take it like medicine, three hours after dinner.

Note: If you have diabetes, consult your doctor before following this advice.

***STEP #5:* Go from white to brown.** Instead of white rice and white bread, opt for brown rice and whole-grain bread. Veggies (including greens) are good, too, as well as whole grains.

***STEP #6:* Cut out added sugar.** Start by saying no to cake, cookies, candy, sweet drinks and processed foods full of sugar. This might sound hard, but since it comes later in the plan, you will be shocked at what a nonevent it is.

Helpful: Don't forget to read food labels since many food products you wouldn't expect contain added sugar.

Key advice: Whole fruit, which contains natural sugars, is fine, but don't overdo it with high-sugar fruit, such as bananas, raisins or figs.

***STEP #7:* Get in touch with your feelings.** Once you're off the sugar roller coaster, it's common to experience emotions that have been masked by your use of sugar. To better understand these new feelings, consider self-help approaches, including guided imagery or meditation, and/or talk therapy.

This plan will remove your cravings. Beyond that, use it as a life skill rather than a diet.

Ouchless Insulin!

Massachusetts Institute of Technology

People with type 2 diabetes may soon be able to forgo insulin shots.

In development: A blueberry-size oral capsule, which contains a single needle made of compressed, freeze-dried insulin that is injected into the stomach wall after it's swallowed. It appears to lower blood sugar as effectively as shots.

Prostate Drugs Increase Diabetes Risk

Ruth Andrew, PhD, chair of pharmaceutical endocrinology, University of Edinburgh, UK.

Men who took *finasteride* or *dutasteride* (drugs for enlarged prostate) were 26% to 32% more likely to develop diabetes, respectively, than those taking *tamsulosin*, a medication with a different mechanism of action, according to an 11-year study of more than 50,000 men with an enlarged prostate.

Reason: Finasteride and dutasteride alter the actions of steroid hormones, which affect how the body handles sugars and fats.

Negative Personality Traits Up Diabetes Risk

The study "Personality Traits and Diabetes Incidence Among Postmenopausal Women" was published in *Menopause*, the journal of The North American Menopause Society.

All those "Negative Nellies" out there may have more to worry about than frown lines. Researchers digging into data from the Women's Health Initiative (WHI) recently identified an association between personality traits (such as negativity, pessimism and hostility) in postmenopausal women and a higher risk of developing type 2 diabetes.

The good news is, a sunnier disposition, including optimism, may help protect against diabetes. *Here's what the researchers found—and what's being recommended…*

Study details: Nearly 140,000 postmenopausal women who did not have diabetes completed a self-administered questionnaire that assessed their personality traits and their health behaviors, such as diet, exercise, smoking and drinking alcohol. Over the next 14 years, 19,240 (about 14%) of the women developed diabetes.

Those who scored highest for hostility (highest quartile) had a 17% increased risk of developing diabetes compared with those in the lowest quartile for hostility.

Those who scored highest for negativity had a 9% increased risk of developing the disease compared with those with the lowest negativity scores (lowest quartile).

For unknown reasons, the link between hostility and diabetes risk was not as pronounced in women who were obese compared with women who were not—though obesity remains a major risk factor for the disease.

Now the positive side: The study participants with positive personality traits characterized by high optimism, low negativity and low hostility had a 12% lower risk of developing diabetes compared with those who were least optimistic.

"Personality traits remain stable across one's lifetime," explains JoAnn Pinkerton, MD, executive director of The North American Menopause Society. For that reason, Dr. Pinkerton says, this new finding could help doctors identify women who may be at a higher risk for diabetes so that they can tailor prevention and treatment strategies to each woman's personality.

Takeaway: If you're a postmenopausal woman—especially if you have risk factors for diabetes, such as being overweight or obese… low physical activity…and/or a family history of the disease—discuss with your doctor whether your personality may be putting you at even greater risk. Knowing where you stand is the first step to protecting your health!

Feet Feeling Pins and Needles?

Janice F. Wiesman, MD, FAAN, clinical associate professor of neurology at NYU Grossman School of Medicine in New York City and author of *Peripheral Neuropathy: What It Is and What You Can Do to Feel Better.*

Are you feeling "pins and needles" on the soles of your feet? What could be causing this?

There are two main culprits…Peripheral neuropathy (PN), a nerve disorder, often causes numbness, weakness, pain and tingling in the extremities. Common causes of PN are nerve damage caused by diabetes...heavy alcohol use...and medications, including certain chemotherapy drugs, cholesterol-lowering statins and fluoroquinolone antibiotics. Vitamin B-12 deficiency or excess levels of vitamin B-6 also can lead to PN. Some supplements and energy drinks have very large amounts of B-6. Impaired kidney function and bone marrow cancer are less common causes of PN.

With spinal stenosis, another possible culprit, arthritis causes overgrowth of the bone that surrounds the nerves, compressing them as they exit the spinal cord and run into the legs, then feet.

See your primary care doctor. If PN is suspected, blood work will help identify the underlying cause. Your doctor also may order an electrical test of your nerves and muscles. If more testing is indicated, you'll likely be sent to a neurologist. Spinal stenosis is typically diagnosed with a spine MRI and treated by a neurologist.

Depending on the cause, treatment may include an anti-inflammatory, such as *ibuprofen* (Motrin)...*gabapentin* (Neurontin), an anticonvulsant also used to treat pain...and/or *duloxetine* (Cymbalta), an antidepressant that can be used for pain. Controlling an underlying cause of neuropathy, such as diabetes, or changing a drug identified as a possible cause will also give relief.

Eating a well-balanced diet and getting regular exercise will help deliver nutrients and oxygen to nerve endings in your feet, easing symptoms.

Also helpful: A vibrating foot bath. Some people find that acupuncture helps, too.

CHAPTER 7

Diet and Fitness

The Healthiest Diet

The best nutrition advice sounds surprisingly simple—eat whole foods, preferably plants. But it gets tricky...once you consider that some whole foods are better than others when it comes to fighting major killers such as heart disease, cancer, diabetes and infections. For example, did you know that blueberries and blackberries far outperform other fruits as sources of antioxidants—substances that protect your cells from all sorts of damage?

Here's the clincher: Before you assume that your diet is "good enough," consider this—the number-one cause of death in the US is the Standard American Diet (SAD), according to research published in *JAMA*. For most leading causes of death, your genes account for only 10% to 20%. So getting your diet in optimal shape should be at the top of your priority list. Of course, fitting in all the nutrients backed by strong scientific evidence can be challenging. But it's doable—if you build your diet around a few key foods.

To keep it simple, nutrition expert Michael Greger, MD, FACLM, has spent more than a decade combing through the evidence to create his daily list of must-have foods...

•**Beans are a go-to source for healthy protein but also offer iron, zinc, fiber and potassium.**

What they do: Help lower cholesterol and high blood pressure and play a role in the prevention of colon cancer and stroke.

Which kinds to eat: Try a variety, including black beans, black-eyed peas, lentils, split peas and chickpeas. Canned beans are fine as long as you choose low-sodium varieties or simply rinse them well before using.

Daily dose: Three servings. A serving is one-quarter cup of hummus or bean dip or one-half cup of cooked beans.

Michael Greger, MD, FACLM, founder of the website NutritionFacts.org and author of *How Not to Die: Discover the Foods Scientifically Proven to Prevent and Reverse Disease.* He is also author of *How Not to Diet: The Groundbreaking Science of Healthy, Permanent Weight Loss.*

Note: I recommend legumes over meat because they are loaded with nutrients—and are naturally low in saturated fat and sodium and free of cholesterol.

•**Berries are the fruits with extra bragging rights.**

What they do: Studies show that berries protect your brain, heart and liver, boost immunity and offer potential cancer protection.

Which kinds to eat: Blueberries and blackberries have the highest levels of antioxidants, as noted earlier, but others, including goji berries and cranberries, also pack nutritional punches.

Helpful: Frozen berries retain most nutrients—if not more—than fresh.

Daily dose: One serving. That's one-half cup of fresh or frozen berries.

•**Other fruits shouldn't scare you off because of their natural sugar.** As long as you eat your fruit whole or blended, with its fiber intact, the sugar is not a health problem.

What they do: Studies show that people who eats lots of whole fruits lower their risk for type 2 diabetes.

Which kinds to eat: Everything from apples and watermelon to avocados.

Daily dose: Three servings. A serving is one medium-sized fruit or one cup of cut fruit.

•**Cruciferous vegetables are nutritional powerhouses that produce a chemical called sulforaphane,** which is linked to a wide variety of health benefits.

What they do: These vegetables may help fight cancer, boost liver function, manage type 2 diabetes and protect your brain and eyesight.

Which kinds to eat: The category includes broccoli, kale, cabbage and cauliflower but also arugula, bok choy, collard greens and even horseradish.

Important tip: Frozen versions will not produce sulforaphane—unless you sprinkle them with mustard powder, which contains the necessary enzyme destroyed in the freezing process.

Daily dose: One serving. That's one-half cup of chopped vegetables, one-quarter cup of broccoli sprouts or one tablespoon of horseradish.

•**Greens.** Dark green, leafy vegetables pack the most nutrition per calorie of any food.

What they do: In research conducted at Harvard and published in *JAMA* and *Annals of Internal Medicine*, each additional daily serving of greens was linked to a 20% reduction in risk for heart attack and stroke.

Which kinds to eat: The list includes many cruciferous vegetables, such as kale, collard greens and arugula, but also extends to other leafy greens such as spinach and mesclun salad mix.

Helpful: If you find greens bitter, try mixing them with lightly sweetened dressings or fruits, such as fresh figs or grated apples.

Daily dose: Two servings. A serving is one cup raw or one-half cup cooked.

•**Other vegetables should be included to get the "rainbow" effect of a bountiful veggie diet.**

What they do: People who eat a variety of vegetables (and fruits) show decreased signs of inflammation and lower rates of type 2 diabetes.

Which kinds to eat: Get a colorful mix including artichokes, zucchini, asparagus, yams, beets and squash. Don't forget onions, garlic and mushrooms (technically fungi). Plain white button mushrooms may offer the greatest health benefits.

Daily dose: Two servings. A serving is one cup raw or one-half cup cooked.

Good rule of thumb: Fill half of every plate you eat with vegetables—ideally, including breakfast.

•**Flaxseeds are potent sources of lignans,** plant estrogens that can dampen the sometimes harmful effects of the body's own estrogens.

What they do: Flaxseeds help fight breast cancer, high blood pressure and prostate enlargement.

What kinds to eat: Grind whole seeds or buy them pre-ground to help ensure that you'll absorb the nutrients. The powder lasts about four months at room temperature and up to six months in the freezer. Sprinkle on oatmeal, salads, soups and other foods.

Daily dose: One serving—one tablespoon ground.

•Nuts and seeds are a perfect snack food.

What they do: Nut eaters are less likely to die from cancer and heart and respiratory diseases, studies show. Nuts also can provide the fat that aids the absorption of plant nutrients.

Which kinds to eat: Almonds, Brazil nuts, cashews, chia seeds, pistachios, pumpkin seeds and sunflower seeds are all good, but the evidence is strongest for walnuts, which are high in omega-3 fats and antioxidants.

Daily dose: One serving. That's one-quarter cup of nuts or seeds or two tablespoons of nut or seed butter.

•Herbs and spices add flavor, color and antioxidants.

What they do: Herbs and spices help control blood pressure when they are used in place of salt. One standout, turmeric, contains a pigment, curcumin, which is particularly beneficial for brain health. Turmeric is linked to reduced inflammation and anticancer effects.

Which kinds to eat: Grate fresh turmeric root to use in cooking or add a raw slice to a smoothie. Sprinkle turmeric powder onto sweet potatoes or roasted cauliflower. Use other spices, from basil to thyme, to flavor everything. Spices make a great substitute for salt.

Daily dose: One-quarter teaspoon of turmeric powder (or one-quarter inch raw), plus any other salt-free herbs and spices you like.

•Whole grains including bread, rice, cereal and even pasta can be part of a healthy diet—as long as they come in whole-grain form.

What they do: Reduce risks for heart disease, type 2 diabetes and stroke.

Which kinds to eat: Branch out beyond wheat, oat and corn to quinoa, amaranth, millet, buckwheat and sorghum. Labels should list whole grains. The best products are high in fiber (at least 5 g per serving) and contain little or no added sugar.

Daily dose: Three servings. A serving is one-half cup of hot cereal or pasta, one tortilla or slice of bread or three cups of popped popcorn.

When to Sit...When to Stand While You Eat

Food doesn't taste as good if we eat it while standing.

Recent finding: The physical strain of standing reduces the body's sensory sensitivity, making tasty foods seem less flavorful. On the other hand, standing helps people better tolerate unpleasant tastes, such as medicine.

Dieters—take note: The study also found that eating on your feet led to less consumption, which might mean weight reduction.

Dipayan Biswas, PhD, professor of business and marketing at University of South Florida, Tampa, and leader of a study published in *Journal of Consumer Research*. USF.edu

Using Only Sea Salt or Gourmet Salt Can Lead to Iodine Deficiency

Neal D. Barnard, MD, is adjunct associate professor of medicine at George Washington University School of Medicine and Health Sciences in Washington, DC, and president of Physicians Committee for Responsible Medicine. PCRM.org

---

Iodized table salt is the most common source of iodine. Deficiencies can lead to fatigue, weight gain, hair loss and goiter. One-half teaspoon of iodized salt per day meets the daily requirement for iodine. Sea vegetables such as nori, wakame or dulse flakes are another potent source of iodine. Have a modest serving two or three times per week.

Why Healthy Poke Bowls Are All the Rage

Janet Bond Brill, PhD, RDN, FAND, is a registered dietitian nutritionist, a fellow of the Academy of Nutrition and Dietetics and a nationally recognized nutrition, health and fitness expert specializing in cardiovascular disease prevention. Based in Allentown, Pennsylvania, Dr. Brill is author of *Blood Pressure DOWN, Cholesterol DOWN* and *Prevent a Second Heart Attack*. DrJanet.com

"Poke Bowl" mania is everywhere—on social media…in your local grocery store… and even at a nearby poke bar. So what are these one-dish wonders? In case you're not quite sure, poke (pronounced "POH-kay") is the ubiquitous rice bowl filled with super-fresh raw fish and other vibrantly colored toppings. *It's not too late to learn how to make your own poke bowl creations…*

A CUSTOMIZED ONE-DISH MEAL

Poke is a traditional Hawaiian dish that dates back centuries. Today's poke bowl is a delicate dish of fresh, diced raw fish (often marinated) and served cold over rice. The rice and fish are seasoned and topped with vegetables and sauces packed with savory umami (the so-called "fifth" taste—after sweet, salty, sour and bitter—that imparts a meaty-type richness).

All ingredients are sliced and diced into bite-size portions. The beauty of a poke bowl is that it is an easily customizable dish, so you can change up the ingredients to your liking. Think of it as the next generation of fast-food sushi, where you can have a complete, nutritious meal ready to eat in minutes, no rolling required. And even if you're a vegetarian, you can create your own fish-free poke bowl.

MAKE YOUR OWN HEALTHY POKE BOWL

At the most basic level, a poke bowl is made up of…

•**The base.** This is typically white rice. To make it healthier, choose brown rice, quinoa, farro or fresh dark leafy greens instead. Arugula is especially healthful, as it is a cancer-fighting cruciferous vegetable.

•**The protein.** Cubed, sushi-grade raw salmon or ahi tuna (yellowfin tuna) is the standard protein. However, if you're worried about eating ahi tuna due to overfishing and/or its high mercury level, choose the salmon sashimi instead. If you don't like raw fish, then cook it to your liking. It will take only a few minutes.

Note: Be sure that you do not marinate the fish in soy sauce or you'll add too much sodium. Remember, you can always opt for some other lean protein, such as hamachi (Japanese amberjack or yellowtail fish)…cooked shrimp, chicken, crab or octopus…scrambled egg…or tofu (as a vegetarian option).

•**The veggies.** Healthy choices include cubed avocado, seaweed, shaved radish, shredded carrots, shredded Napa cabbage, cubed cucumber and edamame.

•**Seasonings.** Instead of high-sodium soy sauce, try a plain (but flavorful) rice vinegar, which has no sodium and is low calorie, with sesame oil. For spice, try sliced jalapeños, sriracha sauce (which contains *capsaicin*, a chili pepper derivative good for metabolism) or wasabi. A sprinkle or two of Eden Shake Furikake Sesame and Sea Vegetable Seasoning (a Japanese seasoning mixture of sesame seeds, chopped seaweed and salt—one tablespoon has 150 mg of sodium) is another healthy option.

•**The toppings.** Cubed mango, sliced pears, scallions, pickled ginger and onions, chopped nuts and sesame seeds are nutrition-packed options for toppings. To keep it healthy, stay away from the fried stuff (such as onions or wonton strips)!

Keep Food Separate

Don't let different foods touch one another on your plate. This will help you to more clearly see how much you're eating and practice better portion control.

Joel Harper, celebrity trainer and author of *Mind Your Body: 4 Weeks to a Leaner, Healthier Life*.

Food Addiction Is Real

Ashley N. Gearhardt, PhD, associate professor of psychology at University of Michigan and director of its Food and Addiction Science and Treatment Lab, both in Ann Arbor. One of the preeminent researchers in the field, she was a principal developer of the Yale Food Addiction Scale, FastLab.psych.lsa.umich.edu.

A lot of people love their junk food—candy bars, potato chips, donuts and greasy french fries, to name just a few. They know all these foods are bad for them, but they just can't help themselves. Are these people "addicted"—the way that others are hooked on alcohol or opioids?

The concept of "food addiction" has been kicked around since the 19th century, but only recently—as obesity has reached epidemic proportions in the US—have doctors and scientists taken it seriously.

Now: With mounting scientific evidence showing that certain patterns of food consumption do have much in common with drug and alcohol addictions, many of the mysteries of out-of-control eating patterns are finally being unraveled.

Are you—or someone you know—a food addict? *What you need to know…*

HOW ADDICTION AFFECTS THE BODY

Doctors diagnose an addiction when the use of a substance, such as drugs or alcohol, or a behavior like gambling is beyond a person's control. When it takes hold, you can't stop your addiction—despite the toll it's taking on your health, work and personal relationships.

Satisfying your "appetite" for the substance or behavior consumes considerable time and energy. You may experience intense cravings for the object of your addiction and suffer physical and emotional pains of withdrawal without it.

On a biological level, the brains of individuals who are addicted to a substance or behavior are different from other people's brains. Circuits that process reward are overstimulated, and those that regulate self-control are less active. In other words, in addiction the strong desire for the drug is coupled with weaker brakes, which makes it hard to stop the behavior even when it is getting you into trouble.

Recent scientific evidence: Using brain imaging and other analyses, researchers have seen similar biological patterns in people whose food consumption fits the "addictive" pattern, according to research published in 2018 in *Nutrients.*

Still, the diagnosis of food addiction remains controversial. Unlike alcohol or painkillers, food can't be an "addictive" substance, some argue, because we need it to survive.

There's some truth to that argument because people don't become addicted to food in general, but almost always to certain highly processed products—typically salty snacks like potato chips and food products that are high in fats and refined carbohydrates, particularly added sugar, and low in protein and fiber. Junk food, in other words.

The simple carbs of these highly addictive edibles hit the bloodstream rapidly to spike blood sugar, and the oral pleasure of high-fat or salty foods further amps up the brain's reward system. Whole foods—or those that are less processed—affect blood sugar levels and the brain much more gradually.

WHO BECOMES AN ADDICT?

Contrary to what many people assume, not all addicts are obese or overweight. In fact, 11% of people whose weight is normal have significant symptoms of food addiction, according to a systematic review published in *Nutrients.*

However, the more you weigh, the greater the risk—among obese individuals, the rate of food addiction is 25%. At the same time, as these figures show, many obese—even morbidly obese—people are not addicts.

As scientists investigate the connection between body weight and food addiction, it appears that being overweight can be a cause—as well as a consequence—of this addiction. There is evidence that obesity changes how the brain's reward system operates, making it necessary to have more food to get the same emotional charge—you need two slices of pizza where one used to do.

Food addiction affects both men and women, although some studies suggest that rates are a bit higher in women. Middle-aged women (ages 45 to 64) are more likely to have food addiction than older women, according to research published in *The American Journal of Clinical Nutrition*. It appears to run in families—children of food-addicted parents are more likely to develop the problem themselves, possibly reflecting the influence of both upbringing and genetics.

THE BIGGEST DANGER ZONES

While the US isn't the only country plagued by food addiction, surveys show that the problem is significantly less common in other countries. Americans live in what many call a "toxic" food environment—junk food is cheap, always available and relentlessly advertised.

What's more, many of these foods are *designed* to be addictive. So-called "Big Food"—the major food manufacturers—invest heavily in research to develop products that have precisely the effects on the brain and body that lead to their compulsive consumption.

The harmful effects of food addiction are, not surprisingly, mainly those that occur with obesity—increased risk for heart disease, diabetes, orthopedic problems and certain cancers. But there is also evidence that the surplus of fat and refined carbs of addictive foods raises cholesterol and the risk for diabetes even if you're not overweight.

Regardless of your body weight, as the continuous urge to overeat addictive foods robs your energy and time, more wholesome activities are neglected, and the out-of-control feeling damages self-esteem. It's common for food addiction to also lead to isolation and depression.

HELP FOR FOOD ADDICTION

You can take steps on your own to improve your relationship to food—especially if your addiction symptoms are not significantly interfering with your daily life. *What to do...*

•**Keep a journal to identify foods that trigger compulsive eating or craving.** Note the situations in which you struggle for control—are you stressed, angry, frustrated or bored?

•**Find nonaddicting foods that you enjoy**—clementines, unsalted nuts, baby carrots, air-popped popcorn and hummus, for example—**and keep them handy.** Whole foods are good choices because they do not have the amped-up reward levels of junk food.

•**Don't miss meals or deprive yourself to make up for yesterday's bingeing.** When we are hungry, it tells our brain's reward system to be extra responsive to food. That's why being really hungry can make us more vulnerable to addictive foods.

•**Be alert for signs of stress and/or boredom, and use nonfood remedies**—take a short walk or listen to your favorite music. When you're hit with a craving, distract yourself. Research shows that even intense cravings often subside quickly on their own.

•**Get professional help.** If preoccupation with food stays out of control and interferes with your life despite your efforts to curb your addiction symptoms, you need more help than you can give yourself. See your doctor for a physical exam—problems like a malfunctioning thyroid can amplify the drive for food.

The field is new, so there are few clinicians who treat food addiction. Your best bet is a therapist who uses cognitive behavioral therapy (CBT) for eating disorders and can adapt it to addiction. To find a CBT professional near you, consult the Association for Behavioral and Cognitive Therapies at ABCT.org.

There is little scientific evidence that 12-step programs, such as Overeaters Anonymous, help with food addiction, but such a program may be worth considering if other options have failed.

Use Some "Flour Power" to Get More Nutrition

Janet Bond Brill, PhD, RDN, FAND, registered dietitian nutritionist, a fellow of the Academy of Nutrition and Dietetics and a nationally recognized nutrition, health and fitness expert who specializes in cardiovascular disease prevention. Based in Allentown, Pennsylvania, Dr. Brill is author of *Blood Pressure DOWN, Cholesterol DOWN* and *Prevent a Second Heart Attack*. DrJanet.com

When it comes to baking, the go-to ingredient for generations of Americans has been all-purpose flour, which is made from wheat. But if you're looking for some variety in taste, an extra boost of nutrition and even some gluten-free options, other flours should be on your radar. Most grocery stores now stock these "alternative" flours, but if yours doesn't, check your local health-food store or shop online. *My four favorites…*

•**Rye flour.** Rye is a very healthy whole grain that's popular in Scandinavia, where their dense, fiber-filled black bread is made of 100% pure rye flour. Here in the US, rye bread is made from a mixture of rye flour and wheat flour. Rye grains are highly nutritious, filled with soluble fiber, vitamin E, calcium, iron, magnesium and potassium. The high levels of magnesium and potassium help lower blood pressure, and the soluble fiber lowers cholesterol. Rye also has been shown to promote weight loss and elimination and to help prevent type 2 diabetes. Rye, which tastes sweet and malty, is sometimes used in baked goods such as piecrusts or crackers.

Note: Rye does contain gluten, albeit less than what's found in all-purpose flour. To bake with rye flour, mix with all-purpose flour—use up to 40% of light rye or about 20% of dark rye/pumpernickel flour.

•**Chickpea flour.** Chickpeas (also known as garbanzo beans) are a legume—not a grain—so this flour is gluten-free. Packed with plant protein, iron, fiber, vitamins and minerals (especially the blood pressure–lowering mineral potassium), chickpea flour is highly nutritious. With a subtle flavor, chickpea flour is a versatile ingredient for use in the kitchen. Chickpea flour, which adds a nutty taste and gives a nice protein boost over wheat, can be used for baked goods such as batter to coat fritters for frying and as a thickener for soups. If you choose to substitute chickpea flour for all-purpose flour, use three-quarters cup of chickpea flour for each cup of all-purpose flour.

•**Almond flour.** Ground almonds are a wonderful way to get your daily dose of heart-healthy nuts. High in protein, insoluble fiber, vitamins, minerals and monounsaturated fat, almond flour gives baked goods a rich flavor and makes them more tender and moist. If you substitute one-to-one for all-purpose flour, use more egg to offset almond flour's density.

•**Oat flour.** One of the healthiest grains on Earth, oats are filled with vital nutrients such as plant protein, vitamins (especially B vitamins) and minerals (especially iron and zinc).

Oats also contain two unique disease-fighting substances—a group of antioxidants known as *avenanthramides* and the powerful cholesterol-lowering soluble fiber called beta-glucan. Unlike all-purpose flour, oat flour is gluten-free. (Just be sure to buy a product labeled as such if you are gluten-free, since contamination can occur during processing.) Oat and wheat flours have a similar taste profile, except that oat flour is sweeter and more dense. Due to the lack of gluten, oat flour will need more yeast for baked goods that rise. Oat flour is best for baking quick breads, pancakes and cookies, which allow for a one-to-one substitution for all-purpose flour.

The Best Protein Powders

Tod Cooperman, MD, president, founder and editor in chief of ConsumerLab.com, a subscription-based website ($47.40 annually) that evaluates consumer products relating to health, wellness and nutrition. ConsumerLab.com recently completed an extensive product review of protein powders, shakes and drinks.

There was a time when bodybuilders and the elderly were just about the only people to use protein supplements. No more!

Now: There's an ever-increasing selection of protein powders available not just in health-food stores but also on the shelves of most US supermarkets and drugstores.

So which products contain the highest-quality ingredients at the best prices? For four top picks, we spoke with Tod Cooperman, MD, president and founder of ConsumerLab.com, which identifies the best health and nutritional products through independent testing.

WHY WE NEED PROTEIN

Our bodies need protein to build and maintain our muscles, bones and skin. Protein also helps keep our energy levels high and promotes weight loss in those who want to drop unwanted pounds.

Protein is especially important as we grow older. With each decade after age 30, we lose as much as 3% to 5% of our muscle mass, leading to weakness that also increases our risk for falls and broken bones. A recent report suggests that people with pronounced muscle loss, a condition known as *sarcopenia*, face more than twice the risk for a fall-related fracture.

Adults should get 0.36 grams (g) of protein per pound, according to the recommended dietary allowance. For example, someone weighing 150 pounds would need to get 54 g of protein daily. But research published in 2019 in *The Journal of Nutrition, Health & Aging* found that 30% of men and 45% of women ages 51 to 60 failed to meet this basic threshold…and 37% of men and 48% of women fell short during their next decade of life.

While foods (such as meat, seafood, dairy, legumes and nuts) should be our main sources of this vital nutrient, more and more people are turning to protein powders and drinks to help them get adequate levels in their diets. Such products are not only convenient, but also are free of the saturated fat and cholesterol that are often found in protein-rich foods.

Caveat: Protein—whether it's from food or a supplement—is not a miracle fix. Regular resistance exercise, such as lifting weights or using weight machines, is also necessary. As part of an overall fitness program, older adults should do strength training two to three times a week. Strength-training regimens may include squats, wall push-ups and exercises, such as biceps curls, that use hand weights.

THE CHANGING FACE OF PROTEIN

The proteins found in powders and drinks are no longer your run-of-the-mill dairy-based products, derived from whey or casein. There's a recent push for more plant-based sources, including pea, hemp, rice, soy or other nondairy ingredients, which work well for people who are lactose intolerant.

Important: Because high protein intake can impair kidney function in people with kidney disease, they should talk to their doctors about how much and what types of protein they should consume. Some doctors advise increasing overall fluid intake when consuming a high-protein diet or protein supplements to help protect the kidneys, but this is probably not necessary if you have normal kidney function. Before adding a protein supplement to your diet, check with your doctor if you have any concerns.

ConsumerLab.com approves protein supplements based on their quality, value, taste and mixability. The products below also did not exceed contamination limits for lead, cadmium, arsenic or mercury. *Among the top low-sugar powders tested by Consumer Lab.com…*

MYPROTEIN IMPACT WHEY ISOLATE

•**Protein source:** Whey.

Price: 52 cents per 20 g of protein.

Why it's a top pick: Low in carbs and virtually fat-free, this whey isolate (it contains only 0.31 g of lactose per serving) has a slight powdered-milk taste and blends well into drinks. It provides 22 g of protein per serving and 12% of an adult's daily value for calcium. It's gluten-free.

NOW SPORTS PEA PROTEIN, NATURAL UNFLAVORED

•**Protein source:** Pea.

Price: 37 cents per 20 g of protein.

Why it's a top pick: Mixing easily and smoothly into liquids, this product enhances the taste of vegetable smoothies and provides 24 g of protein per serving. At 330 mg of sodium per serving, it's slightly higher in sodium than most protein powders but is gluten- and lactose-free.

NUTIVA ORGANIC HEMP PROTEIN

•**Protein source:** Hemp.

Price: $1.04 per 20 g of protein.

Why it's a top pick: With a bountiful 8 g of fiber per scoop—one of hemp's big benefits—this unsweetened supplement also has naturally high levels of potassium, iron, magnesium and zinc. Its complex but pleasant vegetable flavor is offset by a somewhat gritty texture that makes it less suitable for mixing with plain water but terrific in a smoothie. This powder provides 15 g of protein per serving. It has no measurable lactose but is not gluten-free.

GARDEN OF LIFE SPORT ORGANIC PLANT-BASED PROTEIN, VANILLA

•**Protein source:** Mixed.

Price: $1.35 per 20 g of protein.

Why it's a top pick: Primarily pea-based but also containing navy, lentil and garbanzo beans as well as cranberry protein, this powder mixes easily and evenly into water and other thin beverages. It provides 15 g of protein per serving and has a clean vegetable flavor with only a slight artificial-sugar sweetness despite its stevia content. This gluten-free powder has no measurable lactose.

Celery: The Stealth Health Food Worth Getting More of

Janet Bond Brill, PhD, RDN, FAND, is a registered dietitian nutritionist, a fellow of the Academy of Nutrition and Dietetics and a nationally recognized nutrition, health and fitness expert who specializes in cardiovascular disease prevention. Based in Allentown, Pennsylvania, Dr. Brill is author of *Blood Pressure DOWN, Cholesterol DOWN* and *Prevent a Second Heart Attack.* DrJanet.com

---

You might think that celery is just one of those plain-Jane foods that you find on a veggie platter or sticking out of your Bloody Mary. And because celery is emblematic of dieting, you probably wouldn't be surprised to learn that a five-inch stalk has just three calories. But did you know that for those three calories, you also get a whole lot of nutrition? High in fiber, bulked up with lots of zero-calorie water plus a nice dose of disease-fighting antioxidant phytonutrients, vitamins K, C and A, folate and potassium, this fabulous, crunchy, super-low-calorie food deserves a second look—even if you're not dieting. Research suggests that the powerful antioxidants in celery help the body fight off heart disease (by lowering blood pressure)…boost immune function…and lower inflammation.

Some other little-known nuggets about celery…

***FACT #1:* Calories do count.** Some people claim that celery is a "negative-calorie food"—a term that means you will burn more calories digesting celery than it contains, for a net loss. This sounds plausible—in theory—but in reality, even the lowest calorie foods, such as celery, grapefruit and cucumber, still contain more calories than it takes to break down and absorb them in the body.

***FACT #2:* Celery juice is not a cure-all.** Search social media for #celeryjuice, and you will be inundated with gorgeous photos of what is often touted as a miracle green elixir, a drink capable of curing everything from eczema and infertility to cancer and even mental illness. The problem is, there is no scientific data supporting these claims. Plus, when you juice a lot of celery, you concentrate the vegetable, so it's going to be higher in sugars, carbohydrates and calories. With the juicing process, you also strip away the beneficial fiber—the very substance that helps you feel fuller longer, improves your intestinal health and feeds the healthy bacteria in your gut.

***FACT #3:* Raw is best.** Celery often is eaten raw—and for good reason. Blanching or boiling celery causes a significant loss of antioxidants, according to research. When eaten raw (or steamed), celery retains almost all the antioxidants.

It's time to get creative: Celery makes a great addition to almost all salads, and it definitely adds some crunch and pizzazz to the mouthwatering salad recipe below!

COUSCOUS, ORANGE, GRAPE AND CELERY SALAD

1 cup uncooked couscous

1 small orange

2 Tablespoons extra-virgin olive oil

1 Tablespoon white wine vinegar

Dash of sea salt

Dash of freshly ground black pepper

3 approximately 5-inch celery stalks plus ½ cup celery leaves, chopped

½ pound red seedless grapes, halved

Directions: Cook couscous according to package directions. Remove from heat and let cool. Zest the orange peel, and juice the orange. In a small bowl, whisk together one tablespoon orange zest, juice from the orange, extra-virgin olive oil, white wine vinegar, salt and pepper for the dressing. In a salad bowl, mix together the couscous, celery and grapes. Toss in the dressing and serve. Makes two servings.

Nutritional information per serving:
Calories, 250…fat, 15 g…cholesterol, 0 mg…carbohydrates, 46 g…dietary fiber, 2 g… total sugars, 21 g…added sugars, 0 g…protein, 6 g…sodium, 35 mg.

Health Benefits of Lemon Water

Prevention.com.

It *can prevent hunger spikes:* If you feel like snacking soon after a meal, mix one cup of warm water with the juice of a half lemon and a pinch of lemon zest.

It boosts energy: Process a sliced lemon, with the peel, in a blender…freeze in an ice-cube tray…put a cube in water for a quick energy pick-me-up.

It protects your cells: Lemon is a good source of vitamin C—a powerful antioxidant.

It controls bloating: The citric acid in lemons helps your stomach break down food, and lemons contain potassium, which can hold down sodium levels and reduce salt-related bloat.

It can protect against kidney stones: Drink the juice of two lemons diluted in water every day to help block the formation of the painful stones.

That Second Cup of Joe Is OK

Even heavy coffee drinking is good for health. People who drank one to eight cups of coffee a day—or even more—were less likely to die from any cause over a 10-year study period than people who did not drink coffee. The protective effect applied to ground and instant coffee, caffeinated or decaffeinated.

Study of nearly 400,000 UK coffee drinkers by researchers at National Cancer Institute, Rockville, Maryland, published in *JAMA Internal Medicine*.

Vanilla Makes Drinks Seem Sweeter

Study by researchers at Penn State University, State College, Pennsylvania, published in *Food Quality and Preference*.

Vanilla makes already-sweetened milk beverages taste sweeter—so the amount of added sugar can be reduced, possibly by 20% to 50%. It may be possible to produce reduced-sugar, sweet-tasting chocolate milk for the National School Lunch Program. And if you want to try to cut down on drinkable calories, try a bit in coffee or another beverage instead of sugar.

Unusual Caffeine Drinks

Robert S. McCaleb, president and founder of the Herb Research Foundation, a nonprofit research and educational organization based in Boulder, Colorado. He designed the herbal tea component of the World Tea Academy's Certified Tea Professional program.

Do you ever wish you could get a little dose of caffeine but you don't like coffee and are bored with the same old teas? If you're looking for something a little different as far as your caffeination requirements go, you may want to consider yerba maté, guayusa and yaupon.

Made from assorted species of the holly plant, these beverages have been enjoyed by indigenous peoples in South America and Central America and the lower US for thousands of years. In addition to caffeine, they all have lots of vitamins, minerals, antioxidants and amino acids, so you can feel good about indulging in them.

The caffeine levels for these drinks typically are somewhere between those of green and black tea but below coffee. Many people find the energy boost they produce less jittery than coffee, even when comparable amounts of caffeine are consumed.

Yerba maté, guayusa and yaupon are sometimes roasted after harvesting, giving them deeper earthy, toasty, woody tones—something that might remind you a bit of a black tea. And sometimes they're simply dried rather than roasted, resulting in flavors that are similar to green tea—grassy and almost spinachy rather than earthy.

Here are a few options if you're interested in exploring these drinks...

•**Yerba maté is a very popular traditional beverage in Argentina, Paraguay, Uruguay and other parts of Central America and South America.** It's probably the caffeinated holly drink that is easiest to find in supermarkets and tea stores.

Examples: Guayaki Traditional Organic Maté ($17.96 for 75 tea bags)...and Numi Maté Lemon, which combines yerba maté, green tea and lemon myrtle ($5.35 for 18 tea bags).

•**Guayusa grows mainly in the Amazon rain forest of Ecuador.**

Examples: RUNA Organic Guayusa Tea ($19.98 for one pound of loose-leaf tea)...Celestial Seasonings Organic Mint Guayusa ($5.39 for 20 tea bags).

•**Yaupon is made from the only caffeinated plant native to North America.** The yaupon plant grows wild around the Gulf Coast. It has slightly more caffeine than the other beverages listed here, though still only about as much as a cup of black tea. Yaupon was regarded as an unwanted weed in modern times. It was only rediscovered as a beverage in the past decade when a small Texas company called CatSpring began harvesting, processing and selling wild yaupon.

Examples: CatSpring Marfa Dark Roast Black Yaupon or Pedernales Green Yaupon (both $10.99 for 16 tea bags).

That Sounds Delicious!

Bradley P. Turnwald, PhD, postdoctoral scholar in the department of psychology at Stanford University, California, and coauthor of a study published in *Psychological Science*.

Good-for-you-foods that sound indulgent are more likely to be eaten. According to research done at Stanford University and other US institutions, simply knowing that a healthy food is good for you isn't enough to make people choose it. "Taste-focused" descriptions that feature specific flavors and textures excite your taste buds.

Example: The next time you want your family to eat baked squash, tell them it's "herb-crusted roasted squash."

Easy, Healthful Two-Ingredient Breakfasts

Roundup of experts on two-ingredient breakfasts, reported at WellAndGood.com.

Apple slices and nuts—try pecans or walnuts, which go well with apples. *Eggs and salsa*—scramble an egg or two and top with salsa. *Eggs and avocado*—either scramble eggs and mix avocado in, or cook the avocado with the egg cracked and cradled inside it. *Oats with milk*—at night, mix one-half cup of oats with dairy or nondairy milk, then eat it in the morning. *Celery sticks and almond butter*—just spread the almond butter on the celery. *Guacamole toast with seeded rye bread*—the bread provides fiber and the avocado-based guacamole gives healthful fats.

Make-It-Yourself Energy Bars: They're Easy, Nutritious—and Delicious!

Danielle Omar, MS, RDN, a Fairfax, Virginia–based integrative dietitian and founder of FoodConfidence.com.

Store-bought energy bars usually contain 140 to 300 calories each. They often are short on fiber and protein and contain way too much sugar and too many "empty" carbohydrates.

However, the nutritious energy bars described here have approximately 200 calories each (give or take, depending on the ingredients used) but are worth consuming because they are filled with fiber and healthy fats. Each bar also provides about 6 g to 8 g of energy-boosting protein.

To get started, line an eight-by-eight-inch baking dish with plastic wrap, making sure to leave a few inches of overhang.

For each of the recipes in this article, you will press the mixture into the baking dish and chill in the refrigerator until firm (usually about 30 minutes). Once the mixture has been chilled, hold the plastic wrap where it overhangs the dish and pull up to pop out the uncut energy bars.

OAT ENERGY BARS

1 very ripe banana, mashed

1½ cups instant or quick-cooking oats

½ cup shredded, unsweetened coconut

½ cup chopped, unsweetened dried fruit of your choice

½ cup maple syrup, agave or honey

½ cup natural nut butter of your choice (or sunflower butter if you have a nut allergy)

2 Tablespoons ground flaxseed

2 teaspoons ground cinnamon

2 teaspoons vanilla extract

Combine all the ingredients for this recipe in a large bowl (you may find that it's easiest to mix these ingredients with your hands).

For even more protein: Add ½ to 1 cup (depending on taste) of cooked quinoa. Or you can add ½ to 1 cup of a plant-based protein powder. I recommend a "no flavor" protein powder, such as VegaOne.

For extra fiber and healthy fat: Toss in a handful of chia seeds or hemp seeds.

CHOCOLATE QUINOA ENERGY BARS

1 cup cooked quinoa

⅓ cup raw sunflower seeds

1 cup instant or quick-cooking oats

⅓ cup chopped, unsweetened dried cherries

¼ cup shredded, unsweetened coconut

⅓ cup maple syrup

1 teaspoon vanilla extract

2 Tablespoons almond butter

½ cup cacao nibs (for crunchy flavor) or bittersweet chocolate chips

½ teaspoon sea salt

In a large bowl, combine the quinoa, sunflower seeds, oats, dried cherries and unsweetened coconut. Mix well, then stir in the maple syrup, vanilla extract and almond butter. Finally, stir in the cacao nibs or chocolate chips and sea salt. Table salt can also be used, but I prefer sea salt since the trace minerals left behind in the evaporation process provide extra flavor. If you prefer a mild sweet-salty flavor, use salted sunflower seeds.

GUILT-FREE CHOCOLATE CHIP COOKIE DOUGH ENERGY BARS

These grain-free bars contain dates, which give them their sweetness and provide the texture needed to hold all the ingredients together.

½ cup dry-roasted almonds

½ cup raw cashews

2 Tablespoons almond or peanut butter

1⅓ cups pitted dates

½ cup shredded, unsweetened coconut

½ teaspoon vanilla extract

⅛ teaspoon sea salt

2 Tablespoons cacao nibs or bittersweet chocolate chips

½ cup unsweetened dried cherries

Process the ingredients in a food processor until fairly smooth but pasty. Refrigerate—and enjoy!

Fun New Fruit Salad Flavors

Ellie Krieger, RD, author of *Whole in One: Complete, Healthy Meals in a Single Pot, Sheet Pan or Skillet.* EllieKrieger.com

Make your fruit bowl even brighter with traditional flavorings used in untraditional ways…

Balsamic glaze: Buy a bottle of a sweet and tangy balsamic reduction, and use it as a delicious drizzle over fresh fruit. It's especially luscious over berries, cherries and peaches. The thick syrupy texture of the reduction is far better on fruit than straight balsamic vinegar, which is thinner and more acidic.

Chili and lime: Liven up tropical fruit such as mango and pineapple. Toss three cups of cut fruit with a dressing of one tablespoon of lime juice whisked with one tablespoon of honey plus a generous pinch of ancho chili powder.

Creamy lemon-poppyseed: Swirl one tablespoon of lemon juice, lemon zest and a touch of honey into a cup of plain yogurt, then stir in a teaspoon of poppy seed. Add the dressing to your cut fruit for a creamy treat that really pops.

4 Healthy Nighttime Snacks

Janet Bond Brill, PhD, RDN, FAND, is a registered dietitian nutritionist, a fellow of the Academy of Nutrition and Dietetics and a nationally recognized nutrition, health and fitness expert who specializes in cardiovascular disease prevention. Based in Allentown, Pennsylvania, Dr. Brill is author of *Blood Pressure DOWN, Cholesterol DOWN* and *Prevent a Second Heart Attack.* DrJanet.com

Let's be honest—most people love to nosh a bit if they become engrossed in a new TV series or a big-screen film they can finally watch at home. But is it possible to snack healthfully? Yes, it is.

As a nutritionist who has done her own share of late-night snacking, here are my four favorite yummy treats—each under 200 calories…

•**Dark-chocolate covered banana.** Get your potassium from the banana and a heart-healthy dose of dark chocolate with this sinfully delicious dessert treat. Cut a ripe banana into slices and place them on a plate. Melt a tablespoon of dark chocolate baking chips in the microwave and drizzle over the banana slices. Top with a tablespoon of fat-free whipped topping—all for just 190 calories.

•**Pumpkin pie Greek yogurt.** Pumpkin is packed with disease-fighting antioxidants and a generous punch of protein. Plus, it's low in calories and it's filling. A six-ounce serving of plain 0% Greek yogurt contains no fat, about 15 g to 20 g of protein (equivalent to two to three ounces of meat) and 20% of your daily recommended calcium intake.

Directions: Take one small container of 0% fat plain Greek yogurt, add in two tablespoons of pure canned pumpkin…sweetener of choice (to taste)…and one-half teaspoon of pumpkin pie spice. Mix together and top with fat-free whipped cream and one tablespoon of diced walnuts for an approximately 170-calorie sweet treat.

•**Red bell pepper slices with a zesty dip.** Red bell peppers are packed with nutrients such as folate, potassium and vitamins A, B-6, C, E and K. And all this for a mere 30 calories per pepper. Dip the slices in honey mustard for added zip (two tablespoons has 140 calories)…or salsa (nutrient-rich, no fat and about 10 calories in two tablespoons).

•**Cinnamon apple chips.** For a sweet and healthy, high-fiber snack, grab some nutritious apples, add some cinnamon and a touch of sugar.

Ingredients:

3 small Red Delicious apples, cored

1 teaspoon cinnamon

2 Tablespoons sugar (*Optional:* To reduce the sugar and carbohydrate count, substitute one tablespoon of Truvia Baking Blend or Splenda Sugar Blend for the sugar.)

Directions: Preheat your oven to 200°F, and line two baking sheets with parchment paper. Using a sharp knife, slice the apples as thin as possible (leave the nutrition-packed peels on the apples). Place the apple slices on the parchment paper in one layer. Mix the cinnamon and sugar, and sprinkle half of it onto the sliced apples. Bake for 40 to 50 minutes, flip the apples, add the rest of the cinnamon/sugar mix to the other side and bake for another 40 to 50 minutes. The apples will be a golden brown. Remove from the oven and let the chips cool. The chips are best eaten within a couple hours of cooling. Makes two servings (each less than 200 calories).

Cut Out That Snack

William E. Kraus, MD, distinguished professor of medicine, Duke University School of Medicine, Durham, North Carolina.

Cutting just 300 calories per day improves health.

Recent study: Normal-weight adults who ate 300 fewer calories daily for six months significantly reduced their levels of cholesterol, triglycerides, blood pressure and blood sugar. After two years, those who continued the reduced-calorie diet experienced a drop in chronic inflammation linked to heart disease, cancer and dementia.

Takeaway: Skipping one daily snack of a few cookies, a scoop of ice cream or some potato chips could reduce your risk for heart disease, diabetes and cancer.

Sneaky Ways to Get Your Veggies

Janet Bond Brill, PhD, RDN, FAND, registered dietitian nutritionist, a fellow of the Academy of Nutrition and Dietetics and a nationally recognized nutrition, health and fitness expert who specializes in cardiovascular disease prevention. Based in Allentown, Pennsylvania, Dr. Brill is author of *Blood Pressure DOWN, Cholesterol DOWN* and *Prevent a Second Heart Attack.* DrJanet.com

Mom was right…you do need to eat your veggies. They are the crown jewels of a plant-based diet—the scientifically proven prescription for better health and longevity. Of course, not everyone likes the taste of certain vegetables. But fortunately, you can get your veggies and enjoy the flavor of your foods by camouflaging the veggie taste that's off-putting to you or members of your family. Clever ways to "mask" the taste and texture of your veggies…

•**Add canned pumpkin…to pancakes, chili or almost anything.** Pumpkin tastes mild (so it's easily masked) and is naturally orange in color, which means that it contains large amounts of vitamin A to sustain sharp

Don't Let Junk Food Wreck Your Health

Make a plan for how many treats you will allow yourself weekly—sticking to the plan will create a reward in itself to help balance the short-term reward of eating a doughnut or piece of cake. Chew slowly and enjoy the taste of whatever you eat—paying attention will make you appreciate the food more and can lead to consuming fewer calories. Eat junk food when you are almost full, never on an empty stomach—your self-control is lower when you are hungry so you are more likely to overindulge.

Teresa Fung, ScD, professor of nutrition, Simmons University, Boston, writing at Medium.com/popular-science.

eyesight…the antioxidant beta-carotene to help fight cancer…and vitamin C to maintain a healthy immune system.

•**Hide veggies in a casserole.** To add flavor, color and nutrition, get out your vegetable grater when cooking a casserole. Mixing just about any vegetable, such as carrots, celery, asparagus or mushrooms, with a classic cheese sauce and topping with bread crumbs and Parmesan (and perhaps a toasted nut topping) creates a family-pleasing casserole that's a snap to fix and bake.

•**Go for chocolate.** Try puréeing sweet potato, beets or zucchini and add it to your brownies. Or sneak some spinach into your favorite chocolate cake batter. Defrost frozen spinach, squeeze out any excess moisture and put it in a food processor. Add two teaspoons of vanilla and two eggs and purée until very smooth. Add this "wet" mixture to the typical dry ingredients and bake as usual.

•**Make creamy pasta sauce.** Skip the high-fat cream and butter in most alfredo and vodka sauces. Instead, try pumpkin, butternut squash or cauliflower puréed with white beans for a delicious, low-calorie pasta sauce without the veggie taste. Don't believe it? *Try my nutrient-packed pasta sauce recipe…*

CREAMY PUMPKIN PASTA SAUCE

1 teaspoon extra-virgin olive oil

2 shallots, minced

3 cloves garlic, minced

1 15-ounce can pure pumpkin purée

½ 15-ounce can cannellini beans

1 Tablespoon oregano (or mixture of Italian spices)

1 teaspoon cracked black pepper

½ teaspoon sea salt

1 15-ounce can low-sodium vegetable broth

Directions: In a small saucepan, heat the olive oil over medium-low heat, and cook the shallots until soft and translucent (for about 10 minutes). In a blender, add the cooked shallots and the rest of the ingredients in the recipe. Blend the sauce until it is a smooth purée. *Makes eight servings* (one-half cup each).

Nutrition information per serving: Calories, 50...fat, 1 g...cholesterol, 0 mg...carbohydrates, 10 g...fiber, 3 g...protein, 2 g...sodium, 180 mg.

Pick a Healthy Pizza

Prevention.com

Frozen pizzas that are good for you should have crusts made from whole grains, cauliflower or other vegetables...fewer than three grams of added sugar...low sodium...a limited amount of cheese...vegetables, not meat, as toppings.

Worth considering: Caulipower Veggie Cauliflower Crust Pizza...Amy's No-Cheese Roasted Vegetable Pizza...Freschetta Whole-Grain Chicken and Fire-Roasted Vegetables Pizza...Quest Thin-Crust Spinach and Mushroom Pizza...Newman's Own Thin & Crispy Margherita Pizza.

Stop the Media Multitasking

Richard B. Lopez, PhD, postdoctoral research fellow, Rice University, Houston, and leader of two studies of media multitasking, published in *Brain Imaging and Behavior.*

Media multitasking is linked to obesity. People who keep switching among portable digital devices, such as smartphones and tablets, are more susceptible to food temptations and other behavior indicating lack of self-control.

Too Little Sleep Linked to Unhealthy Eating

Thorsten Kahnt, PhD, assistant professor of neurology at Northwestern University Feinberg School of Medicine, Chicago. Northwestern.edu

People are more likely to indulge in unhealthy foods that are high in fat or sugar when they haven't had enough sleep. In a recent study published in *eLife*, participants partook more heavily of an array of unhealthy foods including doughnut holes, chocolate chip cookies and potato chips following nights when they got only four hours of sleep than when allowed a full eight hours of sleep.

Smell, not exhaustion, seems to be at the root of the increased snacking. Brain scans revealed that when someone is sleep-deprived, his/her *piriform cortex*, a region of the brain that processes odor, experiences a heightened ability to identify food smells...while its ability to communicate with the *insula*, a region that processes signals associated with food intake, is diminished.

Net result: Tired people are more likely to succumb to the smell of high-calorie foods, such as doughnuts and potato chips—not just their mere presence.

It's possible (though not yet proven) that sleep-deprived brains intentionally steer people toward high-calorie foods when they're fatigued as a survival strategy. For much of humankind's history, packing on a few extra pounds during stressful times when sleep was in short supply was a prudent precaution. In the past, the problem that was costing someone sleep might make food hard to come by the next day.

What to do: Try to avoid the smell of fatty or sugary foods following nights when you didn't get sufficient sleep. If you can't avoid those tasty smells, remind yourself that you are especially likely to be tempted by these foods when you are tired. This awareness can boost your ability to resist. If you're trying to lose weight, include "get sufficient sleep" as part of your diet plan.

More Alcohol, More Hunger

Two-year mouse study by researchers at Francis Crick Institute, London, UK, published in *Nature Communications*.

The part of the brain responsible for eating—the hypothalamus—is directly affected by alcohol. The alcohol activates hypothalamus neurons called AgRP to increase appetite, decrease metabolism and lower energy levels. So the more you drink, the hungrier you get—which means binge drinking and binge eating are likely related.

Exercise Creates Better Food Habits

Molly Bray, PhD, chair of the department of nutritional sciences, University of Texas at Austin, and corresponding author of a study published in *International Journal of Obesity*.

Young adults who exercised for 30 minutes three times a week at a relatively high intensity—after previously exercising for no more than 30 minutes a week—were more likely to choose lean meats, fruits and vegetables and less likely to opt for unhealthful options. The change happened even though researchers told participants not to alter their diets.

Innovative Calorie Counter

This app photographs the food on your plate to get an estimate of calories, protein content and other nutritional data. Search for Foodvisor at Apple Apps or Google Play.

Foodvisor

Don't Let Cold Weather Sabotage Your Fitness!

Denise Austin, an influential fitness and health professional for 40 years. Known for her at-home workouts, Denise hosted the longest-running TV fitness show in history. She is the author of 12 books on fitness, including *Fit and Fabulous After 40*. The creator of more than 100 workout videos and DVDs, she coined the motto "Progress Not Perfection." DeniseAustin.com

Even though it can be tempting to curl up under a cozy blanket on the couch and hibernate on those cold winter days, you know that will undermine your fitness—and your overall health.

Good news: It takes only a few tweaks to your daily routines (both outdoors and indoors) to stay active during the winter...and even—dare we say it?—make it fun. *What you need to know...*

WHY YOU NEED WINTER EXERCISE

Physical activity is crucial no matter what the season, but wintertime exercise offers unique benefits...

•**Increased immunity.** Research published in *British Journal of Sports Medicine* found that adults (ages 18 to 85) who got about 20 minutes of aerobic exercise (done intensely enough to break a sweat) at least five days a week for 12 weeks had only about half as many colds as those who were sedentary.

•**Reduced risk for lethargy, low mood and irritability.** These are telltale symptoms of seasonal affective disorder (SAD), but getting natural light outdoors helps guard against it.

•**More vitamin D.** Sunshine accounts for up to 90% of our annual intake of vitamin D—a key nutrient for bone health, muscle strength and other vital functions. Even though you'll get more winter sunshine in some southern and western states, exercising outdoors—no matter where you live—allows you to get more vitamin D than you would if you stayed indoors.

THE JOYS OF OUTDOOR EXERCISE

If you live in an area where the mercury plummets during the winter, there's something undeniably invigorating about crisp outdoor air. Classic winter sports, such as skiing and ice skating, are great heart-pumping, muscle-strengthening forms of exercise.

But if you're not keen on hitting the ski slope or ice rink, there's an alternative that works for most people, regardless of their fitness level. You guessed it…good old-fashioned walking. It's a convenient way to get both a cardio workout and weight-bearing exercise for stronger bones.

My advice: During winter, walk at least 20 minutes a day to promote circulation and burn fat.

Note: To warm up your muscles, do your favorite stretches and light arm pumping and walking inside your house, or march in place, for three to five minutes, before going outdoors.

Helpful: Listen to your favorite music if you like, but stay alert to your surroundings. I like upbeat songs like "Walking on Sunshine."

If walking doesn't excite you, liven it up by grabbing a neighbor or friend to join you for a brisk jaunt. Or if solitude is more your thing, head for a state park, where the beauty of a recent snowfall or the glint of winter sunlight can enrich the experience.

STAY SAFE OUTDOORS

While outdoor exercise has undeniable benefits, it can be dangerous if you don't do it correctly. If you have any lung problem (such as asthma), heart disease, diabetes or any other chronic condition, check with your doctor before exercising outdoors in cold weather. *In addition…*

•**Wear moisture-wicking fabrics closest to the skin when layering your clothing.**

Also: Forgo cotton—it stays wet if you perspire.

•**Avoid tight clothing.** It can inhibit blood flow and lead to loss of body heat.

•**Cover your head, ears and fingers.** Your body focuses on keeping your core warm, so your extremities are vulnerable. Also, you never want to walk with your hands in your pockets—that can throw off your balance. And don't forget sunglasses—especially in snow, which reflects more UV rays.

•**Opt for bright colors so that you stand out in cloudy, gray or dim surroundings.** Fluorescent yellow-green is the safest choice for daytime exercise.

•**Don't wear sneakers made of "summer" fabrics (such as mesh material).** Instead, choose sneakers made of heavy, heat-trapping material with rugged soles for traction.

•**Moisturize exposed skin (such as on the face and lips) to prevent chapping, and don't forget sunscreen.**

SNEAK IN SOME INDOOR ACTIVITY

Don't miss opportunities for indoor activities, too. *If you're tired of the usual options, such as gym workouts, yoga, dance classes or even mall-walking, try these moves (several times a day)…*

•**Do leg squats for a minute or so while brushing your teeth or blow-drying your hair.** If you have bad knees, do mini-squats while gripping a counter.

•**Do push-ups against the kitchen counter while waiting for your coffee to brew.** Aim for 15. If you have wrist problems, try arm scissors—extend your arms in front of your body and parallel to the floor. Then, scissor your arms horizontally. Aim for 30.

•**Lift hand weights while talking on the speaker mode of your phone or watching TV.** Work your triceps (hold one hand weight with both hands behind your head with your elbows bent at 90 degrees, then straighten your arms to bring the weight over your head)…and biceps (hold a hand weight in each hand down at your sides with your palms facing up, then

A Little Bit of Exercise Could Save Your Life

Regularly participating in running—even once a week—is associated with up to a 27% reduced risk for death from any cause...up to a 30% lower risk for death from cardio-vascular illness...and up to a 23% reduced risk for death from cancer. The percentages were those of runners from an analysis of 14 previous studies, comparing their death rates with the death rates of people who did no running.

Željko Pedisic, PhD, associate professor of public health, Victoria University, Melbourne, Australia, and leader of a meta-analysis of studies involving 232,149 people, published in *BMJ*.

curl both weights to shoulder height). Repeat each exercise for at least one minute.

Helpful: Start with light hand weights and work up to a weight that's comfortable for you.

•**Do the stairs.** Instead of walking up (or down) your stairs once, go up and down four times. If you're concerned about your balance, use a handrail.

Get a Full-Body Workout with this Modified Plank

Tehrene Firman, fitness blogger writing at MSN.com.

A bear plank is an extra-challenging but stationary full-body exercise. Start on all fours with your shoulders lined up with your wrists and your knees at a 90-degree angle. Keep your back flat. Lift your knees so they hover a few inches off the floor. Flex your core and hold the position for up to a minute—be sure to keep breathing regularly. Slowly bring your knees back down to the floor. Rest for 10 seconds and repeat.

Do More Than HIIT

Brock Armstrong, fitness coach based in Vancouver, Canada, writing at QuickAndDirtyTips.com.

Do not rely on high-intensity interval training (HIIT) by itself. HIIT involves brief periods of high-intensity exercise—30 seconds to five minutes apiece—alternating with shorter rest periods, during a single exercise session. Proponents say that it provides full workouts that are shorter than those using moderate intensity but with the same or better aerobic results. However, doing HIIT on one piece of equipment, such as an exercise bike, is not enough—exercise must be structured to work out the whole body in multiple ways. It also should be combined with walking, strength training, flexibility exercises and recovery days.

Get Fit Together: The Benefits of Exercising as a Couple

John S. Raglin, PhD, sports psychology researcher, professor in the department of kinesiology and director of graduate studies at the School of Public Health at Indiana University–Bloomington. He is author of a published paper titled "Factors in Exercise Adherence: Influence of Spouse Participation" and dozens of other studies on sports psychology.

You know all about the motivational advantages to working out with an exercise buddy, but are they the same when the buddy is your spouse or life partner? The answer is yes and perhaps more so. Working out with your spouse or partner can strengthen your relationship along with your muscles. Here's how to start off on the right foot.

COMMIT TO AN EXERCISE PLAN

Sticking with an exercise program isn't easy. The average dropout rate is 50%, most often after just a few months. But exercising with your significant other can change that. I studied married people who joined a fitness program by themselves and as a couple. After 12 months, the couples had a better-than-90% adherence rate—that's remarkably high when you consider average adherence is about 50% after 12 months for people joining without their spouse. Most interesting was that they didn't need to be doing the exact same exercise program, provided they went to the gym together, so the issue of "he's stronger than I am" or "I don't like the same machines" doesn't matter. You don't have to work out side by side—you just have to make the commitment to exercise at the same time and place.

For busy working couples, it even can create date-night closeness. It's a terrific alternative to sitting silently in a movie.

KEYS FOR EXERCISE SUCCESS

•**Account for your differences.** Most couples have different fitness levels, and you need to create a plan that accounts for those. If you're working out with machines in a gym, it's easy to simply go together for a set period of time or go to a class together. But if you want to go running or biking together and one of you can handle a greater pace and distance than the other, you'll have to make accommodations.

Try this: Agree to separate distance goals. Start off together at the same speed, but pick a point where the person with less stamina will stop and allow the other to continue or where the one who is in front will pause and wait for his/her partner.

Hint: Make your route a repetitive loop that goes past your car or your home to make it convenient for one person to stop if needed. Don't put yourselves in the position of having to navigate differences on the fly when one of you suddenly runs out of gas at the midway point of the route.

•**Introduce your partner to the workouts you like.** If you are already in a class and want your partner to join (kickboxing, for example), make sure he will feel comfortable joining. If your partner thinks of the activity as being for the opposite sex, don't force it. On the other hand, if your spouse is open to trying it, help him avoid feeling awkward with the activity itself. Do this with a preview—demonstrate how to do key moves and use any equipment. It's like hosting friends in an unfamiliar city—you make the right introductions and give them the lay of the land so that they'll be more comfortable and confident.

•**Create a backup plan.** People drop out of fitness programs for many reasons—from a brief illness to changes in work schedules. To avoid getting derailed, preemptively take steps to create work-arounds should speed bumps occur.

Example: If one spouse has to miss a week of exercise for a business trip, agree that the other will do it alone rather than sit it out—it's easier for one partner to rejoin activities than for two people to both do a reboot. And if one continues on his own, the other will be more likely to jump back into the routine. Have a list of alternate activities in case neither of you can get to a scheduled class. Switch to an after-dinner walk, for example.

•**Set and reset goals.** Initially, your shared aim might be to exercise a certain number of times a week for a certain length of time. After a while, each partner might add individualized goals. Maybe one wants to build more muscle, while the other wants to boost cardiovascular fitness. That's all OK. In fact, it gives each partner an additional opportunity to be supportive—cheer each other on and celebrate as you reach personal goals. ("Show me your muscles!") Just remember that if you get to your goal first, take time to reinforce all the progress your spouse has made, too. Being at different fitness levels becomes a problem only if one partner feels inadequate or believes that he is falling too far behind. Note that classes in gentle disciplines such as yoga and tai chi will have you both going at the same steady pace, no matter what your respective fitness levels are. Spin and Pilates also allow for different levels in the same class.

•**Consider a personal trainer.** If you're having trouble coming up with a fitness plan, consider signing up with a professional trainer who can take each partner's skill set into account, as well as make adjustments so that you're both doing the same type of program but at your own pace.

Important: Shop around for a trainer who has experience working with couples—ask friends, the manager at your gym and coaches at your local schools for recommendations.

•**Train together for an event.** When you set a competitive goal, such as running a 5K, you train harder and more regularly, and you can revel in the accomplishment of the goal. This can be very exciting for both partners. If you won't be side by side during the actual event, you still will be able to support each other before and after the event.

Lunges: The Ultimate Exercise for Your Workouts

Joel Harper, a New York City–based personal trainer whose clients include several Olympic medalists. The creator of the PBS DVD *Joel Harper's Firming After 50*, he designed all of the personal workout chapters for Drs. Mehmet C. Oz and Michael F. Roizen's YOU series of books and accompanying workout DVDs. He is also author of the Bottom Line blog "Your Personal Mind-Body Coach." JoelHarperFitness.com

Want a simple and effective exercise that has a slew of benefits, including improved balance and greater core strength?

Just put one foot in front of the other…and do a lunge! That's right—one of the best exercises you can do requires no equipment and can be done just about anywhere you have a few feet of floor space.

Why you need to do this exercise: Lunges increase the strength of your glutes (butt), quads (front thigh) and hamstrings (back thigh)—a powerful muscle trifecta that's required for walking, climbing stairs and maintaining the good balance you need to prevent falls. Strengthening these muscles also helps prevent hip and back pain. Building the muscles targeted by lunges is crucial because most people lose more strength in their lower extremities over time than in the upper part of their bodies. When done correctly, the lunge is among the best exercises for slowing the bone loss that occurs as we age.

Not just for gym rats! To start doing lunges, you don't have to be in tip-top shape. This exercise can be modified to fit your current fitness level…and then tweaked as you get stronger.

TWO-EXERCISE REGIMEN

While the standard lunge involves taking a step forward and dropping the opposite knee toward the floor, I recommend two simple exercises that will give you more benefit than the old-fashioned lunge we all grew up with. *To get started, do…*

•**Knee bounces.** These lunge "prequels" work the entire body, with an emphasis on the quadriceps, but are gentle on your joints and help you build the strength and balance you need to do the lunge that follows correctly.

What to do: Get down on the floor, on your hands and knees (on a carpet or yoga mat), with your hands under your shoulders and your knees under your hips. While keeping your elbows soft, curl your toes under and lift both knees about one inch off the ground. From there, lift your buttocks so that your knees bounce an inch up and then one inch down for up to one minute. Do not let your knees touch the ground.

Next up, do…

•**Concentration lunges.** This modified lunge strengthens the entire leg and improves your balance. I recommend this version because it locks your feet in place and enables you to have perfect form.

What to do: Start by kneeling in an upright position with your knees cushioned by a folded towel. Then step forward with your right foot so that your right knee is directly over your right ankle, and your left knee is under your left hip.

Place your left palm on your stomach and the back of your right hand on your lower back to help you maintain proper posture throughout the exercise. Curl your left toes under, and press into both feet to straighten both legs—quickly, but with control—lifting as high as you can. At the top, bend both knees and slowly drop straight back down, tapping your back knee on the towel. Without pausing, press back up and repeat. Do 25 up-downs, and then switch legs (remember to also switch hands).

Watch your form! Throughout the exercise, keep your knee over your ankle without letting it shift toward your big toe, and keep a straight line from the top of your head to your tailbone. Do not lean forward over your front leg. Push your hands toward each other to make sure that your stomach is taut throughout the move.

To make it less challenging: Do concentration lunges next to a chair, and use the seat for support (hold on to the chair with the hand opposite your forward leg) as you move up and down.

To make it more challenging: Each time you press up, lift off the ground into a soft jump.

Keep it fresh: Once you can comfortably do two sets of concentration lunges (25 with each leg…or as many as you can work up to), you can add hand weights and do arm curls while lunging to create more resistance.

For a well-rounded regimen, combine your lunges with other strengthening moves (such as squats and push-ups) and get at least 150 minutes per week of moderate-intensity (on a scale of one to 10, "moderate" is about a six to seven) aerobic activity (such as walking at 3 mph or faster…bicycling at around 10 mph…gardening…or ballroom dancing).

Important: Done incorrectly, a lunge can strain your knees and back, so always strive for perfect form.* If you feel any tightness or discomfort in your knees, skip the concentration lunges and stick with the knee bounces.

Helpful: A session with a personal trainer to ensure that you're using proper form.

As with all strength training, your body will need two days of rest in between lunge days to fully recover so that you will not cause undue stress to your lower back, knees and calves.

*Consult your doctor before starting this (or any new) exercise program.

The Weighted Vest Advantage

Wayne L. Westcott, PhD, professor of exercise science at Quincy College in Quincy, Massachusetts, and author of 29 books on strength training, including *Building Strength & Stamina.*

Move over dumbbells and resistance bands…and make room for the weighted vest!

This underused piece of exercise paraphernalia is designed to add some heft to a variety of workouts.

Bonus: Even if you're just a casual exerciser, a weighted vest can make your muscles stronger, help you burn more calories and crank up the benefits of your cardio workout.

Important: To make sure that a weighted vest and the workouts described here are right for you, check with your doctor. Use of a weighted vest may not be appropriate for those with osteoporosis, pregnant women, obese individuals and people with orthopedic injuries, especially those affecting the spinal column.

Once you get your physician's go-ahead, a weighted vest can help you…

• **Build lean mass.** A weighted vest is a great tool to combat the age-related loss of muscle mass and strength known as sarcopenia and to preserve your ability to complete activities of daily living, such as climbing stairs and carrying groceries.

• **Burn more calories.** Strap on a weighted vest that equals 15% of your body weight and walk at an easy 2.5-mph pace, and you'll burn 12% more calories than a person not wearing a vest, according to research. Wearing a weighted vest has also been shown to feel less taxing than adding intensity by other means, such as increasing speed or walking on an incline.

• **Retain bone mineral density.** In a Canadian study, researchers found that a weighted vest helped reduce bone turnover (a physiological process that fuels bone loss) while reducing body fat and increasing muscle mass in postmenopausal women.

• **Improve walking ability.** Wearing a weighted vest can improve walking ability in people with gait problems caused by conditions such as Parkinson's disease and certain types of palsy.

THE RIGHT VEST FOR YOU

To choose a weighted vest that's right for you, first look for a form-fitting vest that covers your chest. If it extends down toward the waist, even better. This will better distribute the weight of the vest without affecting your hip movements when walking. Wide shoulder straps are a plus—they don't interfere with your range-of-motion and put less stress on the shoulders than narrow straps. Also look for a vest that offers a relatively even weight distribution for the front and back.

When determining the weight of your vest, start with 5% to 10% of your body weight. For example, if you weigh 120 pounds, look for a vest with a starting weight of six to 12 pounds. Most vests also have pockets that allow you to add weight packets as you get stronger, but don't exceed 15% to 20% of your body weight.

Helpful: Always add weight gradually—for example, by two-pound increments, adding a one-pound weight to both the front and rear vest pockets to prevent injuries.

3 EASY WAYS TO USE YOUR VEST

If a weighted vest is new to you, it's smart to incorporate it into your existing exercise plan. Consider starting with 15-minute endurance training sessions and progressing gradually by five-minute increments to 45-minute sessions. *You can use a vest for…*

• **Warm-ups.** This will help you quickly engage muscle fibers and raise your core body temperature. Walking at a slow pace with the vest on is the perfect warm-up for weighted-vest walking at a brisk pace. While you shouldn't run with a weighted vest (it creates too much landing force), a pre-run weighted-vest walk can serve as an effective running warm-up.

• **Walking.** You can create a cross training–like program by wearing your weighted vest every other day—go at a slower pace for 20 minutes on the days with it and at a faster pace for 30 minutes on the days without it.

Bonus: On the "off" days, you'll feel lighter and find it easier to increase your pace, which is great for motivation.

Note: Weighted vests may be used in other weight-bearing exercise, such as elliptical training, but should not be used in exercises such as running, as mentioned above, and rope jumping that produce large landing forces.

• **Strength training.** Wear your weighted vest to increase resistance for standing exercises done with a straight torso, such as squats and stationary lunges.

However: To avoid overstressing your back, don't wear a weighted vest for exercises that involve bending your trunk forward or backward or that require horizontal body positions, such as planks and push-ups.

A standard strength-training protocol while wearing a weighted vest is to complete a total of three sets of eight to 12 reps with two minutes of rest between each set. Start with just the vest. You should be able to do at least eight reps in good form. Once you're able to complete 12 reps for each of the three sets, you can add weight to the vest.

Important: The additional muscle stress associated with wearing a weighted vest requires at least 48 hours recovery time between successive strength-training workouts. Although endurance training usually requires less recovery time, an every-other-day protocol is recommended to avoid overtraining syndromes.

---

8 Simple and Surprising Ways to Improve Your Posture: You'll Have More Energy and Confidence

Joel Harper, celebrity trainer and author of *Mind Your Body: 4 Weeks to a Leaner, Healthier Life* and the Bottom Line blog "Your Personal Mind-Body Coach." JoelHarper Fitness.com

---

Your posture is not only important for your physical and emotional health—it also sends a message to others about who you are and how you feel about yourself. People unconsciously notice your posture when speaking to you or simply seeing you. Slumped shoulders or a tilted head sends all sorts of negative messages. It says, *I'm tired… I'm not confident…I'm grumpy…I'm not approachable…I'm worn out.* Beyond inadvertently projecting these messages to others, you also are internalizing these messages yourself. Your posture affects your thoughts, your words and your overall energy.

Luckily, there are simple things you can do every day to improve both your posture and the messages that it sends to your mind and spirit…

•**Use a "mental mirror."** Look at all the people around you, and ask yourself, When someone looks at me, how do I look? Seeing yourself in this mental mirror helps you automatically sit up a little straighter, pull your stomach in, drive your shoulders back and raise the top of your head.

•**Look up.** When you walk, do you look down? Most people do. The problem is that when you look down, your shoulders immediately roll forward, putting tremendous pressure on your neck. Whenever you're walking, look straight ahead instead. A lot of people think, *Oh, I'm going to trip.* But you won't because you have peripheral vision that keeps you from tripping and you certainly don't need to look at your feet to know what they're supposed to do. When you look straight ahead, it reduces strain on your neck. If you must look down, do so with your eyes—not with your whole head.

•**Clasp your hands behind your back.** When standing, interweave your hands behind your tailbone with elbows slightly bent. If you have to move your shoulders to do that, then your shoulders were rolled forward. Ideally, if you put your hands behind you, your shoulders shouldn't move at all. This exercise reminds you to get in the habit of thinking about your posture and standing up a little straighter. It's a simple trick that will make a big difference.

•**Find out how tight your neck muscles are.** Put your hands in front of your face with your palms facing you and pinkies linked together. Then put your hands up on top of your head, and gently drop your chin toward your chest using just the weight of your arms. There are certain stretches you shouldn't feel at all. This is one of them. If you do feel it, that's a sign your neck and shoulder muscles are too tight. Do this stretch daily for five deep inhales, and the stretch will get easier. This move allows you to get rid of the tension in your neck and shoulders. If tightness continues, consider getting a massage.

Warning: Stiffness also may be a sign that you are dehydrated. Most people don't drink enough water. You can improve your posture just by drinking more water. To determine how many ounces you should drink through the course of each day, cut your body weight in half and use that number.

•**Put an hourglass on your desk or set an alarm to remind you to move.** This way, you have a visual reminder of when an hour has gone by. A lot of people get lost in their work, and the next thing they know, they've been sitting at a desk for three hours. The hourglass makes you a little bit more accountable for getting up and walking for at least a minute or two—whether it's just to get some water or walk some papers over to another desk.

•**Make sure all your stretches are balanced.** Many people think they should stretch both sides equally, but if one side of your body is tighter than the other, you need to adjust for that and stretch the tighter section more. Be mindful of this imbalance. The goal is that both sides should feel similar when done stretching. Give each stretch a number from zero to 10. Zero means you don't feel it, while 10 means you feel it a lot. If one side is a four and the other is a six, go back to the six side again and stretch until it feels closer to the four. Work gradually, and open up that area so that it's equivalent to the other side.

•**Be aware of what good posture feels like.** Put your back against a wall with your butt flush against it. Position your heels about one inch away from the wall, and keeping your shoulders back, try to pull your stomach back toward the wall as much as you can. Everybody's different. The size of your butt and the arch in your back will determine how close your lower back will be to the wall. While in this position, try to put the back of your head against the wall behind you with your chin straight. A lot of people can't do it because they're so hunchbacked. If you do this move over and over again, it will help you become aware of the right posture and improve it. Once this posture starts to feel more comfortable, it means that the muscle balance in your chest and your back are equal.

•**Start each day more mindful of your posture.** Every morning, before you get going for the day, lie on your back—either in bed or on the floor. Interweave your fingers and put your hands behind your head with your elbows flared to the side. Bend your knees, and with your feet flat on the bed or the ground, drop both knees to the left side. Place your right knee over your left so that your right knee can ultimately go all the way down to the bed or floor, and just relax there. This is a passive stretch. Passive stretching means that you're letting gravity do the work and you're not pressing it, you're not pulling and you're not forcing it. Then switch sides and drop both knees to the right. You want to do this every day to free your back muscles and allow good posture habits.

THE SINGLE BEST STRETCH

Bad posture often starts in the hips. When your hips are out of line, it throws off your back. And if your back bothers you, you tend to compensate with your shoulders and neck.

Try this stretch, which you should feel in your outer hip…

While sitting up straight in a chair, place your right ankle on top of your left knee, and gently press your right knee down, holding for three deep inhales. Do this on one side, then the other side, and then come back and do the tighter side again.

Important: Be aware of which side is tighter. Work gradually, and open up that area so that it's equivalent to the other side.

Stretches for Body Parts You Didn't Know Needed It!

Jessica Matthews, DBH (doctor of behavioral health), a certified yoga teacher, professor of kinesiology at Point Loma Nazarene University in San Diego and 2017 IDEA Fitness Instructor of the Year. She is author of *Stretching to Stay Young: Simple Workouts to Keep You Flexible, Energized, and Pain-Free.*

Even if stretching is part of your regular workout routine, there are probably body parts that need stretching and aren't getting it. But if you want to keep your whole body flexible, energized and pain-free, you need to keep those ignored areas limber, too.

Regular stretching enhances flexibility and range of motion in joints, which helps the body move with greater ease when doing other kinds of exercise as well as during daily activities, while also helping to prevent injuries such as muscle strains and falls. Stretching also can help to reduce pain and stiffness. And when paired with mindful breathing, stretching can help mitigate stress and reduce mental tension.

However, most people tend to leave some muscles out of stretching routines because they're not aware of them, such as the quadratus lumborum and the tibialis anterior…and other muscles they may exercise to strengthen but not know they also need to be stretched, such as the biceps and obliques.

The American College of Sports Medicine recommends that flexibility exercises be performed at least two to three days per week, with daily stretching being most effective. The following passive static stretches should be held to the point of mild tension or slight discomfort to enhance joint range of motion, but never to the point of pain. Each stretch should be held for 15 to 30 seconds per repetition. *Some commonly ignored muscles and the stretches that keep them limber…*

•**Biceps stretch.** The biceps brachii is located at the front of the upper arm and is the primary muscle involved in flexing the elbow and moving the forearm. Biceps exercises tend to focus on concentrically engaging (shortening) the muscles in order to build them up. Even when followed by lengthening motion, the lengthening is created by tension and doesn't really stretch the muscles. Stretching the biceps helps maintain their ideal length and range of motion and minimizes risk for injury.

Bonus: Biceps stretches may support improved posture, countering a rounded shoulder position by also stretching the shoulders and pectoral muscles.

How to do it: Stand facing a wall, as close as you can get to it. Extend your left arm along the wall straight out to shoulder height and place your palm flat against the wall, thumb pointing up. Keep your right arm relaxed at your side. Keeping your left palm on the wall, rotate your body clockwise (to the right) by pivoting on your feet to assume a position with shoulders and hips perpendicular to the wall and your right foot slightly ahead of your left foot. Complete the stretch by rotating your hips and shoulders away from the wall while your feet stay firmly in position. Hold the stretch for three to five breaths (approximately 30 seconds). Switch sides and repeat. Complete two repetitions per side.

•**Quadratus lumborum and obliques stretch ("standing crescent moon").** The quadratus lumborum (QL) is a deep abdominal muscle that connects your lower spine to your pelvis. The QL gets taxed by extended periods of sitting, poor posture and also strain from repetitive day-to-day movements, leading to tightness and pain in the lower back. The obliques—internal and external—are muscles found on the sides of the rectus abdominis (the "six-pack" muscles) and run from hips to rib cage. They help stabilize the spine and aid in flexion (the ability of the spine to bend), lateral flexion (bend to the side) and rotation (twist). Tight obliques can pull the spine out of alignment and lead to poor posture. Research also shows that when lateral flexion is restricted, it increases risk for low-back pain. Lateral flexion of the spine is often neglected in daily exercise routines.

How to do it: Stand with feet hip-width apart, arms at your sides. Keeping your left arm relaxed at your side, inhale and sweep your right arm out to the side and up, fingers pointing toward the ceiling and your palm facing to the left. Next, exhale while reaching your right arm over your head toward your left side, keeping your fingertips pointed out, as you lean your torso to the left to stretch the right side of your body. Hold the stretch for three to five breaths (approximately 30 seconds). Switch sides and repeat. Complete two repetitions per side.

•**Tibialis anterior stretch.** Your tibialis anterior is located on your outer shin and is involved in moving the foot and ankle, specifically pointing your foot up. You're probably familiar with tight tibialis anterior muscles—commonly called "shin splints." Lengthening the muscle helps avoid this potential pain. Exercises that stretch the backs of the legs, such as runners do to warm up, put the foot and ankle in a position that tightens the tibialis anterior. To stretch this muscle, you need to do the opposite—point your toes forward, a move that is not part of many exercises.

How to do it: Stand barefoot next to a wall or chair on your left side with your feet together. Bracing your left hand on the wall or holding a chair for support, bend your right knee and extend your right leg back, pointing the toes of your right foot so that you can place the tops of your tucked-under toes on the floor behind you. Keeping the tops of your toes on the floor, shift your weight slightly forward to create a stretch in the front lower part of your leg (shin). Hold this stretch for three to five breaths (approximately 30 seconds). Switch sides and repeat with your left leg. Complete two repetitions per side.

Illustrations of stretching figures: Copyright © Christian Papazoglakis/Illozoo

Walkers: Try This 100-Step Trick

Catrine Tudor-Locke, PhD, professor of kinesiology, University of Massachusetts at Amherst.

Exercise guidelines call for 150 minutes of aerobic exercise per week at "moderate" intensity or 75 minutes at "vigorous" intensity.

But how do you know if you have reached your desired intensity of exercise?

New finding: In a study of 76 adults, researchers found that counting steps walked per minute (called walking cadence) is the key to knowing how hard you are exercising.

What to do: Wear a watch with a second hand (or set the timer on your smartwatch) and go for a walk. Simply count the number of steps you take in 15 seconds, then multiply that number by four.

Moderate intensity begins at about 100 steps per minute, while vigorous intensity kicks in at around 130 steps per minute.

Note: While the study was conducted on adults ages 21 to 40, preliminary data on older adults suggest the findings will be similar.

10,000 Step "Rule" Revisited

I-Min Lee, MD, ScD, professor of medicine, Harvard Medical School, Boston.

When about 17,000 women (average age 72) wore an activity tracker for seven days as they went about their day-to-day lives, those who took an average of 4,400 steps each day were 41% less likely to die during the four-year follow-up period than women who took fewer than 2,700 steps, regardless of how fast they walked. Longevity continued to improve with more steps taken…up to 7,500 steps per day. There was no further reduction in the risk for death when additional steps were taken.

CHAPTER 8

Emotional Health

Make Stress Your Superpower

A new boss. A letter from the IRS. An ailing parent in need of your help. We all live in a stressful world. While we generally think of stress as bad and something we should eliminate from our lives, there actually is a way to think about stress differently and use it to our advantage.

When you change the way you think about stress, it can become your superpower...

YOUR INTERNAL WARNING SYSTEM

Anxiety is basically an alarm system handed down by evolution that alerts us when there is a threat. Sometimes the threat is on the outside (like an angry driver cutting you off)...and sometimes that threat is on the inside (say, you're torturing yourself about an upcoming presentation).

What if you changed your way of thinking about anxiety-provoking situations and learned to accept your feelings instead of simply running away from them?

In a Harvard University study, participants were placed in a high-stress situation. They had to give a speech in front of a hostile audience, all of whom sat with their arms crossed and brows furrowed. Before giving the speech, half of the participants were told that having a racing heart would improve their performance, while the other half were informed that they should try to ignore anything that made them nervous. The group that had been told to welcome their anxiety found the task to be less demanding and also had a more efficient cardiovascular response than the group who held a negative view of their nerves. Embracing stress had a clear upside and helped people to feel better.

Lisa Damour, PhD, psychologist in private practice and senior adviser to the Schubert Center for Child Studies at Case Western Reserve University, Cleveland. She is author of *Under Pressure: Confronting the Epidemic of Stress and Anxiety in Girls*. DrLisaDamour.com

Stress and anxiety are like fraternal twins—they have a lot in common and often travel together, but they're not the same. Stress usually describes feeling emotional or mental strain or tension, while anxiety is a more dramatic sense of fear, dread or panic. It's time to learn to take control of your stress and anxiety. *Here's how…*

• **Use stress to solve problems.** When we're feeling worried, the question to ask is, *What is making me fret?* Treat your stress not as a problem in and of itself, but as a signal that something is amiss. Try to identify the problem at the root of the stress.

Example: You're scared about losing your job because you heard there might be layoffs at your company.

At the root of the stress: You feel completely out of control and filled with a fear of the unknown.

Solution: Take charge by getting your résumé together or talking to your boss to get more information about the rumor. By looking more carefully to identify the root of your stress, you often can proactively find the solution, too!

•**Let stress spur you to action.** Although it may seem counterintuitive, avoidance and procrastination only increase your worries and make your stress worse.

Example: You get a bill and put off opening it because you are scared to see the damages. In the immediate term, this move feels good. You get a momentary sense of relief. But invariably, over the long term, your distress will build because you know you must pay the bill. There are two reasons that avoidance makes things worse. One is you get trapped repeating this action because the fear continues—so every month you'll get relief by pushing your bill aside…but you never actually feel better, since the problem remains hanging over your head. You are not giving yourself the opportunity to competently manage the thing that you are afraid of—even if the bill is as high as you expected (or higher), you can come up with an actionable plan to address it.

•**View stress as a motivational tool.** When you're stressed, adrenaline surges and gets your body geared up for action. If you're an elite athlete, these physiological changes help spur you to run faster or hit a home run. But even those of us who aren't Olympians can use stress to improve our performance at work, sports or even playing charades.

Example: You are about to be interviewed for a job you really want. Those sweaty palms mean you're bringing your A-game. Try telling yourself, *That's a sign that my body is preparing me to do a great job.* Simply naming it calms you down.

•**If you believe in the power of your stress, it can boost your performance.** In a study published in *Personality Processes and Individual Differences*, one group of participants learned about the many helpful benefits of stress, while the second group was taught that stress is always harmful. Several days later, the participants in the "stress-is-helpful" group reported an upswing in their mood and the quality of their work, while participants in the "stress-is-harmful" group did not.

•**See stress as proof of your resilience and strength.** Psychologists have long recognized that stress has what we call an inoculating function, where people who are able to weather difficult life circumstances—such as overcoming a serious illness—often go on to later demonstrate higher-than-average resilience when faced with a new difficulty.

It's like the saying, "What doesn't kill you makes you stronger." With each stressful challenge that is overcome, you develop additional emotional strength.

•**Deploy stress to shine light in dark corners.** Let's say you're frazzled because you're caring for your children and aging parents at the same time. A lot of that stress actually comes in the form of daily hassles—too numerous to allow you much perspective on the problem.

But stress can work like a flashlight to illuminate the parts of your day that are the toughest. If you notice your tension is heightened around dinnertime, for example, pay attention to that clue. You could choose to order more takeout for dinner and relieve some of the pressure on yourself as you're juggling other obligations.

Remember: You can't always vanquish major stressors, but you can try to reduce the number of everyday irritations.

Note: While stressful feelings are normal, they can cross the line and become a chronic condition. We know when that happens because the alarm stops making sense. Or it goes off all the time, even when there is no real threat. What should you do if your levels of stress are making you feel increasingly miserable or physically sick? If things feel like they are spiraling out of control, call and make an appointment with a mental health counselor. There's a lot he/she can do to help you.

When Anxiety Steals Your Joy

Debra Kissen, PhD, MHSA, clinical fellow, Anxiety and Depression Association of America (ADAA), cochair, ADAA's Public Education Committee, and executive director, Light on Anxiety CBT Treatment Center of Chicago.

Not everyone who suffers from anxiety looks like they're suffering. Some anxiety sufferers might seem outwardly calm, deal competently with whatever life throws at them—and even be quite successful. Yet inside, they're just barely keeping a grip on their fears and worries.

These people have high-functioning anxiety. Their suffering is not as obvious as the paralyzing version—but it's just as damaging. The term "high-functioning anxiety" is relatively new and not currently recognized as a mental-health diagnosis. One reason may be that a diagnosis of anxiety disorder has to meet the criteria that symptoms (such as fear, worry, sleep problems, stress) impair functioning at work, at school or in other critical areas of life.

People with high-functioning anxiety are functioning fine—even brilliantly. But their functioning is at great cost. Constantly suppressing their inner turmoil takes a toll on joy. And the stresses that might stay suppressed (at least for a while) in one area, such as work, tend to pop up somewhere else, such as with family and friends. Also, not dealing with it now can turn anxiety into a full-fledged disorder down the road...and even increase risk for other health issues, such as dementia and heart disease.

HOW TO FIND YOUR ZEN

If you or someone you know fits the description of high-functioning anxiety, here are the strategies that can help...

•**Cognitive behavioral therapy (CBT).** This form of psychotherapy is effective for breaking the cycle of negative thoughts that leads to anxious feelings. Treatment is usually short-term and focuses on learning self-calming skills that challenge negative thoughts.

•**Belly breathing.** Slowing your breathing tells your brain that you're safe. Inhale slowly through your nose, letting the air move down into your abdomen so that your belly expands with your breath. Then let your belly deflate as you exhale slowly through your mouth.

•**Mindfulness meditation.** Mindfulness combines belly breathing with purposeful, focused thoughts on the present—rather than dwelling on problems from the past or worries about the future. Mindfulness meditation has been shown to relieve not just anxiety but also depression and pain.

•**Muscle relaxation.** Physical tension is a hallmark of anxiety. Tensing and then relaxing specific muscle groups trains you to notice when your muscles are tight—and how to release the tension in your muscles, which releases mental tension as well.

•**Yoga.** An ancient mind-body practice that combines deep breathing, physical movement and meditation, yoga stretches and strengthens muscles while improving mental well-being.

•**Healthy lifestyle.** Don't underestimate the anxiety-reducing benefits of regular exercise, proper sleep, limiting caffeine and alcohol, and eating a healthful, balanced diet.

•**Medication.** If the above steps don't give you relief, you may benefit from medication. Certain drugs, such as selective serotonin reuptake inhibitor (SSRI) antidepressants, including *fluoxetine* (Prozac) and *sertraline* (Zoloft), can help ease anxiety.

Finally, bear in mind that some anxiety can be good—if it's not excessive, it can spur you to reach a desired goal!

Tumors Hate Happy Vibes

Feeling good may slow tumor growth. When the brains of mice were stimulated after the animals had cancer cells implanted, they released dopamine, which disabled some cells that promote tumor growth—and the mice's immune systems responded more effectively against the tumors.

Study by researchers at Technion-Israel Institute of Technology, Haifa, published in *Nature Communications*.

Are You Too Agreeable?

Dennis Portnoy, MFT, licensed psychotherapist in private practice in San Francisco. He is author of *The Intrinsic Self* and *Overextended and Undernourished*. DennisPortnoy.com

People rave that you're easy to work with…you're the world's nicest person…and groups get along better when you're around. As glowing as that praise is, if you receive these compliments frequently, it also could be reason for concern. You may be sacrificing your own happiness and success for the sake of keeping the peace—and the effects can erode your self-esteem.

Here's what you need to know about "harmony addiction" if you go to great lengths to avoid discord…

EXCESSIVE PURSUIT OF HARMONY IS NOT ALTRUISTIC

People who chronically set aside their own interests tend to tell themselves that they are making personal sacrifices for the sake of loved ones, friends, coworkers…or total strangers. They may not realize the sacrifices they're making—putting other people first may have become second nature. Harmony addicts often strive to dodge discord even when doing so works against everyone's interests.

Example: A husband never tells his wife when she does things that bother him. He convinces himself that not saying negative things reduces conflict and increases marital harmony. But because he never speaks up, his wife continues to do the bothersome things, leaving him frustrated with her. By avoiding conflict, he inadvertently creates distance.

Why don't harmony addicts speak their mind? Because despite what they tell themselves, they're not avoiding discord for the sake of other people—they are doing so because discord makes them feel anxious or unsafe.

For some, this means staying out of arguments at all costs. For others, even lingering interpersonal tensions or a sense of disengagement is too much.

THE ROOTS OF HARMONY ADDICTION

Adults addicted to harmony almost always faced one or more of these challenges during childhood…

• **They felt they had to act as peacekeepers for parents who argued** (or, less often, for other family members).

• **One or both of their parents were themselves harmony addicts,** and the child learned to imitate this behavior …or one or both parents reacted explosively during disagreements, and the child learned to avoid conflict at all costs.

• **They were regularly punished or admonished for making waves or voicing opinions.** Such children often become adults who are afraid to speak their minds.

• **They grew up surrounded by chaos.** Such kids often prioritize peace and serenity as grown-ups.

• **They felt different from and/or teased by their peers and learned to prioritize fitting in over their own needs and feelings.** This is common among children whose families had fewer financial resources than their peers… and children who are physically different from their peers.

• **The oldest child often has an exaggerated sense of responsibility for others.**

OVERCOMING HARMONY ADDICTION

A three-step plan can help you become aware of your behavior and release its childhood roots…

1. Try being less agreeable for a few days. You don't have to be difficult—just stop saying "yes" to everything. When you have a differing opinion, voice it. When someone needs something that isn't your responsibility, don't volunteer to do it. When you catch yourself monitoring other people's moods and opinions and wanting to keep emotions at bay, stop and consider what you think and want. Harmony addicts often have overactive scanning reflexes—they devote a tremendous amount of time and energy to interpreting the words, facial expressions and body language of the people around them, ready to set things right at the first hint of displeasure.

Warning: Not jumping in to smooth things over is likely to make you feel anxious. Anticipate this and leave the room if necessary. Keep a journal of the times you were not 100% agreeable and how doing that made you feel. What happened? You should begin to see that the world did not come to an end just because you didn't acquiesce to demands. If you felt uncomfortable, that's not a reason to stop—it's a wake-up call that your drive to foster harmony is excessive and likely interfering with your own life. Understand that discord makes you feel anxious or unsafe. On the plus side, you actually may surprise yourself when you stop feeling responsible for things that are outside your realm.

2. Reflect back on your childhood, and consider how your childhood challenges still affect your behavior today. How would it have affected your childhood family life and/or your interactions with your peers if you didn't strive to create harmony when you were young? Would there have been a price to pay? The answer probably is yes. A child whose parents argue takes on the role of peacemaker because the bickering intensifies if he/she doesn't. A child who is admonished for speaking his mind bites his tongue because it's the best way to avoid punishment. A child who feels excluded by his peers puts his peers' priorities ahead of his own because it's better than being an outcast.

But the behavior patterns that helped you survive childhood challenges are probably preventing you from being fulfilled as an adult. An adult has the ability to create boundaries in relationships...to discuss disagreements calmly with other adults. It is important to remind yourself that as an adult, you can now walk away from a heated situation. An adult usually can stand up for

what he believes without being punished. There are times and places where a price must be paid for standing up for one's beliefs—but an adult might decide some of these are worth it. An adult can walk away from friends who don't value and respect him. Be aware of childhood patterns continuing in your adult life, and write about these in your journal. You can decide that being the peacekeeper may not be the best option.

3. Reassure your younger self that you're safe now. Come up with a sentence or two that reminds you of how your current situation is different from your childhood situation.

Examples: "It wasn't safe to speak up when I was young, but now I'm a grown-up and not in danger." Or, "It's not like it used to be. It's not my job to keep everyone around me happy, and it won't harm me if they're unhappy. My opinions are important, and people want and need to hear what I have to say."

Repeat these words to yourself out loud or internally when faced with discord—if possible, multiple times a day. Write them on a card so you can remember them when the world around you becomes unharmonious and anxiety kicks in. Or better yet, use your smartphone to record yourself speaking these words, then listen to them when needed.

Don't expect instant results. Lifelong habits are hard to break, and putting your interests ahead of harmony will feel uncomfortable at first. But each time you do so and the world doesn't come crashing down, you'll be one step closer to achieving a healthy balance between your own goals and the pursuit of harmony.

Take Charge of Your Therapy Session

Ryan Howes, PhD, licensed clinical psychologist in private practice in Pasadena, California. He provides psychotherapy for adult individuals and couples. Howes writes the blog "In Therapy: A User's Guide to Psychotherapy" for *Psychology Today* and writes the "Point of View" column for *Psychotherapy Networker* magazine.

Many people enter therapy with the wrong expectations, the wrong attitude and even the wrong therapist—any of which can result in an unproductive, frustrating or disappointing experience. But you can make it a positive experience if you approach it the right way. Think of it as enrolling in a course where you are the subject matter—if you're curious, teachable and motivated, it can be one of the most rewarding classes you ever take.

FIND THE RIGHT FIT

• **Take inventory of your symptoms.** Is anxiety keeping you up at night? Are you fighting with your partner? Maybe you've experienced a trauma that you can't seem to put behind you? If you've got a specific issue, look for a therapist who specializes in it—whether it's weight loss or post-traumatic stress disorder. Search for names at PsychologyToday.com or GoodTherapy.org.

Note: Think about gender preferences. If your issue is not gender-related, such as fear of flying, it won't matter. But if your issue is a controlling mother, then you might prefer a male therapist. Review bios, specialties and treatment approaches, then set up calls with a few therapists—most will offer a free initial phone consultation.

Helpful: Explain what you're dealing with, and ask the therapist how he/she might treat it. After interviewing a few therapists, trust your gut and select one to see for three or four sessions. If you feel like it's not working, move on to someone else. The type of therapist you choose—psychologist, counselor or social worker—doesn't matter as much as your relationship with that person.

• **Take ownership of your session.** You're there to talk, so take some time beforehand to think about what you want to say.

Helpful: Arrive not just on time, but early. Give yourself 10 minutes in the waiting room to reflect on where you left off last time, what's happened since then and what your priority is today. If you wait for the therapist to steer the conversation, he may never get to what you want to talk about because he doesn't know. In between sessions, keep a therapy journal.

How that helps: You can use it to jot down a few notes after each session, as well as relevant thoughts, experiences and even dreams you've had. When journaling, ask yourself, *What do I want?* and *How do I feel?* Refer to your journal before each appointment so that you can bring up the issues that are important to you.

What not to do: Don't rehash everything that happened since you last saw your therapist. Some clients do this because they don't want to deal with deeper issues, which is missing the whole point of therapy. A little conversation about an outside event is OK if something big happened that directly applies to the issue you're working on, but you need to spend more time on the thoughts and feelings that resulted from it. Otherwise, you won't make progress.

• **Don't expect answers.** Should you break up with your partner, quit your job, ground your teenager? A therapist probably is not going to answer that for you. His job is to give you the tools to answer those questions yourself. If a therapist gives you the answer, you won't be any closer to understanding yourself, and you won't be empowered to handle another situation on your own. Instead, a good therapist will help you understand what's going on inside your head and help you develop the tools and emotional strength to address challenges. He might ask, for instance, "Why do you think you feel suspicious about your partner's phone texts?" or "Why are you having trouble completing that job application?"

• **Tell your therapist if you have concerns about the sessions.** Speak up if you don't like something your therapist says, does or even the cologne he wears. If you bottle up concerns, a rift will build and you won't make progress.

Better: Address any frustrations at the beginning of the session so that you can clear the air and move on. Maybe you're upset because your therapist was late or didn't seem to get your point or his aftershave smells like the one your father wore. By telling your therapist how you feel, you're helping him understand you better. Confrontation is hard, of course, but practicing it on your therapist will help you handle it better in life, too. Start with, "I'm a little uncomfortable bringing this up…" Talking about your feelings builds trust between you and your therapist. Don't worry about hurting his feelings. Most therapists know how to handle confrontation without getting defensive. If yours doesn't, consider choosing a different therapist.

•**It's all worth mentioning.** When you're in therapy, buried or forgotten feelings get dredged up.

Example: If something about your son crosses your mind while you're discussing your childhood, tell the therapist about it. Does your sister's face pop into your head while you're describing a coworker? Say so, no matter how random or insignificant it seems. There probably is a connection to what you're talking about—it's like a gift from the psyche—that can help you and the therapist understand deeper parts of you.

•**Pick a good time for your session.** What is the best time of day for a therapy session? Maybe you're a morning person and will be more talkative then...or maybe you come to life when the sun is going down. But timing also can depend on where you have to be after the appointment. It can be tricky to go back to the office after an intense session or to meet your mother-in-law for dinner (after you were just griping about her). If you can't avoid a schedule conflict, then tell your therapist what is on your agenda, so that he can stop the more intense conversation five or 10 minutes before the session is over. The therapist can use that time to help you make an action plan and "cool down," just as you would after a workout. You also can plan your own cooldown period after the session. It helps to go for a walk or write in your journal before heading to your next appointment. This process is called "containment," and it helps you to more easily reenter the rest of the world. It's like putting your feelings on a shelf until it's time to examine them again. The idea is to let yourself regroup and collect your feelings so that you can get back to your normal routine.

Also: Take care of any housekeeping business—scheduling, payments, insurance—at the beginning of your session, not the end. It's hard to switch gears from raw emotion to a discussion of whether your therapist will take your new insurance.

•**Ask about your progress.** From the beginning, talk about the end. Ideally, that will be when all therapy goals have been met. That may be achieved in 12 sessions—or it may take six months or more than a year. If you'd like to keep to a specific time frame, let your therapist know that up front. Along the way, you need to know you're making progress. There are two clues that things are going well. The first is when you begin to "internalize" your therapist. That means when you are on your own, you start to ask yourself the same questions your therapist would. That shows you're incorporating what you've learned in therapy into daily life. The other clue is when you find yourself saying, "I've never told anyone this before." Your therapist is hearing, *This is a safe place, and this client really trusts me.* Whether it's something bad or just too embarrassing to talk about, opening up is a sign that you're healing. Talking about your progress along the way means that you will be better prepared for when therapy ends—a difficult time for some clients. It helps you tie up the loose ends, clarify takeaway points and go back out on your own with closure.

Affordable Talk Therapy

Roundup of experts on telemedical talk therapy, reported in *Men's Health*.

If your insurance does not cover talk therapy or you are unsatisfied with in-network options, various apps offer e-mail, text, audio or video chats—some for free. *7 Cups of Tea* is a free peer-to-peer network of people trained in active listening, with licensed therapists available for a monthly fee. *Woebot* is a free chatbot, based on artificial intelligence and recommendations by psychologists at Stanford University. *Betterhelp* has therapists with a minimum of three years of experience, offers live phone-chat sessions and costs $40 to $70 per week. *Talkspace* uses therapists with at least 3,000 hours of clinical experience, who are accessible by text, audio or video, for $65 to $99 per week.

What's Your Dating Type?

Sandy Weiner, a Stamford, Connecticut–based relationship coach specializing in helping women over age 40. LastFirstDate.com

People really do have romantic "types" that they date repeatedly. A recent study by researchers at University of Toronto showed a dater's new romantic partner very often shares personality traits with that dater's earlier partners—even if their type isn't good for them. It's tough to shake partner patterns because they're frequently rooted in parent-child relationships. Talking with a therapist or relationship coach can help break unhealthy patterns.

Religion: The Health Booster No One Talks About

Harold G. Koenig, MD, professor of psychiatry and behavioral sciences, associate professor of medicine and senior fellow in the Center for the Study of Aging and Human Development at Duke University in Durham, North Carolina. Dr. Koenig is director and founder of Duke's Center for Spirituality, Theology and Health.

Whether you're being urged to get more exercise, eat better or take your medication, physicians dole out plenty of advice on ways to improve your health. But when is the last time your doctor told you to attend religious services? Most likely, never.

But for people who want to do everything possible to stay healthy, this is a recommendation worth considering.

Even though there's been a steady flow of research linking religious observance to everything from lower blood pressure and less cardiovascular disease to better immune function and higher levels of overall well-being, religion's health-promoting benefits don't get much attention.

Why does religion promote good health... and how can people tap into this remarkable benefit? To learn more, we spoke with Harold G. Koenig, MD, a renowned authority on religion and health.

Do the health benefits linked to religion apply only to certain faiths?

No. Studies finding health benefits have included people of many faiths and spiritual traditions, including Christians, Jews, Muslims, Hindus and Buddhists.

Does it matter how often someone attends services?

Definitely. People who attend services once or more each week see more health benefits than those who attend less frequently. In fact, that's one of the strongest and most consistent findings in studies of religion and health, according to an important research review published in 2017 in *Current Directions in Psychological Science*. One study cited in the review found that regularly attending religious services over the course of a lifetime translated into about seven additional years of life. Other studies suggest that the effects on longevity are as strong as those seen for cholesterol-lowering drugs.

Do some people seem to benefit more than others?

Yes. Studies find stronger associations between religion and health in women and older adults compared with men and younger adults. We also know that women and older adults in the US are more likely to attend services, to pray and to say that religion is important in their lives, according to data from the Pew Research Center.

However, some people with strong beliefs become more distraught if their illness persists or worsens. They may even lose faith if they feel that their prayers have gone unanswered.

How does religion help people deal with chronic illness?

Some of the benefits are social. That's because people who belong to a religious institution have a reliable source of social connection and support—one that will not disappear when, for example, someone becomes too ill to work or participate in hobbies and recreational activities. It helps, too, that most religions put a high value on helping others in distress and have systems in place to assist members in times of need.

People with strong religious beliefs also may find it easier to see meaning and purpose in their illness. They may view it as part of a larger plan and believe that their suffering will be rewarded or will reveal new life lessons. Religious scriptures, from many traditions, provide role models for such fortitude.

Many religious groups also encourage healthy lifestyles—such as not smoking or abusing drugs or alcohol. There is one downside, though, to all those social hall suppers—religious people are more likely than others to be overweight, according to research.

What role does prayer play?

No clear link has been established in the scientific literature between prayer and longevity, though the research could be skewed by the fact that people already battling health problems may tend to pray more. But prayer can be a powerful coping strategy.

One theory is that people who pray may gain an indirect sense of control over their stressful circumstances—by believing that a higher power is in control and that praying can lead to change, the believer may feel more internal control than someone who feels all the power is in the hands of other people, such as doctors.

Should I discuss my religious beliefs with my health-care providers or keep them private?

In an ideal world, your medical providers would ask you about your religious beliefs. One big reason is that your beliefs may affect the decisions you make about your care. You cannot have honest discussions with your doctors if they do not know your values. Your care providers also should know where you get social and practical support. If that includes a house of worship, it should be part of the conversation.

They should also know if you have unmet spiritual needs—and would, for example, like to receive visits from a hospital chaplain. So if religion is important to you, but your providers do not bring it up, you should definitely speak up. That said, don't let any health-care provider try to impose his/her religious views on you.

Is religion ever used as part of formal treatment?

Yes. When patients want such help, some mental-health providers now offer a technique called "religiously integrated cognitive behavioral therapy." The idea is to combine a patient's religious beliefs with evidence-based cognitive behavioral therapy (CBT) techniques to relieve depression or other forms of psychological distress.

When chronically ill patients who were Christian, Jewish, Muslim, Hindu or Buddhist received psychotherapy that incorporated their religious beliefs, it was as effective as conventional CBT in treating depression, according to research published in *The Journal of Nervous and Mental Disease.*

As in other forms of CBT, the goal is to identify and change unhealthy patterns of thinking and behavior. The twist is that therapists ask clients to use passages of scripture from their religious traditions to reinforce those healthier ways of thinking and behaving.

Helpful: If you're interested in religiously integrated CBT, speak to your therapist about using workbooks (for Christians, Jews, Muslims, Hindus and Buddhists) that are available for free from Duke University's Center for Spirituality, Theology and Health. Go to SpiritualityAndHealth.Duke.edu and click on "Religious CBT," then "Therapy Manuals."

What about nonbelievers—can they also get benefits from religion?

Belief in a higher power is not necessary to tap into some of the elements of religion that help people deal with a chronic medical condition, pain, disability, financial strain and the other burdens that can come with illness. Many people can benefit from building strong social connections and doing good for others. Meditation is not exactly the same as prayer, but it can help reduce pain and produce other health benefits, such as reducing anxiety, lowering blood pressure and improving sleep problems.

Likewise, studying philosophy can be as uplifting for some as studying scripture is for others. And of course, adopting healthy habits, such as not smoking, not drinking too much and getting plenty of exercise, requires no religious faith. However, current studies do show that religion offers additional benefits to those who follow these health-promoting practices.

How to Protect Your Own Health When Your Spouse Dies

Leslie Kernisan, MD, MPH, clinical instructor, division of geriatrics, University of California, San Francisco. Board-certified in both geriatrics and internal medicine, she is founder of BetterHealthWhileAging.net, a website that provides practical information for older adults and family caregivers. She has a geriatric consultation practice in the Bay Area and writes about geriatrics and new technologies at GeriTech.org.

Losing a loved one is never easy—whether it's a parent, a beloved aunt or your best friend. But when the person who dies is your spouse, the powerful emotions that so often accompany this particular loss may be even more likely to lead to physical ailments, too.

For example, describing such extreme grief as heartache can actually be quite accurate. The death of a spouse often leads to a release of stress hormones that increases one's risk for serious health problems, including heart attack and a weakened immune system that increases the risk of developing a dangerous infection.

To help protect your health after such a loss, here are five ways to soothe that enormous stress—and one thing you should do your best to avoid...

•**Be honest about your needs.** Soon after your loss, friends and loved ones may bombard you with offers to help. While well-intended, those kind gestures won't do much good if they're not meeting your needs. Go ahead and tell the neighbors not to bring dinner every night if all that food is overwhelming for you. (Or if you don't have the heart to prepare your own meals, ask some friends to pitch in for a time.) And if sitting quietly with a friend instead of talking on a given day is what you need, say so.

•**Continue to exercise.** Try to get outside for a walk or other type of exercise at least once a day, even though you may not feel like it. Moving your body—ideally in the fresh air—promotes well-being much better than cocooning yourself at home.

•**Find support.** Spend time with friends and family, or find a bereavement support group through your local hospital. If you have a spiritual tradition, now would be the time to lean on it.

•**Stay on top of chronic health issues.** Enlist others to help you remember to take your medications and/or pick up the refills from the pharmacy. If you're experiencing any troubling symptoms, don't hesitate to see your doctor.

•**Go easy on yourself.** It's completely normal for you to feel intense grief over the loss of a spouse for six to 12 months. Give yourself time to get through what may be one of the toughest experiences of your life.

Warning: Grieving often disrupts sleep, which is a crucial ingredient for good mental and physical health. However, try to avoid sleeping pills if you can. *Benzodiazepines*, such as Ativan and Xanax, in particular, may relieve anxiety and help you sleep, but they often produce negative side effects (including slower brain function and poor balance)—and the body becomes dependent on them very quickly. If poor sleep is a problem, talk to your doctor about safer ways to improve your sleep and get through this challenging period.

15-Minute Vacation

Meditation is as effective as a vacation for stress reduction and increasing positive emotions. Fifteen minutes of meditation per day brings about as much improvement in these areas as a day of vacation.

Study by researchers at University College Groningen, the Netherlands, published in *Journal of Positive Psychology*.

The Healing Power of a Good Chat

Rebecca Shannonhouse, editor-in-chief, health content, Bottom Line Inc.

Smoking and obesity would top anyone's list of serious health risks. But did you know that research has shown loneliness to be on par with those dangers? It has been linked to high blood pressure, diabetes and cancer. Loneliness also increases one's odds of dying early by 26% and is considered a risk factor for Alzheimer's disease. It's estimated that about 42 million American adults suffer from loneliness.

England, where loneliness also has been identified as a health threat, has been at the forefront of addressing this problem by connecting people to local social groups. Now a new initiative known as "chat benches" in local parks is taking hold there. To promote conversation, a small sign is posted on random park benches, indicating that people sitting there are "happy to chat." This simple idea is scientifically sound. There's strong evidence that face-to-face conversation is particularly powerful in helping people overcome loneliness. *In lieu of a chat bench, you can...*

•**Nurture your existing relationships.** This includes your spouse (if you have one), friends, neighbors, etc. Call them regularly and make concrete plans to get together.

•**Put "friendship reminders" on your calendar.** Remind yourself to take steps to meet new people. Seek out groups of people with similar interests—a class at a community college, a choir group, a political action organization, etc.

•**Pick up the phone.** If you're feeling lonely and don't have anyone to talk to, call 800-971-0016. Someone on the Friendship Line, sponsored by the not-for-profit Institute on Aging, will be happy to chat!

Top Treatments for Body-Focused Repetitive Behaviors

David A. F. Haaga, PhD, professor of psychology at American University, Washington, DC, and a member of the scientific advisory board of The TLC Foundation for Body-Focused Repetitive Behaviors (BFRB.org). He conducts research on smoking cessation, depression and trichotillomania and is interested in cognitive behavioral therapy processes and outcomes.

Uncontrollable hair-pulling, skin-picking or nail-biting can take an emotional and physical toll, but help is here...

Many people bite their nails when stressed or fiddle with their hair when bored. In fact, some studies suggest that more than half of all adults engage in these habits at least occasionally. But for a small minority of people, such body-focused repetitive behaviors (BFRBs) are frequent and uncontrollable—affecting both their emotional and physical health.

The main BFRBs are *trichotillomania* (hair-pulling)...*excoriation* (skin-picking)...and *onychophagia* (nail-biting). Sufferers can spend hours each day pulling, picking or biting. The habits can cause a variety of health problems from skin infections to depression, anxiety and isolation.

BFRBs are a challenge to treat—no single treatment works for everyone. *But there are therapies that help...*

•**Forms of cognitive behavioral therapy (CBT) work best.** CBT attempts to change behavior and associated thoughts. A specialized form of CBT, known as habit reversal, has the strongest support for success in treating BFRBs. Here, with the help of a therapist, patients learn to recognize feelings, such as boredom or stress, and situations that trigger the urge to pull, pick or bite. They then develop strategies, like clenching their fists, that make the unwanted behavior impossible.

Habit reversal is well-suited to those who engage in BFRBs without thinking. It helps patients to be more aware of the problem in time to prevent it. Other patients, however, engage in BFRBs with full awareness, possibly because they believe the behavior will alleviate anxiety or boredom. And some patients are aware of what they're doing at times and unaware at other times. In these instances, other CBT interventions may be needed to supplement habit reversal. These could include acceptance and commitment therapy, which encourages patients to tolerate the urges to pull, pick or bite, without acting on them. Meditation and relaxation exercises are also helpful.

Mental health professionals that are specifically trained to treat BFRBs may be difficult to find. For a directory, go to BFRB.org, click on "Find Help + Support," then on "Find a Therapist."

Several sites offer programs to supplement therapy. Try StopPulling.com or StopPicking.com.

•**Medications** are generally prescribed in combination with psychotherapy to lessen the feelings that lead to BFRBs. Medications for BFRBs include the same selective serotonin reuptake inhibitors (SSRIs) given for depression, anxiety and obsessive-compulsive disorder (OCD). Mood stabilizers can be effective for some individuals.

•**N-acetylcysteine (NAC),** an amino acid supplement, helped more than half of those with trichotillomania, a recent study found. NAC may help those with skin-picking and nail-biting, too.

Note: Check your doctor before starting NAC for instructions on dosage and how to take it.

•**Self-help strategies** from BFRB sufferers and mental health professionals…

•Play with fidget toys, such as a fidget spinner, to keep hands occupied.

•Wear white cotton gloves to prevent skin-picking and nail-biting.

•Handle a piece of velvet as a substitute for picking or pulling.

•Pop Bubble Wrap as a substitute for skin-picking.

•Wear a bandanna or hoodie to bed to prevent hair pulling overnight.

•Pull the bristles out of an inexpensive paintbrush to keep hands busy.

For more self-help tips: At BFRB.org, click on "Treatment" under "Learn," then on "Self-help tools."

New research: The BFRB Precision Medicine Initiative is gathering detailed information from more than 300 people with BFRBs in order to gain clues for better treatment. Also, a clinical trial is currently under way to test the effectiveness of the Comprehensive Model for Behavioral Treatment (ComB) for hair-pulling, a CBT approach that aims to identify the function of the behavior and create a replacement for it. Treatments include a scalp massager, deep breathing and wearing bandages on fingertips.

A Whiff of Joe
Experimental and Clinical Psychopharmacology

Regular coffee drinkers can detect the faintest aroma of their favorite brew—and the stronger their craving, the greater their sensitivity to detecting the coffee odor.

Implication: This finding suggests that sensitivity to smell could be further explored as an element in treatments for addiction, including to cigarettes.

Diagnosing Autism in Adulthood Still Helps

Megan Farley, PhD, licensed psychologist who works with teens and children at the Autism and Developmental Disabilities Clinic, Waisman Center, University of Wisconsin-Madison. She also works with adults on the autism spectrum in her private practice.

If you're in your 40s, 50s or older and suspect that the root of your struggles to get on with people—friends, coworkers, family members—might be autism, you may wonder what's the point of getting tested now? Maybe life hasn't been easy, but you've still made it this far. What's going to change now that you're an adult? The answer is that getting a diagnosis even now can still lead to improvements in your life.

When comedian Amy Schumer publicly revealed that her husband, Chris Fischer, was diagnosed with autism spectrum disorder (ASD) in his late 30s (when they were dating), she also admitted that she wasn't entirely surprised. "I knew from the beginning that my husband's brain was a little different than mine," she explained. Schumer said that she wouldn't change anything about her husband…but added that the diagnosis provided the couple with tools that have made their marriage and lives more manageable.

WHAT ASD LOOKS LIKE

Autism is considered a developmental disability that begins in early childhood and affects a person's ability to communicate and socialize in the same ways most other people do, as well as other behaviors, such as body movements and interests. ASD is considered a spectrum disorder because manifestation ranges from the extreme of being non-verbal, engaging in repetitive behaviors such as rocking back and forth and needing intense caregiving…to having well-developed language and some skill with social interactions, but with differences being more apparent over time or in close, interpersonal relationships. ASD in people who have reached adulthood without a diagnosis is often mild enough to have escaped earlier recognition…but significant enough to have created problems along the way. In fact, many adults seeking a diagnosis report that they have had trouble in a job or relationship, such as…

●**Finding it hard to be flexible.**

Example: A person may have a hard time adjusting to a new process for getting something done at work, especially if the reason for the change does not seem logical to him/her. In a relationship, it may be hard to change a routine to accommodate someone else's needs. For instance, if a spouse is sick, the partner on the spectrum may not take over preparing meals or child care if those are not a part his/her routine.

●**Being perceived as antisocial.**

Example: Because noises and smells can be overwhelming to someone with ASD, the person might avoid hanging out in the lunchroom… leading coworkers to think he's unfriendly. Many people with ASD are very honest when asked for their opinion—such as whether a new haircut looks good—which may be experienced by a romantic partner as rude or too blunt.

●**Other areas of difficulty.**

Examples: Standing too close to other people can give an impression of being weird. Taking too long to answer questions and respond to comments can make someone seem slow on the uptake. Constantly misinterpreting facial expressions and body language or taking words too literally can be confusing and frustrating to family, friends and coworkers as well as to the person with ASD.

Whatever the particular challenges a person with ASD faces, it often feels like he/she has to work much harder than everyone else to achieve the same goals…and as though no matter how hard they try, they don't have much success.

CHALLENGES OF GETTING A DIAGNOSIS

Getting diagnosed with ASD can help in a lot of ways. Disclosing your diagnosis to your human resources department and manager can help you get accommodations at your job—such as a written agenda before meetings and a copy of notes taken afterward…adjusted lighting in your work area or moving to a quieter work area…modified work hours to accommodate problems with sleep that are very common for people with ASD. It can also put you in touch with services, including state programs and benefits for people with developmental disorders, such as help with chronic unemployment or underemployment. These services are typically accessed through state vocational rehabilitation departments and may include help with job training or job development as well as counseling for soft skills (such as workplace social skills) and/or co-occurring psychiatric problems.

Perhaps most importantly, a diagnosis can be healing. It can be a relief to understand that your struggles have to do with how your brain has developed. A diagnosis also can validate your experiences and give you a better understanding of yourself—and help family, friends and coworkers appreciate your differences and be more empathetic.

That said, getting a formal diagnosis can be challenging…and frustrating. *Here are some of the major difficulties and ways to overcome them…*

●**Difficulty finding specialists.** We know more about ASD than we did 20 years ago, but the focus still is mainly on children. There are fewer psychologists and psychiatrists knowledgeable about how autism spectrum disorders play out in adulthood. Compounding the challenge is that the diagnostic tools are largely based on childhood presentations or more severe presentations in adults. One example is the Autism Diagnostic Observation Schedule (ADOS), a semistructured, 45-minute interaction between patient and specialist. Tools for assessing adults exist, but they require someone who understand the tools' limitation and can interpret the results in a way that is helpful for adults—instead of misdiagnosing with some other condition, such as ADHD or anxiety, both of which are common and often also present in people with ASD.

Solution: State universities often have autism centers or clinics and might be able to recommend therapists who work with adults. Check in your own state or a neighboring state by Googling "university autism center" and the name of the state. Local autism societies also keep lists of specialists.

•**A formal diagnosis can be time-consuming and complicated.** Besides the 45-minute ADOS and other assessments, a wide range of information from multiple sources helps get an accurate diagnosis. So the psychologist might want to interview other people in your life…especially those who knew you in childhood and adolescence, when ASD behaviors are more evident. Siblings and aging parents may not remember subtle details of a person's social behavior from 40 or 50 years earlier. Also, even if you find a specialist, you may have to wait several months for an appointment.

Solution: Many people self-diagnose by reading about ASD. The downloadable guidebook for adults from the advocacy organization Autism Speaks is one resource. Knowing how difficult it can be to get a formal diagnosis, the autism community is generally very accepting of self-diagnoses. However, eligibility for services usually requires a formal diagnosis.

•**A formal diagnosis is expensive and often is not covered by insurance.** Testing for autism in adults can range from $1,000 to $5,000. You may be able to get assistance from your state's department of vocational rehabilitation if you are unemployed or job hunting. College students may have options through the school's student health department. University psychology clinics may offer a sliding scale fees for an evaluation…as may individual diagnosticians.

AFTER YOUR DIAGNOSIS

Once you get your diagnosis, formal or not, it's up to you how to proceed. *Here are some options to consider…*

•**Find your "tribe."** Look for local and/or national meet-up and support groups. Google "adult ASD, "high-functioning autism" or "As-

perger's" (the latter two terms are no longer used clinically but still used online). Also check into organizations such as your local autism society or the Autistic Self-Advocacy Network (ASAN).

•**Find help.** Therapists who specialize in cognitive behavior therapy or social skills training can help you navigate particular challenges, such as at your workplace or dating. Someone with expertise in adult autism is best, but a couples' therapist or any therapist who is caring, understanding and willing to learn about autism is a good alternative.

•**Tell people—or not.** Whether to disclose your diagnosis to coworkers or family members, especially far-flung relatives you may not see often, is your choice. If you do decide on disclosure, you may be pleasantly surprised by the positive reactions. However, there's also the risk with disclosing that some people may not believe the diagnosis is accurate, which can add to a person feeling unheard and misunderstood. It can help to disclose your diagnosis first to someone you trust who can talk it through with you and help you decide who to tell and how to respond if the reaction is not supportive.

The great news for the future is that adults with autism are advocating for themselves, promoting that it's okay to be who they are—and many more people know and care about adults with autism and want to support them on their own terms. Yes, "odd" behaviors such as hand flapping to self-soothe may make some people feel uncomfortable or confused—at first. But hopefully greater public awareness will lead to greater understanding and acceptance.

Take a Bite Out of Depression

In a recent study, people who ate dark chocolate daily in any amount were 70% less likely to report symptoms of depression than people who did not eat dark chocolate. Other forms of chocolate were not linked to lower depression prevalence.

Lin Yang, PhD, is an epidemiologist in the department of cancer epidemiology, Alberta Health Services, Calgary, Canada, and coauthor of a study of more than 13,000 people, published in *Depression & Anxiety.* CEPR.ca

Are You Being "Gaslighted" by Your Spouse...or at Work?

Robin Stern, PhD, a psychoanalyst in private practice for more than 30 years and cofounder and associate director, Yale Center for Emotional Intelligence, New Haven, Connecticut. She is author of *The Gaslight Effect*.

Are you in a relationship where you constantly second-guess your actions...keep apologizing profusely for everything you do...are somehow always "wrong" without understanding how that happens? You might be involved with a gaslighter. *Here's how to shed light on what's happening and how to protect yourself...*

"Gaslighting" describes a potentially very damaging form of abuse, where one person in a relationship tries to manipulate the other person's perception of reality. The term was inspired by the 1944 movie *Gaslight*, in which Gregory (played by Charles Boyer) tries to convince his wife, Paula (Ingrid Bergman), that she's going insane by manipulating events through various tricks.

THE GASLIGHTING DANCE

In real life, typical gaslighters aren't as obvious or as malicious as the Charles Boyer character. But they do share the same craving for power and control over the other person in the relationship—and a need to always be right. Often, in order to feel more important, they also make the other person dependent on them. Being the victim of a gaslighter takes a severe toll on mental and physical health.

Gaslighters aren't only husbands—they can be a parent, partner, coworker or friend...and either gender. To stop the abuse, the "gaslightee" needs to recognize his/her own role. Gaslightees have a strong need for approval, which makes them vulnerable under the right (or wrong!) circumstances. They tend to be empathic people who can easily see the other person's point of view and accommodate the wishes of others—frequently at their own expense.

Example: Jeanne, a friendly woman, is married to Roger, who doesn't like her attention diverted away from him. He gets angry if she so much as smiles at someone else, especially another man. And because he told her that this bothers him—and told her that smiling at other men is flirting—he feels his anger is justified. Jeanne explains that she is just friendly and smiles instinctively at everyone. But Roger doesn't like it and tells her to keep her eyes on the ground when they go out.

Jeanne's first reaction to Roger's eyes-down rule is that it's crazy—and she tells him not to be ridiculous. But over time, with his continued insistence and her strong desire to please him, eventually she comes to think, *Maybe he's right.*

TURNING OFF THE GAS

Overcoming this dynamic power struggle isn't easy—especially if the gaslighting relationship is with a spouse or family member and/or has gone on for many years. But you can break this destructive pattern. *What to do...*

• **Listen to friends.** Your buddies might see things more clearly than you can. For instance, if your date accused you of being overly sensitive, your friend can offer a reality check: *Maybe you are sensitive. But that has nothing to do with the fact that he left when you were 10 minutes late without even calling you—and then told you that you're upset because you're too sensitive.*

• **Write it down.** Write down the conversations you have with your gaslighter. Looking at who said what as though it were a script between two characters in a play can help you spot gaslighting patterns. Notice where the conversation veers off to be comments about you and your "flaws," not a response to what you just said.

• **Talk to a therapist.** A trained professional can distinguish distortion from fact and also can be more objective than you. Maybe you are sensitive. But that doesn't mean you have to put up with abusive behavior.

• **Be ready to walk.** Unless your gaslighter is willing to change, the only solution may be to leave. Being clear that you are ready to do that makes an unarguable statement that the gaslighting behavior is unacceptable—but you need to stick to your position, or there are no consequences for your gaslighter and no reason to change.

Note: Be prepared for changes in your behavior to cause your gaslighter to react by expressing even less approval of you. Sometimes, the abuse (name-calling, etc.) may ramp up to the point where you need to leave. If at any time you feel frightened or unsafe, leave immediately. Even if the steps you need to take impact you financially or socially, keeping yourself safe is your first priority.

•**Finally, focus on healing...and self-compassion.** While it's possible for a gaslighter to change a long-standing pattern of manipulation, it is hard to give up control, and especially abuse, without professional help—something the gaslighter will need to want.

But if your gaslighter is committed to changing and you do stay in the relationship, focus on healing...taking responsibility for what you say and do...and being honest. You will need to be disciplined around hot-button issues so that you don't slip back into old patterns. And you will need to apply the compassion you so easily extend to others to yourself as well.

The right words...

•**Go-to phrases that help.** Having specific words and phrases to use when you feel yourself losing the power struggle can keep you from getting pulled back into the manipulative vortex. *Phrases to memorize...*

"I'm not going to talk to you while you're yelling at me."

"I don't want to have this conversation while emotions are so heated. Let's pick it up later."

"I'm going to go have a cup of tea right now. This conversation isn't feeling fair/respectful."

"I won't continue this conversation when you are telling me what's wrong with me."

"We will have to agree to disagree—I just don't see it that way."

Of course, what you say to your boss or to your parent will be very different from what you say to your partner. How easy it might be to leave also will be different.

Examples...

Your dad: Haven't heard from you in weeks. Just like your mother, you're all about yourself.

How Capable Is Your Gaslighter of Relating to You?

If you've involved with a "gaslighter"—a spouse, coworker, family member or friend who tries to control you by manipulating your perception of reality—you need to decide whether to leave the relationship or stay and fix it. A critical factor in that decision is whether your gaslighter wants to change...and is able to. *Here are positive signs to look for...*

Does he/she...

...seem capable of understanding and respecting your point of view?

...at least occasionally key in to your feelings and needs?

...at least occasionally put your feelings and needs ahead of his/her own?

...feel remorse about the times he hurts you—in a way that leads him to change his own behavior?

...show interest in changing for his own reasons, not simply to please you or to prove what a good guy he is?

Excerpted from *The Gaslight Effect: How to Spot and Survive the Hidden Manipulation Others Use to Control Your Life* by Robin Stern, PhD, cofounder and associate director, Yale Center for Emotional Intelligence, New Haven, Connecticut.

(*Reality:* You called him this week and had a conversation...the statement about your mother is gratuitous meanness and not true of you or your mother.)

You: Dad, we don't agree about how often I call you—we will have to agree to disagree. I'm getting a cup of coffee now. Would you like one? (Avoid defending yourself, ignore the insult and "leave" the power struggle.)

Your boss: We need to wrap up this project—are you clueless about that? Where is the document you promised to revise? (*Reality:* He didn't ask for it, and you didn't promise it.)

You: I didn't know you needed it this week. I will have it for you tomorrow. We had agreed that deadlines would be in writing, which I think will be very helpful. Will that be possible next time? (Ignore the insult, bring the conversation back to the topic.)

Your boss: We never agreed to that. You're so forgetful! Are you going through menopause? (*Reality:* You are, but you know you hadn't agreed on a deadline—and he is again deflecting the conversation.)

You: I will take responsibility for sending you an e-mail after our meetings about what work needs to be done and when. In the meantime, I will go back to my office and get you what you need. (Avoid his bait and the temptation to defend yourself and keep the conversation on the topic.)

THINGS YOU CAN SAY TO OPT OUT OF A POWER STRUGGLE

If you're involved with a "gaslighter"—a spouse, coworker, family member or friend who tries to control you by manipulating your perception of reality—the following 16 phrases can help keep you out of his/her destructive vortex. *Memorize the phrases that seem most useful for your own situation so that you can pull them out when you need them…*

• "You're right, but I don't want to keep arguing about this."

• "You're right, but I don't want to be talked to that way."

• "I'm happy to continue this conversation without name-calling."

• "I'm not comfortable with where this conversation is going. Let's revisit it later."

• "I think this conversation has gone as far as it can go."

• "I don't think I can be constructive right now. Let's talk about this at another time."

• "I think we have to agree to disagree."

• "I don't want to continue this argument."

• "I don't want to continue this conversation right now."

• "I hear you, and I'm going to think about that. But I don't want to keep talking about it right now."

• "I'd really like to continue this conversation, but I'm not willing to do so unless we can do it in a more pleasant tone."

• "I don't like the way I'm feeling right now, and I'm not willing to continue this conversation."

• "You may not be aware of it, but you're telling me that I don't know what reality is. And, respectfully, I don't agree. I love you, but I won't talk to you about this."

• "I love having intimate conversations with you, but not when you're putting me down."

• "It may not be your intention to put me down, but I feel put down, and I'm not going to continue the conversation."

• "This is not a good time for me to talk about this. Let's agree on another time that works for both of us."

The above list is excerpted from *The Gaslight Effect: How to Spot and Survive the Hidden Manipulation Others Use to Control Your Life* by Robin Stern, PhD, cofounder and associate director, Yale Center for Emotional Intelligence, New Haven, Connecticut.

Fight Back Against Your Inner Critic

Lisa Firestone, PhD, clinical psychologist and director of research and education at The Glendon Association, a nonprofit mental health organization based in Santa Barbara, California. She is coauthor of several books about psychology, including The Self Under Siege *and* Conquer Your Critical Inner Voice. *Glendon.org*

The voice inside your head that calls you an idiot when you make even the littlest mistake could be standing in the way of your success and happiness. No one is unaffected by this voice. We all hear it—and it's incredibly negative and destructive.

Inner critics can be cruel, harshly criticizing their hosts for imaginary failings and minor faux pas. That isn't just unpleasant—it is counterproductive. Faced with frequent, heartless criticism from within, we may conclude that there's no point making an effort or taking a chance because we'll just mess it up.

Why start a new relationship when the voice in your head informs you that you're incapable of holding on to a partner? Why try to invest for the future when the voice says that you'll just mismanage the money?

This negative voice can become the filter through which you see yourself. It both drives your behavior and then later berates you for it.

Example: The voice seduces you in a friendly-sounding way, telling you to just stay home rather than go out to the party that you planned to attend. Later, the voice screams at you that you're lonely, unwanted and have no friends. In the same way, this ugly voice can drive some people all the way to drugs and alcohol, suggesting that they have another drink or hit…then later criticizing them for their stupidity and weakness in partaking.

But you are not doomed to be beaten down by this voice. *By learning where your inner critic actually comes from and ways to weaken or disregard it, you can release yourself and find happiness…*

THE ROOTS OF AN INNER CRITIC

Your inner critic did not begin inside you—it probably traces back to criticism you heard from someone powerful who was in your life when you were a child, such as a parent, teacher, older sibling or peer. Your interactions with this person left your childhood "self" feeling inadequate. Children also learn through observation—not just words. You may have grown up hearing a parent regularly speaking harshly to himself/herself. Children internalize their parents' voices.

Example: A girl who lived with a mother and grandmother who were vocally critical of their own bodies grew up to be a woman whose inner critic said tremendously hurtful things about her own appearance. A man whose father felt like a failure grew up to view himself as one, too.

OVERCOMING AN INNER CRITIC

You can't silence your inner critic by giving in to it—that just feeds it and makes it stronger. Instead, freedom lies in paying close attention to when it talks to you and then acting against it by taking some positive risks.

Example: The next time you see someone you like, ignore the voice—take a chance and ask the person out. The first time you resist the voice, it may get louder, shouting that you'll fail…but if you persist, eventually it will fade into the background.

These five strategies can help you fight back and find a way to take risks. *You have the power to quiet that inner critic's voice and reduce its impact on your life…*

•**Separate the voice from your own thoughts.** If you had a horribly unpleasant neighbor who constantly criticized you, you wouldn't take those criticisms seriously. You would dismiss him/her with an eye roll. Your inner critic deserves similar treatment. When it raises your fears and lowers your confidence, tell yourself, *That's just my inner critic again.*

•**Give its opinion the weight it deserves—little or none.** It's a vestige of an old self. Think about it—would you run your life or make decisions based on what you thought as a child? Of course not. And yet that's what you're doing when you let your inner critic get the upper hand.

Ask yourself, *What do I really think?* Step outside yourself, and take a "third party" look at what's going on. This further separates your feelings from the inner critic's feelings. Use first person "I" sentences when considering your true opinions but not when reflecting on the inner critic's words.

Example: You miss a flight. Your inner critic tells you that you're disorganized and can't do anything right. After reflecting for a moment on this, you might respond with, I make mistakes like anyone, but I actually get lots of stuff right. In fact, this is the first flight I've ever missed. The lines were longer than normal.

•**Try to identify your inner critic's triggers.** When your inner critic overreacts to a seemingly minor matter, there's a good chance that it actually is reacting to a similar incident that occurred in your past. It helps to identify the root source.

Example: You hear less than full agreement when you voice an opinion at a neighborhood association meeting. Your inner critic tells you, *No one cares about your opinion—it's* *worthless.* Perhaps this overreaction occurred because you were the youngest child in your family and your older siblings never valued your opinions.

•**Learn self-compassion.** People who endure cruel inner critics often believe that self-criticism is a path toward self-improvement and assume that the voice is there to motivate rather than destroy. In fact, harsh self-criticism is more likely to convince you that you are not capable of self-improvement than it is to lead to growth. Self-compassion (the ability to be kind to yourself even when you are suffering and to be nonjudgmental toward yourself) is more likely to lead to self-improvement—but self-compassion is a skill that people with scathing inner critics often lack.

Strategies for developing self-compassion include positive journaling and meditation to focus your attention on where you want to go and who you want to be. With your eyes closed, take a few deep breaths and try to be mindful. Meditation strengthens your ability to stop over-identifying with negative thoughts and feelings. They don't define you.

•**Ask yourself,** *So what's my next step?* Inner critics often focus their gaze backward at their past mistakes, constantly reinforcing their shortcomings. Focusing on a single, achievable next step can kick-start positive momentum and break the cycle of negativity and rumination created by an "error."

Example: You eat a bowl of ice cream when you're supposed to be on a diet. Your inner critic says you're fat and lack the discipline to lose weight. There's no point focusing on the past—you can't "un-eat" the ice cream. Instead, ask, *What's my next step?* It might be to throw away any remaining ice cream...or to plan out all of tomorrow's eating in advance to reduce the odds of impulsive snacking.

Also: Another question that can shift focus from the unchangeable past to a more productive future is, *What would I do differently next time?*

Act Like an Extrovert

Sonja Lyubomirsky, PhD, professor of psychology, University of California, Riverside.

Acting like an extrovert boosts happiness.
Recent study: Researchers instructed 123 college students, who were a mix of introverts and extroverts, to act talkative, assertive and spontaneous (all extrovert traits) for one week and then be deliberate, quiet and reserved (introvert traits) another week.

Result: Well-being scores were significantly higher for participants during the extrovert week and decreased during the introvert week.

Surprising: When "faking" being extroverted, the introverts reported no discomfort.

The Art of Doing Nothing

Sandi Mann, PhD, senior lecturer in the School of Psychology, University of Central Lancashire, UK. She is lead author of the study "Does Being Bored Make Us More Creative?" and author of *The Science of Boredom: The Upside (And Downside) of Downtime.* MindTraining Clinic.com

There's a simple activity that spurs creativity, boosts problem-solving abilities and calms anxieties. This activity might sound like it's really something, but actually it's really...nothing. Just a few minutes spent doing nothing could turn out to be among the most productive parts of your day.

Thanks in large part to smartphones, even the briefest breaks in the day are now filled with checking messages, surfing the Internet, listening to podcasts and playing games. As a result, standing around doing nothing seems wasteful, and many people fear it makes them appear unimportant.

But researchers are discovering that banishing boredom and inactivity does not actually make life better. Studies have shown that brief stretches of mindless activity tend to boost people's creativity and problem-solving abilities.

Example: A study published in *Creativity Research Journal* found that participants did better on the creative task of coming up with as many uses as possible for a pair of plastic cups if they first had engaged in an activity that let their minds wander—the boring task of reading mindlessly from a phone book.

DAYDREAM BELIEVER

Why does doing nothing improve creativity and problem-solving skills? Because your brain isn't actually doing nothing when you do nothing—it's daydreaming. And though daydreaming carries negative associations, it's actually time well spent.

When researchers conducted MRI scans on the brains of people who were daydreaming, they found that multiple parts of their brains were highly active—including the "executive network," which is associated with complex problem solving—according to a study published in *Proceedings of the National Academy of Sciences.*

You likely have had the experience of waking from a deep sleep to discover that your dreaming brain has thought up a useful idea. This is the same concept behind daydreaming—but with less risk that you'll forget the idea.

HARNESSING THE POWER OF DOING NOTHING

The secret to getting something out of doing nothing is to allow your mind to wander without exercising any control over where it goes during this time.

Some people can achieve this dreamy let-your-mind-wander state almost anywhere—if you often catch yourself staring into space in noisy, busy places such as coffee shops or on train platforms, you probably don't need to take

---

Three Do-Nothing No-Nos

Yes, it is possible to go wrong when your goal is to do nothing more than daydream…

•**Meditation and yoga are not conducive to daydreaming.** When people meditate or do yoga, they typically try to focus their attention on a single concept or action. This does have benefits, but it's very different from letting the mind wander.

•**Killing time by browsing the Internet or watching mindless TV is not the right sort of doing nothing.** These activities are doing nothing in the sense that you're accomplishing nothing—but staring at a phone, computer or TV screen tends to inhibit your thoughts from wandering freely.

•**Focused problem-solving is not daydreaming.** If you consciously steer your mind to seek a solution to a specific problem, you will undercut the creative power of daydreaming. Instead, let your thoughts drift wherever they take you. Trust that your mind is aware of the big problem you face and is working on that problem even when you're not directing it to do so.

---

any special steps to daydream. You just need to put away your phone or your book and let it happen. Other people may have to actively seek out conditions that are conducive to purposeful daydreaming.

Even people who don't daydream can get in on the action if they try daydreaming while…

•**Standing in line.** Supermarket and airport lines once were prime daydreaming time before the advent of smartphones with all their distractions. Boring queues can be that again. Direct your eyes up toward a spot high on a wall or in a distant corner of the ceiling to reduce the odds that you'll make eye contact with other people or spot other things that grab your attention. Daydreaming in lines can be an effective anxiety-control strategy, too—when you feel frustration about the length of a line, tell yourself to instead be thankful for the opportunity to daydream. It feels better to know that the downtime actually is a good use of your time.

•**Enjoying quiet time during drives.** Turn off your car's radio, and just let your mind wander during your commute or other drives. Make sure you're still paying attention to the road, of course.

•**Sitting in a spot with a pleasant but not dramatic view.** Gaze out a window at a tree… look into a fireplace with a fire burning…or focus on a pond in a park. Just watch the fire…the water…the wind blowing the leaves…or the clouds floating by.

•**Strolling with or without your dog.** Going for a walk is a good way to get away from the potential distractions of home and the workplace. Walking amid trees or fields tends to be more conducive to daydreaming than walking through neighborhoods or cities because nature provides fewer distractions and irritating noises.

•**Swimming.** Swimming isn't doing nothing—it's great exercise. But some people find that it's an ideal opportunity for musing on things. The water cuts down on outside distractions, and the rhythm of the strokes can be hypnotic.

•**Engaging in an activity that occupies your hands but barely engages your mind.** Knit...doodle...bounce a ball against a wall...or color in coloring books. These sorts of activities can encourage people who find it frustrating and unpleasant to be unoccupied. The activity occupies the hands and mind enough to stave off that frustration, at least for a while, but requires such a minimal amount of brainpower that it doesn't prevent you from getting lost in thought.

•**Letting your mind wander for even just a few minutes can be useful, if that's all the time you have.** But it's best if you can try to find at least a few times each week for extended bouts of daydreaming—target 30 minutes, if you can manage that without frustration setting in. Once frustration starts, productive daydreaming becomes unlikely.

Surprising Way to Reduce Negative Emotions

Fangyuan Chen, PhD, assistant professor, department of management and marketing, Hong Kong Polytechnic University, Hong Kong, and leader of a study published in *Journal of Consumer Psychology*.

Think of bad thoughts as if they were people. For instance, if you are feeling sad, imagine sadness as a person and write down a description of what the person looks like. One group of volunteers did that in a recent study, which was inspired by the Pixar film *Inside Out*, in which a child's emotions are portrayed as humanized characters in her mind. Another group in the study wrote about the emotion itself and how it affects them. The group that imagined sadness as a person reported less sadness when recalling an unhappy time in their lives—possibly because imagining sadness as a person made it possible to think of it as being somewhat distanced and detached from them.

Caution: The same technique was also found to reduce the impact of positive emotions, such as happiness. So it is best tried only with negative feelings.

Don't Be a Pleasure Junkie!

Robert H. Lustig, MD, MSL, professor emeritus of pediatric endocrinology and member of the Institute for Health Policy Studies at University of California, San Francisco, and chief science officer of Eat REAL, dedicated to reversing childhood obesity and type 2 diabetes. He is author of *The Hacking of the American Mind: The Science Behind the Corporate Takeover of Our Bodies and Brains*. RobertLustig.com

---

Your new iPhone makes you happy. Reconnecting on social media with everyone you've ever met makes you happy. Binge-watching the latest Netflix series makes you happy. Guess what? You're not happy—you're addicted to pleasure. Your mind has been hacked by a science engineered to stimulate your pleasure cravings. Like any addict, the cycle of chasing pleasurable moments is a no-win game that leaves people perennially unsatisfied.

PLEASURE IS NOT THE SAME AS HAPPINESS

Pleasure is the fleeting feeling of enjoyment or gratification we get when the reward center, deep in the brain, is activated. We derive pleasure from eating a good meal, watching our sports team win or receiving a lot of "likes" on Facebook. Happiness, on the other hand, is a rich feeling of peace, calm and contentment that comes from things such as a long conversation with your son or daughter. *How to spot the difference between pleasure and happiness...*

•**Pleasure and rewards are short-lived.** The day after the Netflix series is over, you're searching for the next one. Happiness and contentment last longer. After that good conversation, your relationship with your child is deeper.

•**Pleasure is visceral and exciting**—it causes your blood pressure and heart rate to go up. Happiness is ethereal and calming—your blood pressure and heart rate go down.

•**Pleasure occurs when you get something,** such as winning money at a casino or buying a new car. Happiness results from giving our time or money to others or a charity.

•**Pleasure often is experienced alone,** while happiness is likely experienced connected to others.

•**Pleasure often is achieved with substances**—caffeine, cigarettes, alcohol, drugs, sugar—but happiness is achieved with deeds or successes, such as seeing a family enjoy the house you volunteered to help build.

HOW DOPAMINE CAN HURT

The brain's reward centers evolved to help us survive, reproduce and stay fit. But recent research in *The Journal of Neuroscience* has linked the release of natural feel-good hormones in response to pleasure and happiness to the same pathways that cause addiction to drugs. These days, thanks to an ever-increasing number of temptations both online and off-line, we have a near constant stream of opportunities for reward, which "hacks" our brain's physiology.

Here's how: A neurotransmitter is a chemical in the brain that, when released, causes other nerve cells to fire. *Dopamine* is an excitatory neurotransmitter that's released when we feel rewarded by something. That's not necessarily bad. But too much of anything can be dangerous. Jumping from one clickbait online headline to another, for example, is too much stimulation, which can kill neurons. Next time, it takes a bigger hit to get the same rush. Just as with opioids and alcohol, the end point is addiction.

Another impact of excessive dopamine release: Not enough production of the calming hormone *serotonin*. Too little leads to depression. So the more pleasure you seek, the unhappier you become.

Stress is a third ingredient at play here. To protect us from stressors such as injury or an important presentation, we produce the fight-or-flight hormone *cortisol*. In small doses over the short term, cortisol is helpful. When stress is chronic, however, and cortisol remains elevated for long periods, it causes dopamine to fire even more, increasing the cycle of reward-seeking behaviors. Cortisol down-regulates production of serotonin adding to our unhappiness. Cortisol is, in effect, the anti-contentment hormone.

Net result: The cycle of hormone release and suppression caused by our nonstop personal pleasure-seeking is harming our emotions. Fortunately, pleasure addiction can be overcome—if you are willing to fight back. *Here's how...*

THE 4CS OF TRUE HAPPINESS

Though not rocket science, there's a scientifically proven formula that can ramp up your serotonin, tamp down dopamine and cortisol, and improve your mood and your health in the process. But know that this road map to reclaiming your happiness takes some effort and sacrifice because it requires breaking away from your current social patterns. *These are four things we all used to do and need to return to doing again...*

•**Connect.** While it may seem extreme to you, log off Facebook, Twitter and Instagram. Instead, make time every day to interact with friends and loved ones face to face, eye to eye, in real life.

Why: Being physically face to face increases empathy and produces serotonin. Research published in *Child Development* shows that as you interact, you adopt or mirror that person's emotions, stimulating serotonin release. You can't achieve that connection with emojis.

•**Contribute.** Give your time, your money and/or yourself by volunteering, donating and performing tasks that contribute to the greater good. Even simple acts of kindness provide benefits.

Why: Multiple studies show that contributing to others or society at large improves your feeling of self-worth, drives contentment and boosts health by reducing your blood pressure, heart rate and stress levels. Doing good results

Beat the Not-Working Blues

Leaving the workplace can cost retirees (and those who have been laid off) their identity, purpose, sense of self-worth and social circle—all of which can have emotional health benefits. Working just one day a week provides the same psychological benefits as working full time, so a paid part-time job can be a solution.

Brendan Burchell, PhD, director of graduate education in the department of sociology at University of Cambridge, UK, and coauthor of a study of 70,000 people, published in *Social Science & Medicine.*

in a better you, both physically and mentally. *Bonus:* You're likely interacting face to face with others when you volunteer.

• **Cope.** This is all about self-care. You know the drill—get enough sleep, stop trying to multitask, eat well, focus on one thing at a time and exercise regularly.

Why: Taking care of Number One is key to managing stress. Sleep deprivation and trying to multitask drive cortisol and dopamine up and serotonin down. In fact, research shows that attempting media multitasking (watching TV, surfing the web, texting and reading all at the same time) literally shrinks the brain in the area associated with executive function—the set of skills that helps you get things done. Exercise, on the other hand, boosts serotonin production. Combined with mindfulness practices (yoga, walks in nature), it may be as effective at reducing depression as taking medication, according to researchers at Rutgers University.

• **Cook.** Stop eating out and relying on processed foods. Use fresh ingredients to prepare food at home instead.

Why: It's no secret that eating fast food and processed foods, as well as supersized restaurant meals, is a major culprit in the obesity crisis. But your food choices can make you happy or miserable, too. How? Processed food is low in *tryptophan,* an amino acid that is a precursor to serotonin. It's also low in omega-3 fatty acids, and omega-3 deficiency has been shown to inhibit serotonin action. Meanwhile, processed food is high in sugar, which depletes serotonin, ramps up dopamine and increases the risk for a smorgasbord of metabolic diseases such as diabetes, hypertension and cancer. Countless studies show that these foods are addictive and unhealthy.

Hope Aids Recovery from Mental Disorders

Matthew Gallagher, PhD, associate professor of psychology, University of Houston, and leader of a study of 223 adults, published in *Behavior Therapy.*

Among people undergoing cognitive behavioral therapy (CBT) for social anxiety disorder, panic disorder, generalized anxiety disorder or obsessive-compulsive disorder, those who experienced increased hope during CBT had improved anxiety symptoms and were better able to move toward recovery. The study defined hope as the capacity of patients to identify strategies or pathways to achieve goals—and the motivation to pursue those strategies or paths.

Reduce Stress with Forms of Focused Breathing

Laura McDonald, American Council on Exercise–certified personal and group fitness trainer and yoga instructor, writing at BHG.com.

Slow breathing can relieve anxiety. Inhale through your nose for three to five seconds, then exhale at the same rate through your nose or mouth. *Box breathing* can help you refocus. Exhale all air, hold for a count of four, breathe in through your nose for a count of four, hold for a count of four, then breathe out through your nose for a count of four. *Nighttime breathing* is good for unwinding before sleep. Inhale deeply to fill your chest and rib cage for a slow count of five...hold for a count of three...slowly release for a count of five. *Controlled breathing* plus visualizing helps with relaxation anytime. Create a detailed, relaxing mental picture while using any comfortable breathing rhythm and count.

How to Overcome Needle Phobia

James Hamilton, MD, a retired family physician who lives in Durham, North Carolina. His seminal academic paper, "Needle Phobia: A Neglected Diagnosis," published in *The Journal of Family Practice* in 1995, established needle phobia as a formal medical condition and has been cited in hundreds of academic journals, including *British Journal of Anesthesia, Cognitive Behavior Therapy* and *International Journal of Clinical Medical Research.*

D read getting injections or blood tests? You're not alone. A 2012 survey found that around one in four adults experiences "needle phobia," and some research points to rates as high as one in three. This aversion can turn deadly when it makes people avoid immunizations and dental or medical care.

For many needle-phobic patients, injections cause a vasovagal reaction (also called vasovagal syncope)—their blood pressure plummets, their pulse weakens, they feel light-headed, and they even might faint.

What to do: Try the following options until you find the solution or combination of solutions that work for you.

•**Numb your arm.** Hold an ice pack against the skin that's about to receive an injection for two minutes before the shot.

Green Is Good!

Merely having a view of a park or other green space from your home (along with access to gardens) has been shown to reduce cravings for alcohol, cigarettes or unhealthy foods—yet another good reason for cities to invest in healthy natural environments.

Health & Place

•**Confuse your nerves and brain with vibration.** Buzzy, a small battery-powered vibrating device, works when held against the arm receiving the injection or giving blood. The vibrations can block nerves from sending pain signals…and prevent the brain from focusing as intensely on any pain signals that are received. The device works best chilled to also get the benefits of icing, and it may be worth the investment for those who need frequent blood tests or injections. ($44.95 for consumer versions, BuzzyHelps.com.)

•**Pinch yourself.** I find that for some patients, pinching themselves immediately prior to the injection on a different part of the body helps. The brain can't focus on two strong stimuli at once, so there's a good chance that it will ignore the injection.

•**Desensitize yourself to needles.** Desensitization is a well-established technique for phobias.

How it works: Slowly increasing your exposure to needles in a relaxed setting can reduce your reaction to them. Start by just thinking about needles/syringes for a few minutes as you sit in a peaceful spot breathing deeply. Repeat this several times a day until you can do it with no light-headedness or fear, then move on to looking at pictures of needles…followed by looking at pictures of people receiving injections…then videos of people getting injections.

•**Distract yourself.** Any mental distraction can reduce your reaction to an injection—an unrelated conversation with a friend…a video on your phone…looking in a direction other than the needle.

Intriguing: Thinking about something that makes you angry is a good distraction when you're about to get a shot. Anger can trigger the fight-or-flight response, which boosts heart rate and blood pressure—potentially overcoming the vasovagal reflex's falling blood pressure and heart rate.

•**Take it lying down.** If shots make you light-headed, get injections while lying down with your legs elevated and shirt collar and belt loosened. This position can offset the falling blood pressure of the vasovagal reflex.

Have a Better Day

As soon as you put your feet on the floor in the morning, say, "This is going to be a great day." It's a very small thing that can have a big impact on how happy and satisfied you feel in your life.

BJ Fogg, PhD, founder and director of the Behavior Design Lab at Stanford University, California, and author of *Tiny Habits: The Small Changes That Change Everything*.

Stop Your Fear of Flying

Martin N. Seif, PhD, ABPP, licensed psychologist in private practice in Greenwich, Connecticut, and New York City, and coauthor of *What Every Therapist Needs to Know About Anxiety Disorders*. Using techniques he developed, Dr. Seif overcame his own crippling fear of flying. DrMartinSeif.com

Fear of flying is caused by a variety of underlying fears and phobias, which have complex genetic, developmental and environmental causes. In my experience, about 70% of those who have a fear of flying are triggered primarily by feeling trapped on a plane. Others may have a fear of heights, crashing, terrorism, physical harm or even a fear of losing control.

Most people with a fear of flying have had an unexpected episode of panic while flying. This typically first occurs between the ages of 17 to 34 but can happen earlier or later in life. It often occurs during a time of significant change in life—good or bad. Due to the panic episode and possible additional episodes, the individual may start to fear that the scary symptoms will return and begin to avoid flying, which only stokes the fear.

Drugs that treat anxiety and depression can be helpful for some, but they have side effects and don't allow patients to develop coping tools.

Identifying the triggers that produce your anxiety and facing those feared triggers while armed with the right tools are the keys for overcoming the problem.

What helps: Cognitive behavioral therapy (CBT) and group therapy programs tailored to address fear of flying. To find a therapist and fear-of-flying programs, go to ADAA.org and click on "Find Help."

Night Owls: Read This

Elise Facer-Childs, PhD, is Transitional Fellow in Industry at Monash University's Sleep and Circadian Rhythms Program, Notting Hill, Australia, and lead author of a study published in *Sleep Medicine*.

Night owls who reset their body clocks reduce stress and improve performance. In a three-week study at universities in the UK and Australia, participants with bedtimes after 2 am reported lower rates of depression and stress and performed better on cognitive and physical tests after shifting their schedules by two hours…getting to sleep and waking earlier…maximizing exposure to sunlight in the morning…and limiting screen time and light before bed.

Overlooked Suicide Risk

William Vaughn McCall, MD, is chair of the department of psychiatry and health behavior at the Medical College of Georgia at Augusta University and lead author of the study, published in *American Journal of Psychiatry*.

Suicidal thoughts can be reduced with better sleep. Yet insomnia isn't always treated in suicidal patients. The first study of its kind has found that adding a sedative—specifically time-released zolpidem-CR—to treatment with an antidepressant can significantly reduce suicidal thoughts and improve sleep. Researchers found that the more severe the insomnia, the greater the reduction in suicidal thoughts with treatment of insomnia.

How to Remember Your Dreams

Michael Breus, PhD, author of *Good Night: The Sleep Doctor's 4-Week Program to Better Sleep and Better Health.* TheSleepDoctor.com

Even though you may not recall your dreams, you can rest assured that you are dreaming. Everyone does. In fact, research shows that most people dream for about two hours each night.

Whether we recall our dreams appears to be affected by the way our sleep process begins and how we awaken. When people are sleep-deprived and zonk out in less than 15 minutes, they bypass *hypnagogia,* a transitional period between wakefulness and sleep that sets the stage for dreaming. Similarly, if we awaken slowly, we are more likely to remember our dreams.

These processes appear to be affected by our neurochemistry, especially levels of *noradrenaline,* a brain chemical that helps regulate important body functions. When noradrenaline is elevated, we're more likely to forget our dreams. A loud alarm clock that jolts you out of slumber, for example, can cause noradrenaline levels to spike.

To better recall your dreams…

•**Keep the same bedtime every night,** and get seven to eight hours of sleep.

•**Don't set an alarm clock.** Allow yourself to wake up naturally. Or try a dawn-simulation clock.

•**Before falling asleep, spend 20 minutes in bed simply relaxing and/or meditating.** This prepares you to enter the hypnagogic state mentioned above.

•**Just as you're about to drift off, repeat to yourself: I want to remember my dreams…I want to remember my dreams.** For unknown reasons, this seems to help.

•**When you first awaken, stay in bed and let your mind drift for about five minutes.** Then write down anything you remember—even a single image can sometimes trigger greater recall.

With practice, most people start to remember their dreams more completely.

Note: Many of my patients tell me that when they use sleeping pills, they do not remember their dreams.

Contact With Nature Quickly Reduces Stress

MaryCarol Hunter, PhD, associate professor, School for Environment and Sustainability, University of Michigan, Ann Arbor, and leader of a study published in *Frontiers in Psychology.*

Just 20 minutes spent sitting or strolling in a place that lets people feel more closely in touch with nature significantly reduces the body's production of the stress hormone *cortisol.* Regular contact with natural surroundings can be a low-cost solution to the stress-inducing effects of urbanization and indoor lifestyles filled with screen viewing. The time of day does not matter as long as nature exposure occurs during daylight. The study's participants also were asked to avoid aerobic exercise, use of social media, the Internet, phone calls, texts, conversation and reading during their nature experiences.

CHAPTER 9

Family Health and Care

How to Handle an "Impossible" Health Care Decision for a Loved One

Imagine if you were living through one of these medical dilemmas...

Your husband had a massive stroke and is now in the ICU on a ventilator. He is not expected to recover. Doctors recommend turning off his ventilator. You never talked about his specific wishes for end-of-life care, but you feel sure he wouldn't want his life artificially extended when there's little chance of meaningful recovery. You agree with the doctors, but your three adult children say, "No!" What should you do?

Your wife's been devastated by metastatic cancer and chemotherapy. There's an experimental drug that might extend her life a few months, but it could have severe side effects and be very painful. In her late 60s, your wife prides herself on being a fighter... but is more suffering really worth it? What should the two of you do?

These are the types of medical dilemmas that can be planned for in an advance directive—a legally enforceable document that guides family members or health-care proxies in decision-making when loved ones are unable to decide for themselves. (There are two kinds of advance directives—a living will or health-care power-of-attorney.)

Troubling statistics: Only 23% of Americans have put their end-of-life choices into writing.

Yet in the absence of a detailed advance directive, you're not alone when you have to make a life-and-death decision for a loved one. Few people realize that hospital ethics committees exist for these sorts of difficult questions. Ethics

Mark Aulisio, PhD, the Susan E. Watson Professor and chair of the department of bioethics at Case Western Reserve University School of Medicine. He is also director of Clinical and Education Programs in Bioethics at Case Western Reserve University, and director of the Center for Biomedical Ethics at the MetroHealth Medical Center, all in Cleveland. Dr. Aulisio has written extensively on ethics committees and consultation.

committees are usually comprised of health-care professionals including doctors from different specialties, nurses, social workers, clergy members, ethicists, lawyers and others.

Nearly all US hospitals have these committees. In fact, all US hospitals accredited by The Joint Commission—that's almost all hospitals—are required to have a way to address ethical issues related to a medical crisis.

YOU ARE NOT ALONE!

During a loved one's health crisis, it's common to feel frightened, conflicted and alone in the difficult decisions before you. *What you need to know…*

•**The hospital ethics committee is there to help you.** The committee is not the ethics police—it has no oversight or enforcement role. Nor are its members wise sages who always know what to do…and they are not empowered to make medical decisions on a patient's behalf.

Rather, the committee's purpose is to help patients, families or surrogates and health professionals identify value conflicts or uncertainties…and resolve the conflict or confusion, often by building consensus around the values and rights of the patient—putting the patient first.

To initiate a consultation with the ethics committee, approach your doctor, nurse, social worker or hospital clergy, and tell him/her that you want an ethics consultation. Most ethics consult services respond promptly to the request. Some ethics consults can take multiple meetings, while others are resolved within a short time. It depends on the nature of the issue underlying the consult request.

When a request is made, consultants will often get a description of the issue, review the patient's chart for relevant information, interview members of the care team as well as family members and the patient himself if appropriate. Depending on the issue, the ethics consultants or team also may ask to have a meeting with members of the care team and family to clarify the patient's diagnosis, prognosis, range of medically acceptable options as well as the patient's wishes and values.

•**It's always appropriate to ask for help.** Maybe you want help but don't think that your issue is an "ethical" dilemma. For example, you might just want a clarification regarding the differences between a living will and a health-care power-of-attorney or perhaps you (or a family member) are uncertain about your role in decision-making and feel overburdened.

Ask for help anyway! You don't need perfect clarity to request a consultation with the hospital ethics committee.

HOW TO GET THE MOST HELP

To maximize the value you'll get from an ethics consultation, you should…

•**Identify the reason for your consult.** Why do you want the consult? What is bothering you? What are your concerns? Be as clear as possible about the reason for your request. This will help the committee help you.

•**Understand your actual role.** The most common ethical dilemma is end-of-life medical care. This may involve a patient who is too incapacitated to make a decision. In these cases, a spouse, adult child or surrogate is asking for help in deciding whether or not to withhold life-sustaining treatment, such as a ventilator or feeding tube.

This is a burden no one can or should bear alone—thinking it is your responsibility to decide whether your loved one lives or dies. That is not the actual role of the spouse, family member or surrogate at the end of life.

Your role, which you clarify with the help of the ethics committee, is to explore, articulate and advocate for what the patient cares about and values. Even if you never had a specific discussion about, say, long-term ventilator support, your knowledge of your loved one's life, personality and values can help the care team make decisions that respect and honor your loved one.

In the end, most decisions should be focused on the best fit between your loved one's values and the range of medically appropriate treatment options—and you are there to simply discern and implement the wishes of the one you love, in the last hours or days of that person's life.

Helping a Loved One Get Used to Hearing Aids: How to Keep Communication Open

Tina Childress, AuD, CCC-A, audiologist, Association of Late-Deafened Adults, Champaign, Illinois. ALDA.org

Adjusting to new hearing aids is a process. Patience and keeping communication options are key.

Hearing aids make many sounds more audible, including environmental sounds such as traffic noise or a ringing phone. But speech is much more difficult to hear because it's a more complex sound. Sometimes hearing aids aren't enough—you or your loved one may need to use assistive devices to communicate in groups, talk on the phone and watch TV.

For better communication with someone with hearing aids: When you want to say something, give the hearing-aid wearer a tap or slight wave to get his attention and make eye contact before talking to him. It's also helpful to have good lighting and speak face-to-face so that he or she can interpret gestures and use lip-reading clues.

Rekindle Your Relationship

If you've hit a rough patch in your relationship and want to recapture the magic, here are some proven techniques to try. **Think about what you love** and appreciate in your partner. **Define whatever problems you have, and break them down into small, manageable pieces** that you can deal with. **Have sex spontaneously. Write down any lingering grudges** on paper, dwell on them as long as you need to, then burn the paper and let the ill feelings go. **Try writing a eulogy** for your partner—not to be morbid, but to help you focus on the happy memories and pleasant interactions you have had.

Roundup of marriage therapists, reported at Prevention.com.

Be sure to pause between sentences and speak at a normal pace (not too fast or too slow). And don't cover your mouth. Speak in your normal tone of voice, since shouting can distort speech. Moving to a quieter place helps with ease of communication as well. If he keeps misunderstanding something, try different words, which he may be able to hear better.

Writing notes can be another effective way to communicate unfamiliar words that may be difficult to lip-read.

Important: Talk with an audiologist if you have further questions.

Couples: Stop Having the Same Fight Over and Over!

Michele Weiner-Davis, LCSW, founder of The Divorce Busting Center in Boulder, Colorado. She is a TEDx speaker and best-selling author of eight books including *Healing from Infidelity, The Sex-Starved Marriage* and *Divorce Busting.* DivorceBusting.com

Research suggests that more than two-thirds of what couples argue about actually is unresolvable. Whether it's differences in parenting styles or how money is spent, couples will never see eye-to-eye on some issues. But that doesn't stop us from relentlessly trying to persuade our partners that we're right. I call these interactions "More of the Same" fights. Everyone engages in these automatic-pilot tiffs from time to time. They're a waste of time and energy, and they're completely avoidable. *Here's how…*

CHANGE THE PATTERN

To break free from unproductive patterns, you have to change your steps in the dance. When you do, the dance will change.

The next time you find yourself in an old familiar triggering situation, start by taking a deep breath and asking yourself, *What's my goal right now? Is what I'm about to do or say going to bring me closer to that goal?* If the answer is, *No, it will push me further away,* or *It simply will be another round of the same old fight,* then don't do it! No matter how justified you feel, refrain from doing the same old thing. Instead, promise yourself that you will do something different—because anything different can change the outcome.

Example: Sally and Bob have been married for 35 years. Sally, an easygoing woman, was repeatedly upset by her husband's tendency to anger easily when he felt frustrated. They had frequent arguments about this. Each time Bob got irritated, Sally tried to calm him down, which had the unintended effect of infuriating him. Eventually, rather than blame Bob for his behavior, she decided to try a different approach—change how she was handling Bob's anger.

One day, while Bob was working in the den, Sally heard him complaining loudly, "I wasn't at the training. I can't believe my boss expects me to do this assignment. I don't know how!" Although tempted to do the usual—rush into the den to demand that he calm down, which would typically spark an argument—she stormed into the den and shouted, "You weren't at the training, and it's unbelievable that your boss would expect you to know what to do. That's ridiculous!" Dead silence. After several moments, with a stunned look on his face, Bob said to Sally in a reassuring manner, "Don't worry. I'll figure it out. It will be OK." It was the first time Sally realized how her lifelong efforts to calm Bob had actually fueled his fire. In other words, her old solution had become the problem.

WHEN IT'S NOT WORTH FIGHTING

Although sweeping things under the carpet when you have lingering feelings of resentment isn't healthful for any relationship, neither is making a mountain out of a molehill. Your spouse is who your spouse is. And as much as you would like to change certain things about each other, it's not realistic.

Example: My husband believes that only he holds the key to the correct way to load a dishwasher. No amount of discussion over the years has changed his thinking on this. Long ago, I decided that when he corrected me or reorganized the dishes in the dishwasher, instead of standing my ground, I would simply tell myself, It's not about me. It's not that I agree with what I see as his "OCD" tendencies, it's just that I've decided not to sweat the small stuff. And we're both better off because of it.

The key to this strategy lies in knowing the difference between issues that arise that warrant your going to the mat, such as being treated with respect and kindness, versus disliking your partner's style or quirks.

Example: You got married knowing about a difference in tidiness thresholds, but you assumed that it would change. When it didn't, it became a source of frustration. Switching your perspective about those quirks or style differences may put an end to arguments. Ask yourself, *How important is this issue really? Can I let it drop because she's never going to change on this point?* In spite of the popular marital maxim that you should always "speak your truth," in reality, sometimes silence is golden.

TALK LESS, LISTEN MORE

Human beings have a universal need to be heard, understood and validated. Unfortunately, we're often too busy stating our positions to genuinely hear or be curious about our partners' thoughts or feelings. Then, because they feel unheard, they up the ante and more zealously reiterate their opinions.

The key to neutralizing any escalating argument is to stop talking, stop focusing on your retort and instead deeply listen to what the other person has been saying and acknowledge his/her feelings. Agreement is not necessary.

Example: Say, "I honestly see your point. My perspective is different, but I do understand why you feel the way you do. Here's what I hear you saying." And then repeat back what you've heard. It's astonishing how readily people become more conciliatory when they feel that their messages have gotten through.

SHORT-CIRCUIT UNPRODUCTIVE INTERACTIONS WITH A TIME-OUT

There are times when even the simplest disagreement spins out of control, and before you know it, you're fuming. At this point, it's best to pause the debate. When you're agitated, you're far less likely to have constructive conversation and far more likely to do or say something hurtful. *Some signs that you or your partner has reached this boiling point…*

•**Negative body language.** Is one of you sitting with crossed arms, piercing eyes or no eye contact at all? That's a signal that listening has stopped and that further conversation will be fruitless.

•**Feeling hopeless.** You find yourself saying, "Here we go again," or thinking, You always have to be right. There's no point talking to you.

•**Tensing up.** You feel it in your body. Some people describe a tightness in their chests. Others say their stomachs are in knots. Still others say their faces feel flushed, or they experience adrenaline rushes that create extreme emotional states.

These are all signs of a dead-end debate or an argument that can spin out of control. The key to de-escalating lies in your ability to spot these signs early on, before you become emotionally hijacked. Instead, take an agreed-upon time-out.

What is an agreed-upon time-out? It means that the two of you have decided—in advance—that some arguments should be put on pause. Choose a signal such as forming a "T" with both hands, or pick a word that is your "safe" word. Then both partners must honor the request and take a break from each other for 30 minutes. Take a walk. Read a book. Listen to music.

Warning: With emotions riding high, it can take a lot of self-control to pause the conversation. Remember past experiences when taking a break has been successful to break the cycle of anger. If you haven't tried it yet, then remind yourself how not taking a break has only escalated the disagreement up until now.

After 30 minutes, reconvene and decide whether or not you need to revisit the conversation. If one partner feels "unfinished," it's important to re-up the discussion. If, however, both partners wish to drop the issue, that's perfectly acceptable. Or if emotions still are running high, agree to a time later when the conversation can be completed.

Mistake: Confusing an agreed-upon time-out with a walk-out. Some of my clients say, "Oh, I do that by leaving the room, but my spouse follows me and keeps on arguing." It's important for you to realize that a unilateral decision to end a discussion by leaving the room or shutting down emotionally is entirely different from having a prearranged mutual agreement to take a breather. Unilateral decisions to exit a conversation, although perhaps helpful to the "leaver," often feel like abandonment to the spouse who wants to resolve matters. Agreeing to reconnect and re-up the conversation, if necessary, after the break makes honoring a time-out much more feasible.

A REMINDER

Although "circuit-breaker" skills minimize the damage of pointless fighting, they're no substitute for intentionally investing time and energy into maintaining the love and passion you share. In today's high-pressured and heads-to-the-screen society, it's increasingly common for couples to feel disconnected even when they are in the same physical space. A foundation based on shared positive experiences—having date nights, engaging in meaningful conversations and a satisfying sexual relationship—creates strong bonds that, in turn, help couples weather rocky times, and remember, *This too shall pass.*

Create "Touch Points"

Julie Morgenstern, author of *Time to Parent*, quoted at Prevention.com.

Keep your relationship strong by creating daily "touch points" with your partner. At least three to five times a day, use a quick call or text, or a short chat at the end of the workday, to help ground your relationship. The frequent contact shows each of you that the other one understands your day-to-day existence and the pacing of your life. This also means that you will need less catching up when you are both home in the evening.

Stepping into the Caregiver Role

Connie McKenzie, RN, CMC, director of Firstat RN Care Management Services, West Palm Beach, Florida. She is on the board of the National Association of Professional Geriatric Care Managers. FirstatHealthCare.com

As your parent ages, you may find yourself acting as his/her spokesperson and health advocate. He may have an increasing number of health issues leading to complicated conversations with doctors…an array of drugs…plus some possible hearing loss or mental decline—all of which make it challenging for him to navigate doctors' visits alone. There also may be some age bias that leads the doctor to offer your parent too much (or too little) treatment.

Whether you're already involved as a caregiver or just stepping in to this new role, here's how to make it better…

CONVERSATION STARTERS

It's fun to talk about grandkids but not so much fun to talk about your dad's fungal infection. So you both avoid it.

Why that matters: If you are largely unaware of your parent's health issues, you're going to be blindsided when a crisis happens. You might not be knowledgeable enough to answer a doctor's questions in the ER or involved enough to mention an additional symptom your parent forgot. This needs to change.

Start by asking for permission. It's hard to dive right into a health conversation. Lay the groundwork first.

Example: "Dad, I'd like to talk with you about how you're feeling. Any health concerns?" You also can add, "It's not that I think you can't handle things yourself. But if I ever have to step in and be your advocate in an emergency, I really want to know this information so that I can best support you."

Additional benefit: If you make it clear that you want to understand and support him, it helps remove the concern that he's burdening you.

Once understood, suggest that you begin to attend doctors' visits with your parent. Before the first agreed-upon appointment, go over your parent's health complaints.

Ask about what you've heard or observed: "Mom, you told me that you don't like this drug you're taking. What effects are you noticing?" Make a written list of her concerns.

SCHEDULING SMARTS

Assuming that it works for your parent, request a morning appointment, when the office is more likely to be running on time and the doctor and staff are likely to be fresher and more attentive. Or ask for the first appointment after the office's lunch break.

Why that matters: It's not just the annoying wait and your parent's exhaustion that are problems. The doctor is not in top form either. According to a study published in *JAMA Network Open*, in the afternoon doctors may not order as many screening tests as they should—a result, in part, of decision fatigue.

Additional benefit: If there are tests ordered, you may be able to have them done the same day.

Note: For an older adult, his routine (including using the toilet) tends to be paramount, and late risers may not be up to an early doctor's visit.

BE ORGANIZED AT EVERY APPOINTMENT

Bring the list of health concerns to the appointment. It's easy for you or your parent to forget to mention something. At a routine checkup, prioritize the most important items at the top. There often isn't time to deal with everything, and this will ensure that the doctor will hear the most pressing problems. Review the list with your parent on the way to the office so that it's fresh in your minds.

When you arrive at the appointment, make sure that the doctor's office has any necessary paperwork needed to allow you to speak on your parent's behalf. Take notes that you and your parent can refer back to.

AVOID MEDICATION MIX-UPS

Be sure the list of your parent's medications and supplements is up to date.

Physically go through all drugs—prescription and over-the-counter—as well as vitamin/mineral and herbal supplements before the appointment. Create an updated list or take photos of the labels on each drug to ensure accuracy—and then review them with the doctor. Many medications need careful monitoring and dosing adjustments.

Additional benefit: As you go through the medicines, you could discover that your mom has an unopened drug or an empty bottle in need of refill. If you notice your parent is confused by his medications, you may need to start helping to organize his meds every week—or arrange for someone else to do so. A weekly phone call to fill the pill box together is a good way to ensure accuracy.

MAINTAINING THE RIGHT FOCUS

Avoid the trap of doing all of the talking to the doctor yourself—even if your parent is sitting right there, especially if your parent has trouble hearing.

Why that matters: It undercuts your parent's involvement in his own health care and makes it easier for him to ignore advice when you're not around.

How to do it better: Be mindful not to answer questions for your parent. After mentioning a few health issues, turn the focus to your parent.

Example: "These are the things Mom would like to discuss, and she would like to share with you some of the symptoms she's experiencing." Don't hesitate to prompt your parent—"Remember, Mom, you told me about the pain you're having in your feet. Can you describe it to Dr. Brown?"

Also: Take notes while they talk. It's very common for a doctor's advice to go in one ear and out the other—in a survey reported in *Journal of the Royal Society of Medicine,* patients who had just left their doctors' offices forgot 40% to 80% of the medical information provided.

Better: At the end of the appointment, read back from your notes and ask if you missed anything.

FOLLOW-UP PLANS

Let your parent know that you will help keep the care plan on track.

Why that matters: Seniors often assume that their doctor will handle follow-up. If your parent is homebound and you can't drive him to get tests, ask the doctor's office if someone there can arrange for a lab tech to visit your parent's home and draw blood there. For test results, arrange for someone from the doctor's office to call you as well.

Also helpful: Find a pharmacy that delivers prescriptions so that your parent gets needed meds in a timely manner. Or use an online or mail-order pharmacy. You also can ask the pharmacy to "reconcile" your parent's various prescriptions so that they are filled on the same date and with the same supply time frame to simplify things.

Caregiver's Checklist

Amy R. Ehrlich, MD, associate chief of the division of geriatrics and medical director of Montefiore Home Care at Montefiore Health System and professor of clinical medicine at Albert Einstein College of Medicine, both in New York City.

Whether or not you're new to caregiving, it's a good idea to have these items in place.

•**Get a health-care proxy or durable health-care power of attorney.** The health-care proxy appoints you as the one who will carry out wishes and make health-care decisions if/when the person becomes incapable of doing so. It also gives you legal standing with the medical team. AARP provides free forms, organized by state. Go to AARP.org and search "advance directive forms."

•**Compile a complete health-care folder.** Include the advance directive…power of attorney…Social Security number…patient insurance ID number…complete contact information for doctors, pharmacy and close relatives…health records…lists of all medications and supplements, including why they're taken and the dosages.

●**Access to online electronic patient portal.** If available, these secure medical- and hospital-network websites allow you to view test results, ask questions of affiliated doctors, make appointments and pay bills. Get a proxy access request and authorization form from the medical network, and ask the patient to sign it and submit it.

●**Stay on top of drug risks.** Keep the list of medications and supplements up to date. Review side effects with the doctor at each appointment and question possible interactions if a new item is prescribed. For at-home research, AARP's free online drug-interaction checker can aid in identifying potential risks. Health Tools.AARP.org/drug-interactions.

●**Locate additional resources.** Community-based organizations are essential for support and resources for families of elderly people. State offices for the aging are located in towns and counties throughout the country. Go to the Department of Health and Human Services website, HHS.gov/aging, and click on "Resources Near You" to find a link to your state's offerings.

Help a Loved One With Dementia Be Comfortable at Family Gatherings

When planning a get-together, think about what he/she would enjoy or enjoyed in the past and try to plan something suitable. Consider a brunch or lunch rather than a later gathering—some people with dementia become confused or fatigued later in the day. Interact directly with the person, not just with his caretaker. Listen patiently when he speaks—he may need extra time to figure out what to say. Invite him to help in a non-stressful way, such as by setting the table or folding napkins, if he is capable of this. Be sure there is a quiet place where he can go if need be.

Be realistic about your expectations: As dementia progresses, he may become less able to interact with people, and a big family group may be overwhelming.

Suzanne Schindler, MD, PhD, instructor in neurology, Washington University School of Medicine, St. Louis, quoted at NextAvenue.org

Dementia Affects Vision, Too

Teepa Snow, OTR/L, FAOTA, an occupational therapist and dementia-care educator who works with caregivers and professionals worldwide through her company, Positive Approach to Care, based in Efland, North Carolina. She has a clinical appointment with Duke University's School of Nursing in Durham, North Carolina.

When a loved one has Alzheimer's disease or another form of dementia, you expect changes in memory and thinking.

But did you know that the brain changes that accompany dementia, combined with aging, can literally change how people see the world?

Four vision changes seen in people with Alzheimer's and other forms of dementia—and how to help them…

●**Poor depth perception.** People with dementia can lose the ability to perceive dimension and see the world in all its 3-D glory. That can affect their ability to judge distances. They might not perceive, for example, that a fan spinning six feet above their heads is too far away to turn off by hand.

Or a picture of an apple may be mistaken for a real one. That can lead to behaviors that caregivers mistake for signs of hallucinations—such as reaching for that fan or trying to take a bite of that apple. It also can lead to accidents, especially with stairs or curbs.

How you can help: You don't have to correct every misperception. In fact, you can build trust by going along with the harmless ones. Let your loved one enjoy the puppies on that YouTube video he/she keeps watching, even if he thinks they are in his yard. But eliminate or lessen hazards, like that ceramic apple he might bite or the bottom step he might miss.

Helpful: Mark the edge of the top and bottom steps with bright tape. Avoid a dark throw rug on a light background—it can look like a hole or step down.

•**A shrinking field of vision.** As we age, everyone loses some ability to see things off to the side, over and under our point of focus. For many people with dementia, this loss of peripheral vision is accelerated and can be severe. In fact, someone with dementia can have a field of vision that is only 12 to 18 inches across, as it takes all the person's ability to take in that amount of visual data and try to figure it out.

How you can help: When approaching a person with dementia, do so from the front—and, if possible, catch his gaze. Put important things, such as food and drinks, right in front of your loved one. Offer guidance in situations where a person with dementia might not see what's obvious to you, such as a handrail on the stairs.

•**Poor color and contrast perception.** A loss of ability to distinguish color and contrast can happen in the earlier stages of dementia, leaving someone unable to tell colored pills apart or respond quickly to traffic signals, especially at sunrise or sunset, when it is dimmer. People with dementia also can have trouble making out objects with inadequate color contrast—an all-white bathroom, for example, can be a nightmare to navigate.

How you can help: Put a colored seat on the white toilet. Make sure food items stand out from the plate—for example, mashed potatoes on a white plate will get lost. One study found that presenting food on a red plate resulted in greater intake for people living with dementia.

•**Need for brighter light.** To see well, people in their 60s need light three times brighter than what's needed by those in their 20s. Someone dealing with vision challenges linked to dementia can have even greater trouble than a similarly aged healthy person in a dim environment.

How you can help: Provide bright light (over 100 watts, in general), but be careful to choose bulbs and fixtures that keep the lighting diffuse—no exposed bulbs or lights that will shine directly into eyes. Use "full-spectrum" bulbs that mimic sunlight. That will help people stay alert and on task.

Important: Vision changes are a primary and early symptom of some types of dementia. In one rare type, called *posterior cortical atrophy,* people may have little memory loss but serious difficulties with vision, including trouble identifying common objects such as the handle versus the blade of a knife. Vision changes and visual hallucinations also are common early-stage symptoms of a condition known as *Lewy body dementia.* For these reasons, you should always report changes in vision to your healthcare providers.

Smart Ways to Deal with Your Loved One's Doctor

Charles B. Inlander, consumer advocate and healthcare consultant based in Fogelsville, Pennsylvania. He was the founding president of the nonprofit People's Medical Society, a consumer-advocacy organization credited with key improvements in the quality of US health care, and is author or coauthor of more than 20 consumer-health books.

If you're a caregiver—whether you're the spouse, a family member, friend or someone who's been hired—dealing with the "patient's" doctor can be a problem. Due to a patient's advanced age or disability or the nature of his/her illness (such as dementia), he may not be able to communicate effectively with the physician. All too often, however, caregivers are not exactly sure what their rights are when it comes to dealing with the doctors caring for their loved one or charge. *What helps…*

•**Start with the patient.** Assuming that the person being cared for needs help at the doctor's office and/or interacting with the doctor, the caregiver (and possibly other family members) should gently explain to the patient that the caregiver will help with all medical issues. This typically includes accompanying the patient to appointments…asking questions…taking notes…and discussing with the doctor related issues, such as symptoms to watch out for or the need for home-care services. The patient should also be reassured that the caregiver will be there to help with—but not dominate—the patient's interactions with the doctor. The patient should feel that he and the caregiver are a team.

•**Get the paperwork in order.** Under federal law, including privacy rules found in HIPAA (Health Insurance Portability and Accountability Act), patients have the right to designate whomever they wish to receive medical information from their doctors or hospitals. But the patient must complete the relevant paperwork with each doctor or hospital. A person also can be designated by being named in an "advance directive" (such as a living will or health-care power of attorney), which states who can receive the patient's health information and who can make medical decisions if the patient is unable or unwilling to do so. Printable advance directive documents (customized for the state in which the patient lives) are available at AARP. org/caregiving/financial-legal/free-printable-advance-directives. Even without these documents, patients have the right to have anyone they wish accompany them during their physician appointments or hospital visits.

•**Make the most of the doctor appointment.** Begin by writing down a list of questions before the appointment. Tell the doctor as soon as you and the patient enter that you have questions that need to be answered before you leave. Also, for each doctor appointment, don't forget to take an up-to-date list of all the medications the patient is taking. Because patients so often see multiple health-care providers, one doctor may not know what another has prescribed.

Important: Even if you are asking the questions or are the person who will implement the doctor's instructions, be sure the doctor speaks directly to the patient. Too often, doctors ignore the patient. Also, if you are not clear about what the doctor is saying or prescribing, ask him to slow down and explain it again and perhaps even write down instructions for you to follow. Don't be rushed. Remember, you are responsible for the patient's care once you leave the office.

Emotional Rescue

Mark Goulston, MD, host of the My Wakeup Call podcast. Dr. Goulston speaks globally on teaching people throughout the world to listen to one another. His books include *Talking to Crazy: How to Deal with the Irrational and Impossible People in Your Life* and *Just Listen: Discover the Secret to Getting Through to Absolutely Anyone.* MarkGoulston.com

It's painful to watch someone you care about when he/she is upset, anxious or having an emotional meltdown. These situations come in all sizes and shapes—your teenage daughter just broke up with her boyfriend…your spouse is panicked about an upcoming presentation at work…a friend's job interview was a disaster. You may find yourself scrambling for the right words, but somehow what you say only adds fuel to their fire.

When nothing you say seems to help, that's a good time to try this calm approach developed by psychiatrist—and former hostage-negotiation trainer—Mark Goulston, MD, to support people through a crisis.

WHY LOGIC DOESN'T WORK

First, you need to know why what you normally do doesn't work. When we see that someone is upset, a common—but ineffective—reaction is to appeal to logic and try to convince the person that everything will work out. Unfortunately, well-intentioned comments such as, "Calm down, it's not so bad" or "There's nothing to worry about," are heard by him/her as, *Your problem is inconsequential or unimportant.* Even our instinct to offer multiple solutions to the problem likely will backfire. That's because the person is in the grip of the fight-or-flight response. The amygdala—the part of the brain that plays an important role in processing emotion—is flooding the bloodstream with stress-related hormones such as cortisol, making clear thinking difficult to impossible. Appeals to reason while he is so emotional just add to the person's upset.

In contrast, identifying with what another person is feeling through empathy creates a sense of connection. It is basic to human relationships. When someone nonjudgmentally acknowledges what is going on with us, that feeling of being understood creates a powerful sense of acceptance and relief. And that can diffuse a tense situation.

My technique of targeted empathy goes even farther, inviting the person in pain to go deeper into the emotion he is experiencing—and allowing him to feel profoundly seen and heard. As a result, defenses relax and the person becomes more open to alternative ways of seeing a situation.

6 STEPS TO TARGETED EMPATHY

Targeted empathy involves a series of six steps. You may not need to follow all the steps, but you should attempt them in order, since each one builds on the next. By going through the steps and taking time to understand the person instead of rushing to fix the problem, you empower him to engage the part of the brain that excels at problem solving... and to create meaningful solutions.

STEP 1: **Listen for hyperbole.** As the other person talks about what is upsetting him, listen for extreme words such as awful...impossible... never again...hate.

STEP 2: **Pause for three seconds after the person has finished speaking.** Not only should you be careful not to interrupt, but allow for some silence before you say anything back. This response communicates the fact that you are seriously considering what he has said.

STEP 3: **Ask about one of the extreme words or phrases the person just used.** Say, "Tell me more about..." or "Say more about..."

Example: Your spouse says, "This project at work is hopeless. I was crazy to agree to work on it." You reply, "Tell me more about what makes the project seem hopeless."

This approach is the opposite of what many of us instinctively do. Typically, we try to reassure by saying, "It's not hopeless" or "You're not crazy" or "Why don't you ask your boss for more time?" Someone in crisis isn't ready to believe those words and is more likely to feel dismissed and misunderstood. In contrast, by encouraging the person to express—and explore—his strong feelings, you create an environment of acceptance and safety.

Once the person begins to tell you more about his feelings, you may notice that his whole perspective is beginning to shift, and he is calming down.

STEP 4: **Give voice to deeper emotions.** To further validate the person's experience, state three to five words that seem to describe how he may be feeling and ask him to pick one.

As a way of introducing this step, you can say, "I want to really understand what you're going through. Let me run some words by you, and you pick the one that connects with you the most."

Examples: For a heartbroken teen, you might offer hurt...crushed...lonely...angry...confused.

For an anxious spouse the night before a presentation, offer overwhelmed...burned out... worried...distracted.

For a friend beating himself up after a bad job interview, perhaps discouraged...embarrassed...pessimistic...frustrated.

This simple approach is more effective than directly asking, "Are you angry?" or "Are you hurt?" A direct question can come across as confrontational and put the person on the defensive. By offering a choice of named feelings, you are keeping the lines of communication open.

STEP 5: **Keep exploring those feelings.** Once the person has chosen a word or words, help him explore those words. Repeat them back by saying, "Tell me more about that" or "Tell me about another time you felt like this." The more he talks as you listen empathetically, the calmer and less alone he is likely to feel.

STEP 6: **Facilitate his problem-solving.** Once you feel he has calmed down and is ready to address the problem, you can begin to ask constructive questions about past situations that might be relevant, such as, "What was your impulse in a past similar situation?"..."What did you end up doing in that situation?"..."What are one or two things you did that worked?" These questions move the person toward a solution— but one of his own making, not yours.

Ask: "In this current situation, what's something you might try now?"

MANAGING YOUR EMOTIONS

Engaging with someone at this deeper level takes commitment and courage. Maintaining your sense of calm and safety can be challenging when someone else is so miserable. Yet if you get upset on the person's behalf or overly anxious, you cannot help the other person.

To keep from getting "hooked" by the other person's words or behavior, focus on being curious about the event that has caused the distress. Genuine curiosity will reduce the temptation to interject your own opinions or talk him out of what he is feeling.

What You Can Do to Help a Loved One at Risk for Suicide

Daniel J. Reidenberg, PsyD, executive director of Suicide Awareness Voices of Education (SAVE), managing director of the National Council for Suicide Prevention and general secretary of the International Association for Suicide Prevention. Based in Minneapolis, he also is the former chair of the American Psychotherapy Association. SAVE.org

---

Kate Spade. Anthony Bourdain. Jeremy Richman (father of a Sandy Hook victim). These tragic, high-profile deaths shine a light on the frightening, rising trend of suicides. According to the Centers for Disease Control and Prevention (CDC), the rate of suicide in the US has increased by 31% between 2001 and 2017, with approximately 47,000 people taking their own lives in 2019. For men it increased 21%, and for women a shocking 50%.

More sobering statistics: The suicide rate for females is highest among those ages 45 to 64, and the highest increase in suicide is in men who are age 50 and over. We don't have any definitive reasons why middle age is such a vulnerable time, but multiple factors likely play a role—excessive stress at midlife, financial challenges and better reporting of suicide numbers.

Losing a loved one is always devastating, but in the case of suicide it's even more so because it theoretically didn't have to happen. Survivors of suicide—the partners, family members and friends left behind—often are tormented by guilt about what they might or should have done: *If I had seen the signs more clearly, acted faster, would he/she still be alive?* The answer may be no—suicides can and do occur without warning—but in many cases, there are red flags. And there are steps you can take to keep someone from suicide.

RISK FACTORS IN PLAIN SIGHT

Not surprisingly, some estimates suggest that up to 90% of suicides occur in people suffering from psychiatric issues. They may have bipolar disorder, schizophrenia, dementia, anxiety disorder or post-traumatic stress disorder or they may abuse substances, particularly alcohol. If you know a loved one who suffers from any of these, you likely already understand the importance of watchfulness. Likewise, if someone you know suddenly becomes overwhelmed by a death, job loss or a chronic or terminal illness, you should be on alert for trouble.

But what about those problems you can't see? Many psychiatric issues are undiagnosed—it's estimated that only half of Americans experiencing major depression receive treatment, yet research consistently shows a strong link between depression and suicide. There are many other risk factors, as well, that may be hidden from your view. *Examples…*

•**Being a victim of trauma or abuse**—experiences some people may never share—increases the odds of suicide.

•**Taking a medication**—one that you don't know someone is on or that you are not familiar with—that puts a person at risk. More than 200 commonly used prescription medications have been linked to increased suicide risk.

According to a recent study, more than one-third of Americans take medications that may increase their risk for depression, and close to one-quarter take drugs that list suicidal symptoms as a side effect. As you might expect, medications to treat mental health issues, such as some types of antidepressants and sedatives, can fall into this category. But so do some birth control pills, steroids, beta-blockers, anticonvulsants, proton pump inhibitors, some antibiotics (including fluoroquinolones) and medications for acne, asthma, allergy and smoking cessation.

Before someone you love starts a new drug, have him/her ask the doctor about risks or side effects and double-check with the pharmacist. If suicide is a potential side effect, have a discussion with the doctor about getting a different prescription. If suicidal thoughts are a possibility, be on the lookout for out-of-character behavior, including withdrawing from routine activities or changes in sleeping and eating patterns.

WATCH FOR RED FLAGS

When someone is suicidal, it's unusual if there aren't any warning signs, but it can be difficult to see them. Everyone is busy with his own life and may not pick up on red flags. It may be months between visits with a friend, sibling or college-age child, making it hard to see a trend. The person considering suicide also is likely to hide his thoughts because of the stigma and shame associated with them. Someone who commits suicide may even have seemed "fine" the day before.

That's why it's important to recognize clues that are a cry for help. *The consensus-based list of warning signs, according to Suicidal Awareness Voices of Education are (in order of risk)…*

- **Talking about wanting to die or to kill oneself**
- **Looking for a way to kill oneself**
- **Talking about feeling hopeless or having no purpose**
- **Talking about feeling trapped or being in unbearable pain**
- **Talking about being a burden to others**
- **Increasing the use of alcohol or drugs**
- **Acting anxious, agitated or reckless**
- **Sleeping too little or too much**
- **Withdrawing or feeling isolated**
- **Showing rage or talking about seeking revenge**
- **Displaying extreme mood swings.**

THE CONVERSATION YOU MUST HAVE

If you see any of the red flags listed, you're going to need to talk with the person. A common misconception is that just mentioning suicide can put the idea into someone's head, but that couldn't be further from the truth. Your willingness to talk actually can prevent a death. It's certainly not an easy conversation to have,

but providing support and connectedness with others during a difficult time are what therapists call "protective factors" because they make someone less likely to engage in suicidal behaviors. *Still, what you say and how you say it can help or hurt the situation…*

- **Avoid making the person feel guilty about his thoughts.** Saying, "You wouldn't be thinking about hurting yourself, would you?" sends the message that you really don't want to hear what's going on with that person, and his response likely will be to shut down. Nor should you minimize what the person is going through by referring to it as a "rough patch" or saying "Things aren't that bad" or "You have everything to live for." These statements reinforce the idea that the person is weak, increase feelings of guilt and hopelessness and make him think that he can't tell anyone how he feels.

- **Bring up your concerns honestly and openly.** Say, "I'm genuinely worried about you. Can we talk?" Start by asking, "Do you feel so bad that you think about committing suicide?" If the answer is "yes" or "sometimes," follow that with, "Do you have a plan to kill yourself?" With each successive "yes" or "maybe," gather as much information as you can while keeping the conversation going—"Have you thought about what method you would use?" "When are you thinking about doing this?"

Note: Even though it may be uncomfortable, it's important to use the word "suicide" in the conversation. This person's brain is focused on death and dying, and that's what you need to connect with. Talking about it in a nonjudgmental, nonconfrontational way is more likely to make him accept help.

Surely, you'll be frightened if presented with affirmative answers or actual plans. Know, however, that there are immediate steps you can take to help…

- **Acknowledge what the person has said to you.** Say, "I'm glad you shared that with me."

Other helpful statements: "You don't have to go through this alone" or "Treatment does work."

- **Ask who else he has talked to.** If your loved has not already reached out to a doctor or a crisis hotline, suggest doing it together—"I'm worried about what you're saying. Let's call the National Suicide Prevention Lifeline at 800-273-TALK (8255) right now."

•**Do some research together.** Go online and look at the suicide warning signs together, just as you would do for any sort of ache or pain, to help minimize the stigma of mental illness. Hopefully, this exercise will convince the person that it's time to get help.

•**Make an appointment.** If the person doesn't seem to be in imminent danger, reassure him that suicidal feelings are treatable. Together, call and set up a time for the person to see a mental health professional as soon as possible. Be tenacious about following up. If necessary, make the appointment yourself, and go to the appointment with him.

•**Recognize an emergency situation.** If you suspect imminent danger, call 911 or take your loved one to a hospital emergency room. Don't leave someone alone if he seems to be at high risk. If he storms out or locks himself in a room, you may have to call for help.

Important to know: Firearms are the most commonly used method of suicide among men in the US, and poisoning (including pills) is the most common method among women in the US, so also explain that you are removing access to these—or another method the person might have told you about.

Organic Foods Best for Kids

Children's risk for depression appears to be increased by exposure to certain pesticides. The pesticides, which include *organophosphates* and *carbamates*, are used in commercial agriculture. Some, such as the organophosphate *malathion*, are sold for residential use, too, under brand names such as Ortho Malathion or Spectracide Malathion. Buy organic produce or submerge produce in a mixture of one teaspoon baking soda and two cups of water for two minutes before consumption.

José Suárez-Lopez, MD, PhD, assistant professor in the department of family medicine and public health at University of California, San Diego. Health.ucsd.edu

Inserting yourself into someone else's life this way is difficult, but—when it comes to suicide prevention—it's necessary. Never worry about being intrusive or overbearing. Finding support, staying connected and limiting isolation can help save a life.

Suicide-Related ER Visits Have Increased

Brett Burstein, PhD, associate investigator, McGill University Health Centre Research Institute, Montreal, Canada, and lead author of a research letter published in *JAMA Pediatrics*.

Kids' suicide-related ER visits doubled between 2007 and 2015. There were 1.12 million suicide-related emergency-room visits by US children ages five to 18 in 2015 (latest data available) compared with 580,000 in 2007. Nearly 45% of the visits were for children ages five to 11.

Should We NOT Give Kids Milk?

Lisa R. Young, PhD, RDN, nutritionist in private practice, adjunct professor of nutrition, New York University, New York City. She is author of *Finally Full, Finally Slim: 30 Days to Permanent Weight Loss One Portion at a Time*.

Humans have been drinking milk for millennia, and it's a dietary staple in many parts of the world. But recent concerns about health risks, such as from growth hormones, antibiotics and saturated fat, have raised questions about whether drinking milk is a good idea—especially for children, who are at a vulnerable stage of their development.

Milk has long been considered by many to be a wholesome source of nutrition—particularly calcium, vitamin D and protein—for not many calories. Children in particular are urged to drink it as one of the best ways to ensure strong bones in adulthood.

It's true that many of the essential nutrients children need for optimal growth and development are available in other foods. However, unless a child is vegan, lactose-intolerant or willing to down large quantities of Swiss chard and sardines, milk is probably the easiest, most concentrated way to get those vitamins and minerals into his/her growing body.

MILK FOR STRONG BONES?

As for milk being the dietary guardian of our bones, that claim has been revised. A recent large study from Harvard University found that higher milk consumption during adolescence did not, in fact, decrease risk for hip fracture in later adulthood. We now know that healthy bones depend on many diet and lifestyle factors of which dairy can be a part, but it is not the only player.

The bottom line is that even though milk doesn't merit perfect food status, neither should it be demonized. Whether to give dairy to children or not is really a matter of preference. *As long as a child doesn't have an allergy or intolerance, it's fine to include an appropriate amount of dairy as part of a varied, healthy diet—with one important exception…*

• **Children under age one should not consume cow's milk.** Infants' digestive systems haven't matured sufficiently to handle cow's milk proteins. Cow's milk can irritate infant intestinal linings and cause bleeding, putting young babies at risk for developing iron-deficiency anemia. The American Academy of Pediatrics (AAP) recommends that babies be breast-fed for the first six months or given formula…and given breast milk or formula to drink until age one. (Formula based on cow's milk is OK because the milk has been altered to mimic breast milk.) Once a child is able to eat finger foods, it's usually OK to introduce yogurt or cheese—separately. But hold off on milk until age one.

• **Don't let milk replace other foods.** Kids have tiny tummies, and filling up with milk means less room for leafy greens, fruits, legumes, nuts and other sources of protein and other healthy foods. Also, drinking too much milk may lead to the calcium in milk interfering with iron absorption. Finally, too much milk can lead to excess weight gain. A study of nearly 9,000 four- and five-year-olds from University of Virginia found that children who drank three or more servings of milk daily were more likely to be overweight than children who drank up to two daily servings. But too much of any food can lead to weight gain.

• **Low-fat milk vs. whole milk.** Because developing brains need a certain amount of fat, including saturated fat, AAP recommends that one-year-olds should drink whole milk. AAP then recommends switching to reduced-fat or skim milk at age two to reduce risk for obesity and elevated cholesterol.

However, whether whole milk or low-fat/reduced-fat milk is better for young children is still under debate. Several studies, including one from University of Virginia School of Medicine that looked at two-to-four-year-olds, have found that children who continue drinking whole milk tend to be slimmer. The thinking is that whole milk makes children feel more satisfied, which results in them consuming fewer calories overall. A 2016 study of 2,745 children ages one to six from University of Toronto published in *The American Journal of Clinical Nutrition* found that those who drank whole milk had lower BMIs and higher levels of vitamin D than those who drank 1% milk.

In the end, whether a child gains too much weight depends on what is eaten in the whole diet. So either kind of milk can be OK. A good compromise may be choosing reduced-fat milk.

• **Include varieties of dairy.** Yogurt contains probiotics, which have many health benefits, and cheese is a good concentrated source of protein. So the two to three daily servings of dairy that a child needs (depending on age) might be one-half cup to one cup of milk for breakfast…a cheese stick at lunch…and one-half cup to one cup of plain or low-sugar yogurt for a snack. Opt for milk and dairy products that are free of rbGH, a synthetic growth hormone (also called rbST), if possible.

CAN'T DRINK MILK?

Children who are allergic to dairy, lactose-intolerant or vegan can still get their calcium, vitamin D and protein from other foods. Just keep in mind that milk provides eight grams (g) of protein and 300 milligrams (mg) of calcium per cup, so you'll need to replicate that.

Plant-based milks—such as almond, oat and rice milks—should be avoided, as they are less nutritious than cow's milk and often contain added sweeteners and artificial flavorings. Even if these milks are fortified, it is not known if the added nutrients are as absorbable as they would be when naturally occurring. The exception is soy milk, which is the preferred alternative for children who can't drink cow's milk. But be sure to choose a brand that is unsweetened.

•**Nondairy sources of calcium.** Swiss chard (101 mg calcium/cup), broccoli (31 mg calcium/ ½ cup), sardines (with bones, 92 mg/two sardines), canned salmon (with bones, 78 mg calcium/ounce), almonds (75 mg calcium/ounce), chickpeas (77 mg calcium/cup) and dried figs (45 mg calcium/ounce) are all good sources of calcium. Calcium-fortified orange juice provides 500 mg of calcium per cup. Mixing it up is the best way to make sure children get a sufficient variety and quantity of nutrients to support their developing bodies' needs. Canned salmon finger sandwiches, almond butter spread on crackers, broccoli flowerets to dip in hummus and rainbow-colored baby chard salad are great ways to make these foods kid-friendly.

Bottom line: Milk still "does a body good." Kids don't have to have milk, but they also don't need to fear it. Getting the same nutrients from other sources is fine—so long as they get all the nutrients and enough of them.

Infant-Feeding Guides May Lead to Overfeeding

Bruce Y. Lee, MD, associate professor, Johns Hopkins Bloomberg School of Public Health, Baltimore, executive director, Global Obesity Prevention Center, and senior author of a study published in *American Journal of Preventive Medicine.*

Infants whose parents followed guidelines from Children's Hospital of Philadelphia and Johns Hopkins Medical Institutions—intended to help start infants on solid foods—were categorized as overweight within just a few months. The same effect was found when following guidelines issued by formula makers Enfamil

and Similac. Since testing real infants would be complex and involve ethical issues, the findings were based on computer-simulation models. But researchers say that their results appear to reflect real-world conditions. Talk to your doctor about a personalized approach to feeding your baby.

How Well Are You Feeding Your Children?

Study of 150 families by researchers at University of Minnesota, Minneapolis, published in *Journal of the Academy of Nutrition and Dietetics.*

Based only on meals, children ages five to seven had an average Healthy Eating Index score of 55.3 out of a possible 100. But when snacks were included in the analysis, the average score was 57.1. Kids in the study got an average of 1,215 calories a day from meals and an average of 1,581 calories from meals and snacks combined. Children who had snacks appeared to get more fruits and other elements of a healthful diet than kids who did not snack. But they also were more likely to have higher consumption of refined grains and sugar-sweetened drinks. To learn more about the Healthy Eating Index, go to FNS.USDA.gov/ cnpp/hei-resources.

Water Helps Kids Avoid Empty Calories

Asher Rosinger, PhD, director, Water, Health and Nutrition Laboratory, Pennsylvania State University, University Park, and leader of a study of 8,400 children, ages two to 19, published in *JAMA Pediatrics.*

One-fifth of US children do not drink water on any given day. Nonwater drinkers consume almost twice as many calories a day from sugar-sweetened beverages as kids who do drink water. That adds up to about 100 extra calories a day, on average, a difference that can contribute over time to children becoming overweight or obese. (Diet soda, fruit juice and other unsweetened drinks were excluded from the study.) Consumption of sugary drinks among American children has fallen in the last 15 years, but some geographic areas and certain populations still have high consumption.

Preschool Exercise Affects Future Heart Health

Study of more than 400 children, by researchers at McMaster University, Hamilton, Ontario, Canada, published in *Pediatrics*.

Physical activity in children as young as age three improves blood vessel health and cardiovascular fitness—and may help prevent adult heart disease. Arteries begin to stiffen when children are very young—and physical activity slows the process. Intense physical activity—such as playing games until out of breath—is beneficial as well, especially when children are active throughout the day.

Screen Time with the Grandkids

Elisabeth McClure, PhD, research specialist at Centre on Creativity, Play and Learning at the LEGO Foundation in Denmark.

Do you have a long-distance relationship with your grandchildren? Three cheers for video chats!

Although the American Academy of Pediatrics (AAP) recommends no screen media before age two (see next article), it makes an exception for video chatting in reasonable amounts.

Children under six can struggle with traditional phone calls, and toddlers have difficulty engaging with a disembodied voice. With video chat, they can interact in the ways that they interact in person. *Here are specific ways you can engage with your grandchildren via video contact...*

•**Read a book.** Point to the pictures. Use the same warm interaction you would in person.

Mud Pies Keep Kids Happy

Kids who make mud pies may have a lower risk for mental illness.

Possible reason: An anti-inflammatory fat in a dirt-dwelling bacterium. The new finding may explain why childhood exposure to bacteria appears to reduce anxiety and other stress-related disorders.

Psychopharmacology

Note: Schedule reading time for well before bedtime. Exposure to blue light at bedtime may make it difficult for the child to fall asleep.

•**Call at snack time but not formal mealtimes.** Pretend to eat the food your grandchild offers you and enjoy it enthusiastically! Have your own snacks ready to pretend-share back with the toddler.

•**Play a board game.** Once a child is old enough for games such as Candy Land, the two of you can play "together" over video chat, with your grandchild driving the game board for both of you.

•**Ask a physically present caregiver to help.** Recite "This Little Piggy Went to Market" while Dad squeezes each toe in time with your song.

•**Respect moods.** There's no right length for a chat. If you choose a time that works for a child's moods and use these techniques, you'll be surprised how time will fly. In most home observations, calls rarely lasted less than 15 minutes.

More Screen Time, Slower Brain Development

John Hutton, MD, director, Reading and Literacy Discovery Center, Cincinnati Children's Hospital, and leader of a study published online in *JAMA Pediatrics*.

Children ages three to five who spent more time in front of screens had slower mental-processing skills and lower levels of literacy than ones who spent less time with screens. The first five years of life are crucial for brain development—deficits can be made up later, but it is harder for the brain to change as people get older. The American Academy of Pediatrics says kids under 18 months should have no screen exposure other than video chatting...and from ages two to five, screen time should be limited to one hour a day.

Social Comparison Harmful for Kids

JAMA Pediatrics

The more time spent streaming videos or in front of the TV, the greater the risk for severe depression in young people.

One reason: They unconsciously engage in upward social comparison, comparing themselves with other teens with seemingly perfect lifestyles.

Video Gaming Is Not a Clinical Disorder

Andrew Przybylski, PhD, director of research, Oxford Internet Institute, Oxford, UK, and coauthor of a study of more than 1,000 adolescents and their caregivers, published in *Clinical Psychological Science*.

The World Health Organization voted to consider obsessive gaming an international disease, but a new study shows that even when adolescents play video games obsessively, it does not mean that the gaming constitutes a clinical issue. Some gamers use video games to escape underlying frustrations and psychological turmoil in their lives—issues not caused by the games, even when people play them for three hours a day or more. This means some adolescents are using video games as a coping mechanism—and taking the games away out of a belief that game-playing is a mental disorder could leave game players without a good way to deal with depression, anxiety and other conditions.

Constructive Use of Social Media OK?

Sarah Coyne, PhD, professor of family life, Brigham Young University, Provo, Utah, and leader of an eight-year study of 500 young people, ages 13 to 20, published in *Computers in Human Behavior.*

Controversial new finding: Social media does not harm teens' mental health. The amount of time teenagers spend on social-media sites has risen by 62.5% since 2012 and continues to increase. In 2018, the average time spent on social media was estimated as 2.6 hours per day. But worries that this usage is increasing anxiety or depression in teens appear unfounded.

Reason: What matters is how teenagers use social-media sites, not how long they use them. Those who use the sites actively to seek out information, connect with others, and comment and post do not appear to have mental-health issues associated with site usage.

Important for social-media users: Limit use for at least an hour before falling asleep.... consider your motivations for engaging in social media—those reasons are more important for mental health than the amount of time spent.

Teen Drivers With ADHD Have Higher Crash Risk

Allison E. Curry, PhD, MPH, senior scientist and director of epidemiology and biostatistics, Center for Injury Research and Prevention, Children's Hospital of Philadelphia, and leader of a study published in *Pediatrics.*

In the first month during which a teenager with attention-deficit/hyperactivity disorder is driving, he/she has a 62% higher risk for a crash than other teens have. Over a four-year period, the risk remains 37% higher for teens with ADHD.

Also: About 36% of teens with ADHD get traffic tickets in their first year of driving—compared with 25% of new drivers without ADHD.

Eating Habits and Autism

Susan D. Mayes, PhD, professor of psychiatry at Penn State College of Medicine, Hershey, Pennsylvania, and coauthor of a study published in *Research in Autism Spectrum Disorders*.

Quirky eating habits may be an early sign of autism in young children. Children with autism often severely limit their choices to foods such as chicken nuggets, pizza and pasta…cannot tolerate certain textures…pocket food in the mouth…eat inedible substances…and/or stick to one color or shape of food. Unusual eating behavior is present in 70% of children with autism, versus only 5% of typical children. Children with these behaviors should be screened for autism so that they can receive early intervention.

Earlier Autism Diagnosis

Karen Pierce, PhD, codirector, University of California, San Diego, Autism Center of Excellence, and leader of a study published in *JAMA Pediatrics*.

Autism may be diagnosed in 14-month-olds. It typically is diagnosed when a child is age three or four, but diagnoses made shortly after a child's first birthday were accurate 84% of the time when the children were reevaluated at age three. And almost all the remaining 16% were found to have some other developmental delay. Diagnosing autism spectrum disorder as early as possible allows treatment to begin before the brain has fully formed connections—raising the possibility that better connections could be made. However, clinical outcomes from treatment starting soon after a child's first birthday remain unknown.

Alzheimer's Drug Shows Promise for Autism

Sheba Medical Center

When 60 children with autism received an Alzheimer's drug, their language skills improved.

Theory: Alzheimer's drugs, such as *donepezil* (Aricept), increase brain levels of *acetylcholine*, a neurotransmitter that's low in both autistic children and Alzheimer's patients.

The Right Kind of Self-Talk Boosts Math Skills

Sander Thomaes, PhD, professor of psychology, Utrecht University, the Netherlands, and leader of a study of 212 children, published in *Child Development*.

Kids' positive self-talk can boost math success if the self-talk focuses on effort, not ability. Children in grades four through six, ages nine to 13, who had negative beliefs about their math ability and who engaged in positive self-talk about doing their best, did better when tested than kids whose self-talk focused on ability—or ones who did no self-talk.

Help a Child Fall in Love with Reading

Maria Russo, PhD, editor of children's books at *The New York Times* and coauthor of *How to Raise a Reader*.

Reading together is one of the most powerful ways to create an emotional bond with your child or grandchild, and with the right techniques and attitude, it's a way to instill a lifelong love of reading.

•**Choose books for the child, not the child's "reading level."** While it's important not to choose a book that's overly complicated for a younger reader, don't worry if the reading level of the book is a bit above or below where the child is at. Reading at home should be about fun, not about "achievement" or "levels"—leave all that to the child's teachers. The most important thing is to think about what excites the child and what topics will be enriching. Kids who say that they don't like reading usually haven't found something that engages them. Graphic novels, picture books, collections of world records, sports statistics, jokes and/or weird facts all are perfectly good choices for young readers.

•**Get comfy.** You could hold a child on your lap, but some kids prefer sitting by your side—beanbag chairs are great to create a cozy feeling of closeness while reading. And some children may have "ants in their pants." Don't assume that a toddler in motion isn't listening. Let him/her move.

•**Take your time.** Reading to a child isn't about getting to the finish line…it's about engagement. With picture books, a child might look at the illustrations in a different order and at a different pace than the words you're reading. Stay flexible, and let the book take you where the child wants to go.

•**Stay enthusiastic, even when reading the same book for the thousandth time.** Repetition is good for babies and older children. Wanting to hear the same story over and over is a part of cognitive development—they're processing the words and the small details.

•**Enhance reading with conversation.** Reading isn't just about speaking the words on the page. With picture books, children "read" by taking in information from the illustrations. Start a conversation around something that is in the drawings. You might ask, "What do you see?" or "What's happening here?"

•**Laugh off any mistakes you make.** This shows a child that no one is infallible. Once kids start school, they feel so much pressure to be perfect—if they see you aren't, they will feel freer.

•**Create new family reading traditions as your child gets older.** One idea is to have a family book club—everyone reads the same book and gathers to talk about it after every chapter or set number of pages.

Kids Read More When Dogs Are Nearby

Study by researchers at University of British Columbia, Canada, published in *Anthrozoös*.

*R**ecent finding:** When a dog was in the room where a child age six to eight was reading, the child was motivated to continue reading longer and to get through moderately challenging passages. The findings held for children in first, second and third grade. This could open the door to further use of therapy dogs for improving children's reading abilities—some schools already use dogs to try to help children who are struggling to read.

Choosing the Right Foods for a Healthier Dog

Lisa P. Weeth, DVM, veterinary nutritionist at Weeth Nutrition Services in Los Angeles. She helps develop diets for dogs with chronic medical conditions and to optimize the health of healthy dogs. WeethNutrition.com

*P*et owners are willing to pay a premium if they think they are giving their dogs the best food—more than $30 billion now is being spent on pet food in the US annually, and there has been a huge increase in the number of brands and formulations. Knowing what's necessary and what's simply fancy packaging can be a challenge—and you may be spending more than you need to. *Here's what you may not realize when figuring out what to feed your canine companion…*

•**Low-cost dog foods can have high-quality ingredients.** Don't get fooled by expensive foods—they may simply be more steeply priced because people will pay more for their perceived value and not because the ingredients are higher quality or better for your dog. Marketers tout the benefits of their pricey, all-organic food, but the truth is, even the lower-priced dog foods will provide all the nutrients your dog needs without any unnecessary ingredients. The large portion of a dog's diet should be protein, but their food also needs whole grains, fruits and vegetables to provide necessary nutrients and fiber.

•**Rest assured that dog food is held to the same quality standards as human food.** There are strict regulations from the Food and Drug Administration that govern what's put into pet food. Lower-cost foods often just use less expensive versions of the ingredients.

Example: Less expensive dog food might contain more organ meats such as liver and kidneys and less muscle meats, but organ meats still provide plenty of protein for your dog and are a good source of vitamins and minerals to boot.

Note: Ingredients such as cranberries and carrots often are listed to make people feel good. In reality, the amounts are so low and they are cooked at such a high temperature that they're typically not providing any nutrients.

•**For dogs that tend to get constipated, opt for wet food instead of dry.** Canned foods have a higher fat profile that can make a dog's stools a little bit softer than kibble-only diets. It's also OK to feed your dog a mix of both wet and dry, but it's not necessary. Wet food does not lead to tartar buildup on teeth, and dry food doesn't help reduce it. That's because dogs don't really chew the kibble very much.

Note: Fresh commercial pet foods may help reduce the size of your dog's poop—they are more digestible and so more of the food gets into the animal.

•**Don't feed dogs food containing onions or garlic.** If you are going to cook for your dog or offer table scraps, you should know that many ingredients that are fine for humans can be dangerous for pets. Most pet owners already know about the dangers of chocolate, which can cause vomiting, diarrhea and internal bleeding. But it may surprise you to hear that onions and garlic also are dangerous—they contain compounds that can damage your pet's red blood cells and cause anemia if eaten more than once a week. And xylitol, an artificial sweetener common in chewing gum and sometimes in peanut butter and other foods, can be toxic in even small amounts. Other toxic foods include grapes and macadamia nuts. Also avoid fatty leftovers such as chicken skin, as they can increase risk for pancreatitis and diarrhea.

Instead: Try broccoli, zucchini and skinless chicken breast.

•**Offer healthy dog treats.** There are many treats on the market—from peanut butter popsicles to sweet potato jerky—but commercial treats can be calorie dense, and while they're helpful for positive reinforcement and creating an emotional bond, they aren't necessary. Healthy snacks are as close as your cupboard. Cheerios (original variety), plain popcorn and fruits and veggies can be just as delicious—and have fewer calories. Just like with humans, treats can sneak up on your pets, so don't overdo—they can quickly become 20% to 50% of a dog's diet.

•**Be careful about creating your own dog food.** Some dog owners make their own food—but you'll have to ensure that your recipe gives your dog adequate amounts of protein, fatty acids, vitamins and fiber. It's important to work with someone who understands nutrition and can guide you in creating your homemade diet—ideally a veterinary nutritionist. Most homemade diets provide enough animal proteins and calories but are weak at balancing nutrients. Problems from deficiencies may take months or years to surface. Generally, things like a lack of zinc, vitamin E or fatty acids are noticeable from the outside, but a deficiency of calcium or vitamin D can brew under the surface until it is too late. Websites such as PetDiets.com could help you explore a homemade diet, but you also should get advice from your veterinarian.

•**Dogs don't typically need foods tailored to a specific breed.** Dog food marketed to specific breeds is a lot of hype, but there are some notable exceptions. Some longer-coated breeds might benefit from more fatty acids to keep their coats shiny and reduce shedding, while larger breeds may need more fiber in their diet than smaller dogs to keep their gastrointestinal tracts working well. And flat-faced dogs such as pugs may find it easier to eat specially shaped kibble (perhaps a cloverleaf shape) that makes it easier for them to grab it out of the bowl.

•**Skip the senior formula.** Foods for older dogs are more of a marketing ploy than a real need—as evidenced by the fact that there's little consistency in the formulations among the brands. Some reduce the calorie count. Others lower the phosphorus in expectation that a senior dog has kidney disease. Unless your veterinarian suggests a certain diet for health issues, a standard adult food will work fine. If your senior dog needs fewer calories because of a lower activity level, you might be able to bulk up the food with fruits and veggies. However, make sure your dog is still getting at least 80% of calories from a commercial diet to avoid an unbalanced diet that could lead to a nutritional deficiency.

Note: Fish oil can be helpful for dogs with arthritis to help decrease inflammation—and the DHA may help senior dogs maintain their brain health.

•**Feeding guidelines are a good starting point but don't need to be followed exactly.** The suggested amounts for your dog's size and weight may be pretty close for about 90% of the dog population, but depending on your individual dog's activity level, you may need to go lower or higher to maintain a healthy weight for your dog. The easiest way to tell whether your dog is at a healthy weight is to gently run your palms along the sides of your dog's chest just behind the should blades. If your dog is a healthy weight, you should be able to easily feel his ribs. If the dog is undernourished, you'll be able to see the ribs and the spine…the dog is overfed if you can't feel the ribs at all or only if you press hard enough.

•**Make diet changes gradually.** Your dog's digestive system adapts to a particular diet, so making dramatic changes can upset the dog's stomach. Generally, switching flavors within the same brand or type of food won't upset your dog's digestive system, but if you're making a big change—such as from kibble to a wet food or to a different brand of food—do it gradually by slowly adding more and more of the new food to the dog's meals and less and less of the old food over the course of a week to 10 days. That will help minimize the chance that your dog will develop diarrhea or constipation.

Important: Take note if your dog becomes finicky or reluctant to eat or seems to be less

---

Keep Your Dog Happier When You're Not Home

•**PetCube Play** is an interactive two-way camera with night-vision options—you can see and talk to your pet. *Cost:* $199.

•**PetCube Bites** is similar but also lets you give the pet treats remotely. *Cost:* $299.

•**GoDogGo Fetch Machine** is a tennis-ball launcher that can be used to set up an automated game, customized for your dog's size and speed and the size of your yard. *Cost:* $180.

•**CleverPet** is a kind of game console with about a dozen color-, sound- and light-based puzzles for a dog to solve—designed around dogs' limited color-sensing ability. *Cost:* $290.

USNews.com

---

perky and engaged than usual. That can be a sign that the diet is upsetting your dog's digestion. If your dog seems itchier than usual…develops dry, flaky skin…or his coat loses its sheen, it also might be time to change up the diet. Consult your vet.

Dementia Is Common in Older Dogs

Melissa Bain, DVM, professor of clinical animal behavior at University of California-Davis School of Veterinary Medicine.

Canine cognitive dysfunction (CCD) affects 28% of dogs ages 11 to 12 and 68% of dogs ages 15 to 16. Owners should watch for behavior changes such as wandering at night, pacing, staring and becoming more fearful or anxious. CCD is incurable but can be treated. It helps to keep routines. Ask your vet about diets that can slow cognitive decline and about the prescription drug Anipryl.

"Puppy Eyes" Are an Evolutionary Adaptation

Juliane Kaminski, PhD, comparative psychologist, University of Portsmouth, UK, and leader of a study published in *Proceedings of the National Academy of Sciences.*

Those big, pleading-looking eyes with which dog owners are familiar are made possible by a small muscle that lets dogs raise their inner eyebrows. Those muscles are the only significant facial difference between dogs and their wolf ancestors. The inner-eyebrow-raising movement makes dogs' eyes seem larger, like those of an infant, and also resembles a movement that humans make when sad—so when dogs use this muscle, they provoke more of a nurturing response from humans.

Portly Pooches Have Shorter Lives, Too

Journal of Veterinary Internal Medicine

Humans aren't the only ones harmed by obesity. A 20-year study of more than 50,000 dogs found that overweight animals died up to two and a half years sooner than those of ideal weights.

Cats Bond With Their Owners

Study by researchers at Oregon State University, Corvallis, published in *Current Biology.*

Cats bond with their owners despite their reputation for being standoffish. In about two-thirds of cases, cats bond closely—as shown by the way they relax when their owners return after leaving them alone briefly in a strange environment.

Halloween Treat Helps a Cat's Digestive System

Add pumpkin to your cat's diet to keep its gastrointestinal system healthy. Pumpkin's fiber helps relieve mild cases of constipation and can keep things moving in cats that are prone to constipation. Pumpkin also sweeps hair out of the digestive system, reducing hair balls. It is also a good source of vitamins A and C and contains zinc, all of which can help support the immune system. Use pumpkin purée, not pumpkin-pie filling. Mix one to four tablespoons in the cat's food, but cut back if the cat's stool becomes too loose.

Roundup of veterinarians reported on PetMD.com.

How to Make a Shy Cat Feel Comfortable in a New Home

Pam Johnson-Bennett, owner, Cat Behavior Associates, Nashville, writing at ModernCat.com.

- **Limit its space** so it does not feel overwhelmed by openness.
- **Restrict the cat to one room** at first, and as it becomes more comfortable, let it gradually explore other rooms.
- **Lower lights.**
- **Avoid loud music** and loud talking.
- **Offer plenty of hiding places,** including tunnels, open boxes and paper bags.
- **Put towels and T-shirts** near the hiding places so that the cat becomes familiar with your scent.
- **When first offering food, put the bowl where the cat feels most comfortable** and then leave the room.
- **Schedule meals** so your presence becomes associated with food.
- **Use a fishing-pole kind of toy** so the cat can play while keeping its distance from you.
- *Let the cat set the adjustment pace**—do not rush things.

Teach Your Cat to Walk on a Leash

Roundup of experts on feline behavior, reported in *The New York Times*.

Cats may go camping or hiking, or just join their owners on neighborhood outings—all while wearing a harness. Some cats accept training and the restrictions that come with wearing a harness and leash—especially if owners are patient and reassuring at all times. When this works, it helps reconnect cats with their desire to explore, all within an owner's control. But some cats will not accept or adapt to restraints and will become stressed—they may hide when an owner approaches or become hyperactive. Talk to your veterinarian if you would like to try going on outdoor adventures with your cat, and get advice on the best way to introduce new activities and the signs of stress to watch for.

How to Know a Cat Is Angry

Reader's Digest. RD.com

Signs that a cat is angry or upset: Watching from a distance despite normally being playful…growling…avoiding a favorite toy…hiding and refusing to come out…displaying an arched back, fluffed-out fur and bushy tail…having ears flattened back against the head and slightly sticking out…defecating or urinating on the bed, furniture or laundry…biting when being petted…refusing a favorite meal. Even purring may indicate distress—a purr can show happiness but also may indicate anxiety or fear.

CHAPTER 10

Get the Best Care

Get the Attention You Need in the Emergency Room

Your choice of words in the emergency room (ER) could affect the quality of your care—or even your odds of survival. And I don't mean being polite and saying please and thank you to everyone.

Busy ER doctors and nurses make rapid decisions about which patients are top priorities… and what tests and treatments patients require. How patients describe their conditions and concerns is crucial. A few well-chosen words could get one patient the prompt treatment he/she needs, while poorly chosen ones leave another suffering for hours—or facing a dangerous misdiagnosis. Frighteningly, the right or wrong language has been found to be a big factor particularly in women's survival after a heart attack. Women more often report breathing difficulty,

fatigue or dizziness, rather than the classic chest pain, leading health-care providers off track. Of course, what you say and how you say it affects both sexes.

Here's the right language to use…

SPEAKING WITH THE TRIAGE NURSE

The single most important communication in the ER occurs almost as soon as you arrive, when a triage nurse (or other hospital employee) makes an initial evaluation of the severity of your condition, likely with the assistance of patient-evaluation software. This evaluation often takes just a minute or two, but if there are misunderstandings, it could lead to hours of delay if the nurse and the automated software decide that you're not in immediate danger.

Older patients are especially vulnerable during triage because they don't always experience

---

Joel Cohen, MD, former emergency room physician who now is medical director of DoctorCare, a geriatric house-call practice based in Scottsdale, Arizona. He is coauthor of *BoomER: Emergency Room Survival Guide for Baby Boomers and Older Folks*. EndlessKnotPress. com the dramatic symptoms a younger person would in certain life-threatening situations.

Example: A young adult is likely to be in obvious agony when his appendix is about to burst, leading to quick attention in the ER…but older people often experience only discomfort and loss of appetite.

When the nurse asks what's wrong…

•**Briefly describe your one or two most concerning symptoms.** Put these into context using phrases such as "the worst I've ever felt" or "I've never felt anything like this before," if appropriate.

Example: "I'm having upper-abdominal discomfort that's not like anything I've ever felt before." If it's bad, say it's bad.

If you're concerned that your symptoms could be related to a serious health condition that you have (or you had in the past…or your doctor has warned you that you are at risk of developing), mention this as well.

Examples: "I'm worried because the only time I felt something similar is right before my last heart attack" or "I'm worried because my doctor recently warned me that if I felt something like this, it could be a sign that I'm having a heart attack."

What not to say: Unimportant details about your health saga. A busy triage nurse might cut you off before you get to your most concerning symptoms…or get so buried in your details that he/she overlooks your key complaints.

Example: Some patients try to tell the story of how symptoms started small but grew over time—only to get cut off before they get to the part where the symptoms escalate. Get the important facts out fast.

When the triage nurse asks your pain level, likely on a one-to-10 scale…

•**Provide the honest number,** then add a phrase that explains why this number should be taken especially seriously in your case, if appropriate. Pain tolerances vary—one patient's seven might be worse than another's 10. If you have a high pain tolerance, that's something the triage nurse should know.

Examples: "My pain level is seven…but this is the worst pain I've ever experienced."

Or, "I'll say seven, but I said three when I had a broken collarbone—this is bad."

What not to say: "10"—unless you truly are enduring what you believe to be the worst pain possible. When people say 10, triage nurses often are suspicious that they're exaggerators, complainers or pain-medication addicts in search of a fix.

Note: If you are instructed to use a one-to-10 scale, do not provide a number higher than 10 in an effort to express that you're in extreme pain. That just makes you seem like someone who can't answer questions accurately.

When the triage nurse tells you to take a seat and wait (or you're told to follow someone to a treatment room)…

Ask, "What's my triage level?" ERs are not first-come, first-served. Most ERs assign each patient a number from one to five that represents the level of urgency. The higher your number, the longer you're likely to wait. One means that you require immediate care…two means you require care within the next 14 minutes… three means you need care within one hour… four means within two hours…and five means your case is considered "nonurgent" and you can safely be left waiting as long as 24 hours. (These time frames are guidelines, not guarantees—how long you actually wait depends on how busy the ER is.) If the ER waiting room is crowded and your number is five, it's probably smarter to head to a nearby urgent-care facility, where the wait might be shorter.

Warning: Do not leave the ER if there is any reason to suspect that your condition might be life-threatening despite the high triage level assigned to you. If the situation did become a life-threatening emergency, your odds of survival would be much greater in an ER waiting room than in your car on the way to urgent care. If you don't agree with your triage number, politely ask for the physician in charge to do a quick evaluation. You have the right to ask for reevaluation if you feel worse while in the waiting area.

What not to say: "How long will I have to wait?" ER staff have no way to answer this— a dozen urgent cases may be about to come through the door. Asking could get you labeled a pest.

SPEAKING WITH ER DOCTORS AND NURSES

ERs can be hectic, and doctors and nurses rarely know their patients—a recipe for miscommunications, misdiagnoses and other mistakes. *Four things to ask or tell ER medical personnel…*

•**"Who are you, exactly?"** Each time someone new examines you and/or offers a medical opinion, ask who that person is and what his title is. If it turns out it's a student or resident—a doctor-in-training—ask, "Can I speak with the physician in charge after you are done with your evaluation?" You also have the right to ask for a consultation by a specialist such as a cardiologist for chest pain if your problem is possibly serious or you are not improving.

•**"What is this for? Who ordered it?"** Get these details whenever a hospital employee hands you a pill, starts to stick an IV into your arm or says he's going to take you for a test. ER staff sometimes get patients mixed up. If you're told it was ordered by a doctor whose name you don't know and/or it doesn't sound relevant for your health problem, ask, "Can you double-check that this is for me?" For medications, be sure you have alerted everyone to your medications. Confirm that there are no interactions.

•**"It's the worst I've ever felt."** Don't just say this (and/or "I've never felt anything like this") to the triage nurse, say it to doctors, too, assuming it's accurate. It sends the message that you're not a chronic complainer with an everyday issue—this is an extreme situation to be taken seriously.

•**"Could you run this by my primary care physician?"** If you're in the ER during your doctor's office hours, ask the ER staff to call your doctor to discuss their conclusions before sending you home. Most doctors' offices also can be reached after hours. Even an on-call provider should have access to your medical records and be able to offer the ER useful medical history. This is especially important if they're sending you home with prescription medications.

Three things you should not say…

Do not say: "I know which painkillers work best for me." When patients request specific painkillers—especially opioids—it sends up red flags that these patients might be addicts fabricating medical problems to obtain drugs. (If you're allergic to specific painkillers, definitely do say that, even if the allergy is noted in your records.)

Do not say: "I need to see the doctor right now!" or "I'm going to sue!" Being demanding or making threats in an ER will not get you what you want, but it might get you labeled a nutcase or a problem patient—which would make the ER staff even less eager to deal with you. If you must ask for rapid attention—maybe you've been waiting for a half-hour for a bedpan—a polite-but-urgent request to a nurse at the nurses' station is most likely to produce a rapid response.

Example: "I know you're busy, but I just can't bear it any longer, could you possibly…"

Do not say: "Aghhhh." Don't scream or moan audibly if you can help it. ER staff sometimes take such vocalizations as signs that a patient is exaggerating or faking pain, perhaps to get quicker attention or because of a painkiller addiction. A silent-but-pained facial expression is a more effective way. It is best to seek ER care with a friend or relative to serve as your advocate.

Don't Let Ageism Make You Sick

Sana Goldberg, RN, a registered nurse practicing in New Haven, Connecticut. A public health advocate and member of the International Honor Society of Nursing, Ms. Goldberg has published scientific papers in *Neuropharmacology* and *European Journal of Neuroscience*. She is author of *How to Be a Patient: The Essential Guide to Navigating the World of Modern Medicine.*

Older adults spend the majority of health dollars in the US. So you'd think that doctors and other health-care professionals would treat these individuals—their best customers—with lots of care and respect. But that's often not the case…and the consequences can be catastrophic.

Important new finding: When researchers from Yale School of Public Health and Yale School of Medicine looked at national data to assess the health effects of ageism (which their study defined as prejudice against people age 60 and older), the results were eye-opening.

Over one year, ageism played a role in more than 17 million cases of eight health conditions, including cardiovascular disease, diabetes, chronic respiratory disease and musculoskeletal disorders such as arthritis, according to their research, which was published in *The Gerontologist.* Ageism is estimated to drive up health-care costs by an astounding $63 billion a year.

The good news is, there's plenty you can do to protect yourself—or a loved one—from the perils of ageism.

A DANGEROUS BLIND SPOT

Most Americans have a blind spot when it comes to ageism. People usually don't recognize when they're being ageist…or when ageism is happening to them. *What to watch out for—in others and yourself…*

•**Second-rate treatment.** Age discrimination often shows up as inferior medical treatment.

Example: When you describe a new health problem, the physician says: "It's just your age" or "That's a normal sign of aging"—and doesn't adequately investigate or treat your problem.

A personal story: Not long ago, my mother—who is 65—was walking around for several months with severe pain in her upper thigh.

The doctor she talked to about the problem didn't believe she was in as much pain as she said she was. He chalked it up to arthritis and prescribed a course of steroids. Finally, she went to the emergency room—where X-rays showed that she had a broken femur (thighbone)!

•**Harmful stereotypes.** In the health-care setting, ageist stereotypes—that is, negative beliefs about an older person or older people in general—can be the driving force behind disrespectful treatment from doctors and other medical personnel.

Example: A doctor thinks all older people are somehow impaired in mind and body—and talks to you in a patronizing way, speaking in high-pitched, loud tones as if you were a child.

This type of treatment is more than a mere annoyance. In a study published in *Psychology and Aging,* people age 61 and older who were subjected to patronizing speech performed more poorly on a cognitive test and had higher levels of cortisol, a stress hormone that can trigger high blood pressure, headaches, weight gain and insomnia.

•**Negative self-perceptions.** Surprisingly, older adults often view old age and the aging process negatively themselves.

Example: You think aging—including your own old age—is inevitably associated with forgetfulness, incompetence, decline and disease. And there's significant harm associated with that mind-set.

What the research shows: In a series of studies, people with self-directed ageism were found to be twice as likely to develop cardiovascular disease…have poorer day-to-day function…be less likely to follow health-promoting practices such as eating a balanced diet, exercising regularly and taking prescribed medications…be less likely to seek care for debilitating back pain…and be at greater risk for depression.

PUT A STOP TO AGEISM

Even though health-care ageism is usually deeply ingrained, there are ways to counter it. Once you recognize that older adults are likely to encounter biases when interacting with health professionals, you've taken the first step to overcoming it. *Additional steps…*

•**Be honest about your own attitudes.** Are you guilty of self-directed ageism—for example, do you assume, on some level, that disease and decline are just a "normal" part of aging? If you do, you need to know that such assumptions may not be true, particularly with the advances of modern medicine. Even though health problems are more common in older adults, when you have a condition that interferes with a full, active, fulfilling life—get the care you need and deserve.

•**Stand up for yourself.** Older adults should never be submissive at the doctor's office or the hospital. Don't seek conflict—but don't avoid it either. Give yourself permission to challenge health-care providers who are not meeting your needs.

And if a concern you've raised is dismissed, say something like: "This one thing is really important to me, so I want to make sure we discuss it."

•**Find the right advocate.** Whether you're going for an annual physical, major surgery or anything in between, get an advocate to go to the appointment with you. This will help ensure that you get top-notch treatment.

Helpful: Be choosy about your advocate. You want someone who is dependable, conscientious, loyal and sharp. Before an appointment, ask this person to help you practice the story you plan to tell the physician about your health problem and the questions you'll ask. And don't be shy about telling your doctor any details (even embarrassing ones) that might help you get the best care.

•**Don't wing it.** Many people don't take their doctor appointments seriously enough. You should always ask questions and, of course, write them down in advance.

Examples: What are my treatment options, and which one do you think is the most effective? What are the benefits, risks and side effects of the medicine you are prescribing? Are tests necessary? What will they show and how will they affect treatment? What costs can I expect, and does insurance cover them? If there is no one to take notes, you may want to record the conversation during a doctor appointment on your smartphone. If you do, just be sure to ask the doctor first.

•**Think ahead.** Before you leave any medical appointment, make sure you know the next steps for your care.

Ask questions such as: How long should it be before my next visit? Are there symptoms that mean I should return sooner than planned? How will I know whether this medication is working? What is the best way to reach you if needed?

•**Make sure you're seeing the right type of doctor.** After age 65, your primary care provider should be a geriatrician—a specialist in aging. This doctor will coordinate your care with other specialists, such as a cardiologist or neurologist. The geriatrician also may oversee your care in a hospital setting if he/she has privileges at the hospital.

•**Ask for a reference from your primary care physician.** Or consult the American Geriatrics Society's HealthinAging.org website to find a geriatrician in your area.

Your Doctor's Overconfidence Can Lead to Deadly Medical Errors...

David E. Newman-Toker, MD, PhD, professor of neurology and director of the division of neuro-visual and vestibular disorders at The Johns Hopkins University School of Medicine in Baltimore. He is also director of the Armstrong Institute Center for Diagnostic Excellence in Baltimore.

I n the work world and in life, confidence is a highly appealing trait. But when it goes overboard, it can be dangerous—especially when it's a doctor who is wielding an infallible, all-knowing attitude.

A growing body of evidence suggests that diagnostic errors—diagnoses that are missed, wrong or delayed—may cause as much death and disability as all other types of medical errors

Timing Your Doctor Visit

Patients who see their primary care physician later in the day are less likely to be sent for a cancer screening than those who go earlier. For example, colonoscopy and other colon cancer screenings were ordered more frequently when patients were seen at 8 am (37%) versus at 5 pm (23%).

Theory: Doctors—and patients—suffer from "decision fatigue," where they are less inclined to make new choices after a long day.

Mitesh S. Patel, MD, MBA, MS, director, Penn Medicine Nudge Unit, University of Pennsylvania, Philadelphia.

combined. And a common cause of these errors, research shows, is an overconfident doctor.

Sobering study: To understand how doctors' confidence levels sync up with their accuracy in diagnosing medical conditions, 118 internal medicine doctors in the US were given diagnostic cases to solve online—two that were easy and two that were difficult. The doctors were given the patients' medical profiles (histories, physical exams and diagnostic tests) and could ask for additional resources if they needed help. The doctors got the right diagnosis in 55% of the easy cases, but in only 5.8% of the hard ones, according to the research, which was published in *JAMA Internal Medicine.*

The doctors then were asked to rate their confidence level for each diagnosis on a scale of zero to 10. For the easy cases, the average confidence level was just over seven. For the hard ones—the ones they got right only 5.8% of the time—the confidence level averaged 6.4, hardly dropping at all.

To learn how physician overconfidence can contribute to diagnostic errors, we spoke with David E. Newman-Toker, MD, PhD, a leading expert in patient safety.

How does doctor overconfidence contribute to diagnostic error?

There is a lot of research showing that people who have the highest confidence levels are less competent than their peers who are a little less confident. So having a little uncertainty is a good thing—you're less likely to assume that you're right, and it gives you some motivation to learn and improve. This is now being recognized in medical schools and residency programs. In the past, confidence and quick decisions were valued in medical training. Today, there is more of an emphasis on a willingness to express uncertainty. Doctors who get more help and more information become better doctors.

We can think of overconfidence as a special type of "cognitive bias" that makes us unaware of the risk we might be wrong. Bias happens to everyone—all people rely on past experience to make new decisions, and our brains often take "shortcuts" or go on "autopilot." But this can be a trap for doctors with years of medical experi-ence. They may substitute past experience for critical thinking and that can be dangerous.

What other factors can lead to overconfi-dence?

The biggest issue in overconfidence is a lack of feedback. When a doctor makes the right diagnosis, the patient comes back and gives thanks and praise. When a doctor makes the wrong diagnosis, however, the patient often moves on to another doctor, and the first doctor never finds out.

For an emergency room (ER) doctor, overconfidence could be a factor when he/she, say, orders a CT scan for a patient with new dizziness to rule out a stroke. If the scan is normal, the ER doc may confidently dismiss it—and miss the diagnosis of stroke. A neurologist would know that an early CT scan (especially in the first 24 hours after symptoms begin) will miss at least 85% of the most common type of stroke, the type caused by a blood clot in the brain. An MRI would miss only about 15% to 20%. The ER doctor may have been overconfident because he did not know what he didn't know.

How can you spot an overconfident doctor and protect yourself from a medical mistake?

The three most important things patients can do is come prepared…ask the right questions…and stay vigilant. *When you have a new problem…*

•**Write down all of your symptoms on a sheet of paper in the order they happened—make a timeline if you can.** Take your time and include all the things that could be important. Giving your doctor a good starting point saves time and helps your doctor focus on your problem.

•**Write down key questions to ask.** If your doctor gives you a diagnosis, ask what else could be causing your symptoms. Ask what your doctor is most worried about. What is the worst thing that could be causing your symptoms? Why does your doctor think that condition is not the problem?

•**Stay vigilant.** If your doctor starts treatment and you are not getting better, don't assume it's just the wrong medication. It could be the right medication for the wrong diagnosis.

Instead of accepting a change in medication or a higher dose, it's OK to question the diagnosis. Don't be afraid to ask for a consult with a specialist or a second opinion. If the doctor seems upset when you ask questions or the treatment being proposed is risky, consider getting that second opinion even before starting treatment.

Some situations are riskier and more error-prone than others. High-risk situations occur, for example, when your doctor is really busy and seems to be in a hurry…if you've been seen multiple times for the same symptoms without a clear diagnosis being made…and if your symptoms are new and serious enough that you've gone to the ER.

Finally, look out for overconfidence "red flags." If your doctor does not give you enough time, does not listen to your questions or gets in a huff when you ask for a consult or second opinion, get another doctor. If you do find out that your doctor made a mistake, let him/her know. That type of feedback may help your doctor avoid the overconfidence trap in the future.

Is That Newly Approved Treatment Really Safe?

Vinayak K. Prasad, MD, MPH, associate professor of medicine and public health at Oregon Health & Science University in Portland. Dr. Prasad is coauthor of *Ending Medical Reversal: Improving Outcomes, Saving Lives.* VinayakKPrasad.com

---

Every year, many new drugs and other medical treatments are approved after rigorous research studies and get adopted into practice. Some of the new treatments are then hyped by the companies that produce them and become very popular.

But here's the problem: Many of these treatments will be found to be ineffective or even harmful when further testing is done years later—this is known as medical reversal. Among established practices tested in studies that were published in top journals, up to 40% have been reversed.

Why medical reversals happen: Early research with a small number of participants may show that a new treatment or medication is bet-

ter than existing treatment. The study seems sound, and the drug or therapy is widely adopted and heavily marketed to doctors and patients. But years later, when many patients are using the treatment, larger studies show that the therapy does not stand the test of time…and/or that the original results were misleading.

Case in point: In 2008, the FDA approved the drug *bevacizumab* (Avastin) as an add-on to standard chemotherapy for advanced breast cancer. Early studies found that it slowed the growth of breast cancer tumors by more than 20%, but follow-up studies found that the tumors eventually grew back and women did not live longer or better. After three years, bevacizumab was withdrawn by the FDA as a treatment for breast cancer.

Other reversals: Sometimes a therapy is taken off the market, but there are plenty of treatments that have been reversed in studies yet continue to be used in practice. *Examples…*

•**Heart stents are commonly placed into the narrowed coronary arteries of people experiencing chronic stable angina,** at a cost of at least $10,000, with the hope of preventing heart attacks, improving symptoms and lengthening life. However, since 2007, studies show that stents do not reduce the risk for heart attack or lengthen the lives of these individuals. These patients can avoid the risks of the procedure and do just as well with medications.

Note: Stents have been shown to help patients who are having a heart attack.

•**Arthroscopic knee surgery is one of the most common orthopedic procedures.** Millions of these surgeries have been performed costing billions of dollars. The procedure repairs the cartilage that cushions and stabilizes the knee with the hope of reducing pain. Tears in this cartilage due to aging are very common in people over age 50. However, since 2013, studies have found that when the tear was not caused by an injury, this surgery is no better than physical therapy.

To learn about many other medical reversals, go to MedicalReversal.com, a site run by a team of researchers.

To protect yourself: For any proposed new treatment, ask your doctor probing questions. *Examples…*

•**Is this treatment supported by a randomized clinical trial?** The most reliable studies are randomized clinical trials (RCTs). RCTs randomly assign patients to the new treatment or the standard treatment and compare results.

•**Was the study sponsored by a drug company or performed by independent researchers?** For more reliable results, look to studies done by reputable independent researchers such as the National Cancer Institute or the National Institutes of Health.

•**Will this treatment relieve my symptoms or help me live longer?**

•**How long have you been using this treatment?**

•**Are there follow-up studies that find that this treatment may not work?**

•**What did you recommend before this new treatment was available?**

•**Is there an older, less expensive treatment that is effective and has stood the test of time?**

•**Does the condition I have need to be treated now?** Could a wait-and-see approach be an option?

If your doctor dismisses your questions, find a new doctor or get a second opinion. Also, you can research clinical studies on a specific treatment on your own online. A summary of the study (called the abstract) will be more readable than the full description.

Helpful website: PubMed.gov.

---

10 Ways Your Pharmacist Can Help You…

Heather Free, PharmD, practicing pharmacist in Washington, DC, and spokesperson for the American Pharmacists Association. Pharmacist.com

If you count on your pharmacist only to count your pills, you're missing out on an important medical ally. Pharmacists are highly educated about medications and the human body. And they tend to be a lot more accessible than doctors. You usually can consult with a pharmacist for free simply by showing up at a pharmacy—no need to be filling a prescription at the same time. These days, many pharmacists can provide a range of health-care services, thanks in part to changing state and federal laws.

Also: Technological advances are freeing up pharmacists to spend more time with their customers. *Ten things your pharmacist might be able to do for you…*

PRESCRIPTION-RELATED ASSISTANCE

•**Find cheaper options on prescriptions.** Your doctor likely has no idea how much the pills that he/she is prescribing will cost you. Pharmacists not only see how much you must pay out of pocket—if appropriate, they can recommend low-cost generic drugs that may work just as well as the pricier name brands…advise you when paying out of pocket for a drug is cheaper than your insurance or Medicare co-pay…and/or offer money-saving pill-splitting strategies. Your pharmacist can call your doctor's office on your behalf to work with the doctor to find a more affordable but still effective medication, including to confirm whether it's OK to substitute a generic for a name-brand product.

Even if your pharmacist has not done this for you in the past, it's worth trying again. Legislation passed in late 2018 banned the "gag orders" included in many pharmacy/insurance company contracts—clauses that prohibited some pharmacists from sharing money-saving advice with their customers.

•**Prescribe certain medications.** Pharmacists in a few states are allowed to prescribe certain medications, saving patients the time and cost of seeing a doctor. This is most common with birth control pills (in California, Colorado, DC, Hawaii, Idaho, Maryland, New Mexico, Oregon, Tennessee, Utah, Washington and West Virginia, according to the National Alliance of State Pharmacy Associations)…tobacco-cessation products (in Arizona, California, Colorado, Idaho, Indiana, Iowa, Maine and New Mexico)…and the opioid overdose treatment naloxone (in most states).

In Idaho, pharmacists can prescribe drugs for a much wider range of common health issues, including strep throat and urinary tract infections…and Oregon has a formulary of drugs that pharmacists can prescribe, including diabetic testing supplies, inhalers and epinephrine injectors. Visit the National Alliance of State Pharmacy Associations (NASPA.us) for more information on resources available in your area.

•**Sort your pills into pill packs or other dose-by-dose dispensers.** Some pharmacies can, upon request, package pills in dose-by-dose blister packs or another system designed to make it easy to remember which pills you're supposed to take when. These packs also help you monitor whether you've already taken a day's dose. This service might be offered for free or for a fee.

•**Reduce pharmacy trips by coordinating prescriptions.** Many pharmacies offer "medicine synchronization"—they'll work with the insurance company to shift the refill dates of multiple ongoing prescriptions so that the customer has to stop by only once or twice each month to pick them up. That isn't just convenient…it reduces the odds that the patient will forget to refill a prescription and miss doses.

•**Review what you take to make sure they all work well together**—including prescription and over-the-counter (OTC) drugs and herbal and vitamin supplements. The typical person age 65 or older fills 20 or more prescriptions each year—and some of those drugs could impact the effectiveness of others. It isn't just prescription drugs that can be problematic—OTC drugs and herbal supplements can cause dangerous interactions as well.

Example: St. John's wort, a medicinal herb commonly taken for depression, can decrease the effectiveness of some blood pressure medications.

Your pharmacist likely can conduct a free "medical reconciliation" upon request, reviewing the drugs you're taking and confirming that they're compatible with one another and appropriate for your current medical conditions. It's worth having this done—the Institute of Medicine has estimated that at least 1.5 million preventable adverse-drug events occur

each year due to a lack of review by medical professionals. Many doctors are specialists and aren't necessarily looking at the big picture when they prescribe. The same goes for walk-in clinics that you may go to once for a specific problem. You could ask your doctor to review your medicines, but a study published in *American Journal of Health-System Pharmacy* found that the reconciliation process is more accurate when a pharmacist conducts it. If you use OTC drugs or herbal supplements—and/or fill prescriptions at multiple pharmacies (which is not a good idea)—bring a list of these or the pill bottles themselves when you ask your pharmacist to conduct a reconciliation. Your records in the pharmacists' computer systems likely list only prescription drugs that you obtain at that pharmacy (or at other pharmacies in the same chain).

BEYOND PRESCRIPTIONS

•**Administer vaccinations.** Flu shots are not the only vaccination offered by many pharmacies. Details vary by state, but often vaccinations for diphtheria, hepatitis A and B, human papillomavirus, pneumonia, shingles and tetanus are available as well, plus vaccinations for international travel. While you may still pay a co-pay for the vaccine, you avoid the cost of an office visit.

•**Perform an annual wellness visit.** Some pharmacies now offer "wellness visits" that are just like the wellness visits provided at doctor's offices—only without the long delays often required to get on a doctor's schedule for a nonemergency appointment. During the visit, a pharmacist would take basic health measurements, such as blood pressure…ask a series of health-related questions…and do basic screening for signs of cognitive impairment. This wellness visit would be conducted by a pharmacist or potentially by another health professional employed by the pharmacy such as a nurse practitioner. Results are sent to the primary care physician for follow-up.

•**Conduct cholesterol, blood glucose, flu, HIV or hepatitis tests.** Some pharmacies now conduct tests such as these on a walk-in basis, no appointment or prescription necessary, often for just $10 to $30, which can be less than the co-pay that often must be paid to have these tests done at a doctor's office. Occasionally pharmacy tests are completely free. Pharmacies usually do not report these test results to doctors, but patients can use the results to determine whether they should see their doctors. If you are reactive to the flu test, the pharmacy can provide treatment.

•**Provide guidance with the selection and use of OTC drugs.** Pharmacists aren't just experts in prescription drugs—they're knowledgeable about OTC drugs. Unfortunately, few pharmacy customers bother to ask for their guidance before picking medicines off shelves.

Tip: Always ask a pharmacist's advice before choosing a cough-and-cold medication. Many of these feature a cocktail of drugs, some of which you might not need…or might have side effects that you don't expect.

•**Provide specialized knowledge about specific health needs.** Like doctors, pharmacists can have board-certified specialties including cardiology, geriatrics, oncology, organ transplant, pediatrics and psychiatric drugs. If you have health needs related to one of these specialties, it could be worth seeking a pharmacist in your area who has that certification—he/she would be ideally suited to offer medicine-related guidance to patients in this area.

Example: A pharmacist certified in geriatrics will be well-versed in age-related decline in liver and kidney function and what that means for older patients' ability to process medicines.

Ask local pharmacies if they have a pharmacist who is board-certified in the specialty relevant to your health. You also can look for local pharmacists certified in this area on the Board of Pharmacy Specialties website (BPSweb.org). This site lists pharmacists by specialty, name and town but not by pharmacy. Enter the names of pharmacists you find listed here into a search engine along with your state and the word "pharmacy" to determine where these local specialists work.

Take Photos for Better Care

Study by researchers at Queensland University of Technology, Brisbane, Australia, published in *Journal of Medical Internet Research.*

Patients' medical photos empower and reassure them and can improve the patient-doctor relationship, leading to better care.

Examples: Parents took pictures of their children's surgical wounds after laparoscopic appendectomies so surgeons could review healing. Parents felt more confident with the medical service, and taking photos also was a good reminder to check how the surgical site was healing. A woman who felt doctors were not listening to her complaints about her six-week-old baby took a video of the child's constant vomiting, and the doctor who saw it recognized that the infant needed surgery. Both clinicians and patients benefit when patients provide visual material to doctors and the doctors take the time to review it and incorporate it into medical records.

Look to Your Nails for Clues About Your Health and for Better Diagnoses

Dana Stern, MD, assistant clinical professor of dermatology at Mount Sinai Medical Center in New York City. As one of the few dermatologists in the US specializing in the diagnosis, treatment and surgery of the nail, she also has a private practice in New York City and Southampton, New York.

Though small in size, your fingernails can offer important clues that point to larger underlying health problems, such as lung disease, diabetes…and even cancer.

Nail changes may be among the first symptoms of an undiagnosed condition. That's because conditions that affect your entire body often alter blood flow to your nails, leading to changes affecting their color, shape, thickness and texture. Paying attention to these digit-protectors could help you get an early diagnosis.

Nail changes to watch for…*

CLUBBED NAILS

Clubbed nails look like upside-down spoons. The fingertips may be swollen underneath. Some people are born with clubbed nails, but clubbing that appears later in life, called acquired clubbing, is almost always health-related.

What it could mean: Eighty percent of people with acquired clubbing have an underlying lung disorder, usually lung cancer, chronic obstructive pulmonary disease (COPD) or some other lung disease. This nail condition also can occur in people with an infection of the lining of the heart chambers and heart valves (*infectious endocarditis*).

For unknown reasons, these lung and heart conditions can cause the connective tissue near the fingertips to grow abnormally fast, and the nail must change shape to accommodate the bulging tissue underneath. The medical conditions that accompany acquired clubbing usually reduce the amount of oxygen in the blood.

Getting diagnosed: If you notice clubbing (that you weren't born with) but haven't been told that you have a lung or heart problem, mention it to your primary care physician.

Your primary care physician should take a full history that includes details of any past or current smoking. He/she should also order a cardiopulmonary workup, including a chest X-ray. Once the underlying cause is treated, the clubbing should disappear.

WHITE NAILS

Healthy nails feature an all-pink to beige nail bed with longer nails also having a white tip. However, a condition known as Terry's Nails occurs when more than two-thirds of the nail— the part closest to the cuticle—appears white, and the remaining band, close to the tip, is pink or red. The lunula (the half-moon shape at the base of the nail) usually disappears.

What it could mean: Terry's Nails often accompanies cirrhosis of the liver, diabetes or congestive heart failure. The condition tends to occur on both hands and is often more pronounced in the thumbs and index fingers.

*Before having your nails examined by a doctor, always remove any nail polish.

Safer GI Procedures

Ask for a disposable scope for GI procedures. Current reusable models of duodenoscopes—used for diagnosing and treating diseases of the pancreas and bile duct—cannot be sufficiently sterilized and have been known to spread infections from one patient to another. The Food and Drug Administration (FDA) recently approved two disposable duodenoscopes for gastrointestinal use. Tell your doctor that you are aware of the FDA recommendation, and request that a disposable scope be used.

Roundup of experts on medical devices reported in *The New York Times.*

Getting diagnosed: See your primary care physician, who will conduct a full history and physical.

DARK STREAKS

A dark streak in your nail could be harmless—an injury, such as a door slam, can "wake up" pigment-producing melanocytes in the nail, causing a brown streak to appear. These harmless streaks are common in people with darker skin. Up to 80% of African-American adults can develop these benign pigment bands.

What it could mean: The streak could be subungual ("under the nail") melanoma, a potentially deadly form of skin cancer resulting from melanocytes below the nail growing in an uncontrolled fashion. Compared with Caucasians, melanoma in African-Americans, Asians and Native Americans is more likely to affect the nails, palms and soles. Nail melanoma usually appears as a single brown or black band running lengthwise along the nail and is most common in the thumb, index finger or big toenail.

Getting diagnosed: Not every dark streak is a melanoma, but it's always prudent to show your dermatologist. People tend to dismiss these streaks (or disguise them with polish), so nail melanoma is often diagnosed late. Caught early, it is treatable. A dermatologist will examine it and order a biopsy if needed.

Colonoscopy Alternative

Thomas Imperiale, MD, is a research scientist at the Regenstrief Institute, Indianapolis, and lead author of a study published in *Annals of Internal Medicine*.

Avoid colonoscopy by using an at-home stool test if you're at average risk. A meta-analysis of 31 studies provides the strongest evidence to date that an annual fecal immunochemical test (FIT), which detects hidden blood in stool, is 75% to 85% effective at detecting cancers. If blood is found, a follow-up colonoscopy is needed. If no blood is found, the test is repeated yearly. Only about 65% of adults ages 50 to 75 comply with screening recommendations. The FIT could boost that.

Heal Faster from Surgery with This Plan

Michael Englesbe, MD, professor of surgery at University of Michigan, Ann Arbor, and founder of Michigan Surgical Home and Optimization Program.

When you're having surgery, you might think your only job is to show up at the right time. The rest is in the hands of the doctors and nurses, right? Wrong. You hold the key to having a successful surgery and faster recovery. The secret? You have to train for surgery—physically and mentally.

Surgery is tough on your body and spirit. I have found that physically, major surgery—one where you receive a general anesthetic—is as hard on your body as running a 5K race. You wouldn't run a race without taking steps to get in shape for it. Along the same lines, you need to prepare and get your body in shape for your operation. Most surgeries are elective, and you and your surgeon can pick a date a few weeks to a month out, giving you time to prepare.

Your whole body—not just the one spot where the surgeon cuts—is affected by the strain. A training plan that includes physical, spiritual and practical preparation has had great success at University of Michigan, where I started a program called Michigan Surgical Home and Optimization Program. We found that patients who got wellness coaching and followed the plan before surgery had shorter hospital stays and were more likely to go home and not to a nursing home. *Here's the plan…*

1. Get walking. Simply walking more before surgery can reduce your hospital stay by one day.

Don't worry if you're not currently fit or active. In my clinical experience, only about 5% to 10% of people having surgery are. What's important is improving your current level, not reaching a particular step goal. Walking is crucial because it strengthens muscles and bones and increases cardio fitness and endurance. The goal is simply to increase the number of steps you can currently walk. If you start with 1,000 a day, maybe you can soon do 1,200 or more.

If walking is hard for you, it's fine to do a half-hour a day of another activity, such as swimming. But the reason we stress walking is that walking is important in getting up and moving after surgery, so it's good to practice.

2. Don't try to lose weight—but do eat a protein-rich diet.

Good news: Unless your surgeon tells you otherwise, you don't need to go on a diet. In fact, it's not the best time to stress your body by cutting calories. Instead, focus on eating healthier before surgery. It's especially important to eat enough lean protein—especially skinless chicken breasts, turkey, fish and beans—because it helps build muscle mass, keeping you in optimal shape. It's not new information, but it bears repeating—eat at least five to seven ounces of protein a day.

Beyond that, opt for a whole-foods–based diet, with five to seven servings of fruits and vegetables a day and whole grains. Limit saturated fats like the kind you get in bacon and butter. Cut back on chips, cookies and other processed foods. The goal is to reduce the unnecessary work your body has to do before and after surgery.

3. Make sure your doctor knows as much as possible about you. Surgery is intimate. It's really important that your surgeon knows and understands you. If your doctors and nurses don't ask you questions, proactively tell them about yourself, including your profession, hobbies, travel plans. Doctors want to know ahead of surgery how we can help you fully enjoy your life.

Why that matters: Some big operations aren't for everyone, and the marginal benefits they'll give may not be worth the other issues surgery creates.

Example: My father is an 80-year-old guy with minimal health problems. One procedure a doctor suggested for melanoma would prevent him from ever playing golf again. He lives to play golf. Because my dad said, "One of my most important goals is continuing to play golf every day," the doctor knew that this procedure might not be right for him, especially because less invasive options for his care were available.

Sharing personal details and your hopes for how life will be after this procedure will remind everyone that there's a real person under the surgical robing. When I'm doing a liver transplant, it helps if I can say to the team, "That's Mr. Smith. He's a retired first-grade teacher. He really wants to get home in the next two weeks so that he can go to his daughter's wedding. That's his goal."

4. Come clean about your medications —all of them. Your surgical-care team will go through exactly which medications and supplements you should stop taking and when. For instance, you have to avoid fish oil supplements because they thin your blood and can increase bleeding. The problem is that patients don't always tell the whole truth about all that they take, either out of embarrassment or fear. You'd be shocked to know how many people lie about taking opioids for pain and benzodiazepines for anxiety. You need to be up front with your doctor because it's dangerous to abruptly stop taking these medications on your own. You can get really sick from withdrawal, and your doctor won't know what's wrong with you.

Important: Be honest about your alcohol consumption, too. If you drink every day and find that you get tremors when you don't drink, then you can't just stop cold turkey—your doctor needs to know so that he/she can come up with a safe plan for you.

5. Line up your support team. The biggest thing people do wrong before surgery is trying to go it alone to spare their loved ones ("I don't want to bother anyone, so I'll just take a taxi to surgery"). That's a dangerous mistake that hurts everyone involved, but especially you. Having a support system actually helps you heal. Most of us get much of our energy and our fuel from our relationships.

You actually get better care when you have family members in the hospital. They can advocate for you and help you feel comfortable at a vulnerable time, including getting assistance for you if the nurses are busy. They can think to ask the questions that your postsurgery brain doesn't think of and they may better remember the information and recommendations from the doctors. Happily, hospitals now make it easy for guests to visit and stay longer hours.

6. Optimize your attitude. I'm a conventional doctor, but I've come to realize that the secret sauce in having a great surgery is a combination of spiritual factors—including an all-around positive attitude and a feeling of empowerment. A study in *JAMA Network Open* looked at almost 7,000 people over age 50 and found that the ones who have a lot of goals and a strong life purpose live a lot longer than the ones who don't.

One of the simplest things that you can do to improve your attitude before a health procedure is to focus on gratitude. Practicing mindfulness with techniques such as deep breathing and meditation also can help. Sooner or later, we all may face a health challenge such as surgery, but training with these mind/body tools can help you feel stronger, calmer and more empowered.

Get Blood Cultures Before Sepsis Treatment

Matthew Cheng, MD, clinical instructor in infectious diseases, Brigham and Women's Hospital, Boston.

Among 325 patients admitted to the hospital with sepsis, those who had blood drawn before starting an antibiotic had more microbial pathogens needed to accurately identify the infection, compared with patients who had blood drawn within two hours of starting an antibiotic.

Takeaway: Treatment should begin as early as possible for potentially deadly infections, but determining the bacteria prior to treatment is also critical in identifying the most effective antibiotic.

The Truth About Cementing Spinal Fractures

Alan Hilibrand, MD, orthopedic surgeon specializing in surgical and nonsurgical care of the spine based in Philadelphia, and spokesperson for the American Academy of Orthopaedic Surgeons.

Study titled "The Efficacy and Safety of Vertebral Augmentation: A Second ASBMR Task Force Report," by researchers at Monash University, Australia, published in *Journal of Bone and Mineral Research.*

People with osteoporosis are prone to painful spinal compression fractures. Standard routine care is frequently surgery—either *vertebroplasty* or *kyphoplasty,* procedures that literally glue the bones back together. However, which is better...and whether either is any better than more conservative therapies...has not been clear. An international task force of orthopedic specialists now has answers.

Roughly 750,000 US adults suffer from vertebral compression fractures most of which are caused by osteoporosis. In fact, these kinds of fractures are the most common complication of osteoporosis and can result from such simple activities as a minor fall, carrying something heavy or even bending the wrong way. *Kyphosis* (curving of the spine) and/or loss of height are often used to detect that such a fracture may have occurred. One-third of compression fractures cause acute and chronic back pain.

Unfortunately, there aren't many treatment options for spinal fractures. Among them are two surgical procedures, where bone cement is injected into the broken vertebrae to stiffen up the bone in the hope that stopping it from moving will reduce or eliminate the pain. *Percutaneous vertebroplasty* involves injecting bone

Don't Let Your Surgeon Double-Time You

Surgeons doing double duty increase certain patients' risks. Lead surgeons sometimes schedule several procedures at the same time, moving between operating rooms as others handle routine parts of the surgeries. A new study suggests that this usually is safe, but it increases the odds of complications—and death—with coronary artery bypass grafts...and for elderly patients or those in poor health. In these cases, patients should ask for nonoverlapping surgery...or consider choosing a different surgeon.

Eric Sun, MD, PhD, assistant professor of anesthesiology, perioperative and pain medicine at Stanford University Medical Center, California, and lead author of a study published in *JAMA.*

cement directly into the injured vertebra. *Balloon kyphoplasty,* a newer procedure, involves inserting a balloon into the crushed vertebra and inflating it to expand the bone to its original shape before injecting the cement.

Because there is no consensus among surgeons as to which procedure is better—nor any agreement as to whether either is better than less invasive approaches—The American Society for Bone and Mineral Research recently created a task force to look into the effectiveness of vertebroplasty and kyphoplasty, as well as other treatments for spinal compression fractures. An international team of researchers looked at 28 studies that addressed the effectiveness of either procedure, as well as other treatments for spinal compression fracture, based on improvement in pain, mobility and/or quality of life.

Results: Compared with placebo (sham surgery without the injecting of the cement) vertebroplasty was no better at improving pain, mobility and quality of life. Kyphoplasty may be marginally better, but the procedure is newer and there were no placebo-controlled trials.

The researchers do not suggest completely ditching vertebroplasty and kyphoplasty for spinal compression fractures. These procedures may still help some people when nothing else does. What the task force recommends is trying more conservative approaches—such as bracing, rehab exercises to strengthen the trunk and offload pressure on the spine, anti-inflammatory drugs and/or painkillers—before going for surgery. In fact, time itself will help your body heal.

Faster, Better Recovery from Hip and Knee Replacement

Daniel Wiznia, MD, orthopedic surgeon who specializes in reconstructive surgery of the hip and knee and associate professor of orthopedics and rehabilitation at Yale School of Medicine, New Haven, Connecticut.

Since most knee and hip replacements are elective surgeries, you have the luxury of taking your time to choose the right doctor and hospital, as well as the time to optimize your presurgical health, all of which can make a big difference in your recovery. *My inside secrets on how to do both…*

CHOOSE THE RIGHT TEAM

It may be convenient to have your joint replacement done at the local community hospital, but a large orthopedic hospital or university teaching hospital is a better option. These doctors perform many more surgeries, plus these centers are where the thought leaders are, so you can benefit from the latest advances, state-of-the-art equipment and a team of specialized professionals.

PRESURGERY PREPARATION

Patients who are the healthiest going into surgery have the best outcomes, so you want to do everything possible beforehand to make yourself a safe candidate. While that can take several months for some, it's worth it to reduce the risks. *At Yale Medicine, we have a checklist of modifiable risk factors that we use to help patients overcome, including…*

•**Excess weight.** Being overweight or obese increases your risk for complications, such as infection and delayed wound healing during surgery and postsurgery, and simply makes re-

covery more difficult. We like patients to have a body mass index less than 38. For patients at an unsafe weight, we provide nutrition counseling to teach them to eat healthier and drop pounds gradually for sustainable weight loss. For patients unable to exercise due to severe arthritis pain or who struggle to lose weight through diet alone, we might recommend bariatric surgery.

•**Poor diet.** Even if you're at a healthy weight, we want to optimize your diet. Adequate nutrition and vitamin reserves sourced from protein, fruits and vegetables help you recover faster and heal your incisions. I have my patients eat an egg every day for two weeks prior to surgery to ensure that they have enough protein stores. If you suffer from anemia, low blood counts or low iron, we may also suggest that you take some vitamins to improve that, such as iron, folate, B-12, calcium, vitamin D and vitamin C, and perhaps a protein supplement. Any supplements should be coordinated with your primary care doctor.

•**Exercise.** Conditioning with a physical therapist before surgery helps strengthen muscles and improve balance so that you recover faster. This is especially important if you are using a cane, walker or wheelchair before surgery. Increasing your mobility presurgery helps reduce your risk of falling and improves postoperative pain control.

•**Substance use.** Patients need to wean off narcotic pain medications, alcohol dependency, tobacco and other recreational drugs prior to surgery, and we provide counseling for that. Tobacco use increases your chances of postsurgical lung complications and infection and delays wound healing. Patients must stop smoking for at least eight weeks before surgery.

Even if you drink alcohol only in moderation, you should avoid it altogether two weeks prior to surgery. Alcohol increases your risk for complications.

•**Dental care.** Have a checkup, cleaning and any necessary dental work done prior to your surgery. Bacteria in your mouth can travel through the bloodstream and would be attracted to your joint implant, increasing your risk for infection. Patients should wait around six months after their joint replacement to have any other dental work.

BE PROACTIVE POSTSURGERY

Many knee- and hip-replacement patients go directly home the day after the surgery—and some even go home the same day. We have found that patients recover faster, have fewer complications and are happier if they are discharged to home rather than a rehabilitation facility. A strong support system also promotes healing.

•**Physical therapy.** Getting moving again is the most important thing you can do to reduce inflammation, swelling and pain. You'll start with a walker and progress to a cane. Usually patients do away with these devices by about four weeks. The physical therapist at the hospital will teach you specific exercises. Depending on your insurance, you will continue with physical therapy either at home or at an outpatient rehab facility. For the fastest and best recovery, perform your routine for 20 to 30 minutes two to three times daily. You'll also need to walk (with your walker or cane as needed) another 60 to 90 minutes daily. Don't worry about distance—the number of times you walk is more important than how far.

•**Pain relief.** Less pain helps you heal faster, but at Yale and other leading surgical centers, we champion a narcotic-sparing approach due to the dangers of opioid pain relievers. We use peripheral nerve blocks during surgery to help reduce pain afterward and give acetaminophen (Tylenol) intravenously, which provides better pain relief than taking it orally. Once home, patients may be prescribed acetaminophen, a nonsteroidal anti-inflammatory (such as ibuprofen) and *gabapentin* (Neurontin), a non-narcotic neurological medicine that can help reduce pain for two to three weeks. Your goal should be to taper off narcotic medication by the end of the second week after surgery and take acetaminophen or an NSAID only as needed.

•**Diet.** Follow the same high-protein, fruit- and vegetable-loaded eating plan as you did before surgery. It can be hard to eat while you're in pain, but your body requires adequate calories to help it heal after surgery. Avoid sugar and refined carbs, both of which can increase inflammation and slow healing.

Skip the Catheter for Faster Joint Replacement Recovery

Michael A. Charters, MD, orthopedic surgeon, Henry Ford Health System, Detroit.

People undergoing hip or knee replacement traditionally have received a Foley urinary catheter prior to surgery because it was thought to prevent postoperative complications.

Recent study: There was no difference in urinary complications, such as incontinence, in those who had a urinary catheter inserted prior to surgery and those who didn't, according to a study of 335 patients. Also, infection rate was higher in some patients who got the catheter.

Bonus: Catheter-free patients were able to get up and walk sooner.

Your Death, Your Terms: Don't Let Your Final Wishes Be Ignored

Barbara Coombs Lee, PA, JD, FNP, attorney and president of Compassion & Choices, a nonprofit organization that works to improve end-of-life care and expand end-of-life options. She is author of *Finish Strong: Putting Your Priorities First at Life's End.* CompassionAndChoices.org

Maria had lived a good life. The 81-year-old Californian raised a family, enjoyed a happy 50-year marriage and ran a secondary school. But now she was suffering from crippling arthritis and congestive heart failure. She signed legal documents declining resuscitation efforts and extraordinary life-sustaining measures.

A year later, Maria was sleeping in a hospital bed—she was receiving treatment for a stomach problem—when her heart and breathing stopped. It was the peaceful death she had hoped for...until the hospital staff shocked her heart back to life and put her on a mechanical ventilator, despite her wishes. Unable to speak, Maria expressed her desire to be taken off the machine through a series of yes/no hand squeezes with her son, but the hospital persisted. Maria eventually died after more than a week of suffering. The hospital staff ignored Maria's legal documents because those documents began, "If I am terminally ill…" and the doctors said she had a slim chance of survival. They ignored her hand-squeeze instructions because they thought Maria was no longer competent to make her own decisions.

Most people have thoughts about how and where they would prefer their lives to end. And more than one-third of American adults have proactively formalized their end-of-life preferences in legal documents known as "advance directives." Yet, like Marie, many of these people will unnecessarily endure deaths very different from what they desired.

Here's how to increase the odds that your priorities will be honored when the end approaches…

THE LIMITATIONS OF ADVANCE DIRECTIVES

Advance directives typically include a living will, which lists health-care treatments you would and would not want and a durable medical power of attorney, also known as a health-care proxy, which empowers a trusted loved one to make medical decisions on your behalf.

These documents are supposed to let people dictate the medical treatments they will and will not receive when they cannot speak for themselves. But the documents typically take effect in only two very specific situations—when someone is terminally ill…and/or when he/she is permanently unconscious. Doctors often are unwilling to conclude that either of these conditions applies, holding out hope that there's still a sliver of a chance that the patient could pull through and, in turn, discouraging families from enacting the patient's wishes, thereby negating the advance directive. As with Maria, occasionally doctors ignore advance directives even when it's clear to others that these documents should apply.

Advance directives also can go unheeded because either no one knows about them or they are inaccessible.

Warning: A widely used DIY living will called "Five Wishes" includes the phrase, "I do not want anything done or omitted by my doctors or nurses with the intention of taking my life." That can be interpreted as contradicting attempts elsewhere in the living will to decline life-extending treatments under certain circumstances. Be sure all instructions are consistent and clear. Working with a knowledgeable attorney is the safest way to do that…or use Compassion & Choices' free End-of-Life Decisions Guide & Toolkit (CompassionAndChoices.org/end-of-life-planning). You also can fill out an advance directive form at PrepareForYourCare.org.

IMPROVE THE ODDS YOU'LL GET THE END OF LIFE YOU WANT

In addition to having an advance directive, you also need to…

•**Be sure your documents are accessible.** File copies of advance directives with your local hospitals. Give copies to family members. Ask them to store copies on their mobile phones for easy access in an emergency. Make sure your preferences in these documents are clear.

•**Tell your loved ones what you want—repeatedly.** Initiate conversations with your close relatives about your end-of-life priorities. Do not be deterred by relatives who insist that you still have many years left…or that it's not an appropriate moment for such a macabre conversation—their discomfort with death doesn't make these discussions any less important.

•**Do this on multiple occasions to ensure your words are remembered.** Include all of your descendants, plus your siblings, your spouse and any other close relatives in these conversations—ideally while everyone is together—to reduce the odds that one of your relatives later misrepresents your end-of-life priorities. Be clear with your family who your designated health-care proxy is, as well as his back-up, so that there is no confusion or argument if he is called on for decisions. Your family's knowledge and unanimous support of your end-of-life wishes increase the odds that all will honor your advance directives.

Warning: Don't exclude adult children who live far away from these conversations. Far-off offspring are likely to insist that health-care providers take unwanted life-prolonging measures.

These descendants are especially prone to want to extend their parents' lives because they feel guilty about not being around at the end.

•Gauge your doctor's willingness to respect your decisions. Share your end-of-life priorities with your doctor, then ask for his feelings on the matter. The doctor should voice respect for your priorities. If he does, ask him to add your advance directives to your medical file. If he dismisses the topic or expounds on his own end-of-life philosophy, it might be time to look for a different doctor.

Example: It's a troubling sign if your doctor dismisses the topic with, "We'll deal with that when the time comes" or "Let's hope that never happens."

•Film yourself explaining your end-of-life preferences. Look directly into a digital video camera, such as the one in a smartphone, and calmly and clearly explain what's most important to you in your life—being capable of thinking clearly enough to have coherent conversations with my friends…living in my own home…enjoying meals with my family…reading and understanding the newspaper or works of literature…being fit and mobile enough to enjoy the outdoors…being present enough to watch my loved ones enjoy their lives. Note whatever it is that you cannot live without and what you hope will be done if you can no longer do these things. Let several trusted loved ones know how to gain access to this video in your records when the time comes…and e-mail copies of it to those loved ones, including your health-care proxy and your estate attorney. This video won't carry the legal weight of your advance directive, but it will have a very real emotional weight—it's very difficult to ignore someone's deeply held desires after looking into his eyes while he explains them. Instruct family members to play the video for any family members, friends or medical professionals who attempt to contradict your wishes.

•Dig for the truth about your actual medical situation. Often people don't get the end of life they want because they agree to medical treatments that contradict their own priorities. Why would they do this? Because of poor communication, patients frequently don't fully understand their medical conditions or the treatments they are agreeing to.

Example: A doctor tells his patient that her condition is "treatable." The patient agrees to the treatment he recommends because, like many patients, she thinks "treatable" means "curable." What the doctor fails to explain is that treatable doesn't mean curable—it only means that there is a course of treatment that can be applied.

If you have health issues serious enough that end-of-life decision-making could be a factor, ask your doctor the following questions when he recommends a treatment or refers to your condition as treatable…

"What's the likelihood that this treatment will cure me?"

"What are the odds that it will prolong my life?"

"How long is it likely to prolong my life?"

"What will my life be like during that remaining time? What will I be able to do or not do?"

"What's the reasonable goal of this treatment?"

Ask these questions even if you are repeating a course of treatment you have gone through in the past—the answers might be different this time.

Example: When cancer returns after a period of remission, an oncologist might prescribe a new round of chemotherapy. But often chemo is less likely to produce a cure—or even an extended stretch of good health—when cancer returns.

•Sign up for hospice care if your condition is terminal. Hospice care helps make the patient as comfortable as possible during end of life with pain-relief and other palliative treatments. It often can be provided in the patient's home, and it is well-covered by Medicare Part A as long as the patient's life expectancy is six months or less. Private insurance generally covers hospice, too. Find local hospice providers in your area at Medicare.gov/HospiceCompare.

CHAPTER 11

Infectious Diseases

Strengthening Your Gut Microbiome in the Era of COVID-19

At the time of writing this, COVID-19 has swept the globe, infecting millions of people worldwide and killing hundreds of thousands. While we've done plenty to mitigate our risk of infection—from practicing social distancing to perfecting personal hygiene to focusing on immune health—one factor may be overlooked by many: Bolstering the health of our gut microbiome to avoid an inflammatory storm.

Consider this: Some people infected with COVID-19 show no signs and some have only minor flu-like symptoms. Others who contract the novel coronavirus—people with conditions such as diabetes, hypertension, kidney disease or those at an advanced age—can have an acute systemic inflammatory response that may re-

sult in death. And others still, including people between the ages of 20 and 60 who become infected but have no known underlying medical conditions, "develop serious illness requiring intensive care treatment," the Lippincott Nursing Center reports. What dictates the severity of responses?

One theory that's currently being investigated is the concept of an inflammatory or cytokine storm—in short, an excessive immune response to potential danger. A surge in an immune response can lead to the fatal shut down of multiple organs.

As you may know, your immune system is your body's natural defense system against infection and illness, and includes two main parts that work in concert with each other—your innate immune system (which you are born with) and your adaptive immune system (which, as

Laurie Steelsmith, ND, LAc, licensed naturopathic physician and acupuncturist in private practice in Honolulu. She writes Bottom Line's "Natural Healing Secrets for Women" blog and is coauthor of three books—*Natural Choices for Women's Health, Great Sex, Naturally* and *Growing Younger Every Day*. DrSteelsmith.com

Johns Hopkins Medicine puts it, "you develop when your body is exposed to microbes or chemicals released by microbes"). Other than your nervous system, your immune system is the most intricate network in your body, working tirelessly at patrolling for invaders. But when it goes into overdrive in an attempt to keep you healthy, it can get stuck doing so—failing to shut off.

This occurs in your innate immune system, which holds a multi-protein complex, known as the NLRP3 inflammasome, that instigates an inflammatory form of cell death and triggers the release of proinflammatory cytokines. While researchers are still learning more about this phenomenon, it's believed that this happens when the immune system encounters a new pathogenic trespasser, which then causes cytokines to surge—and we all know now that COVID-19 is heretofore unknown. (Indeed, cytokine storms are thought to explain the devastating effects of the 1918 Spanish flu pandemic.)

So how can you do all that you can to help your body have a proper immune response to infections, rather than an extreme, possibly deleterious reaction? Part of this may rest in the health of your gut microbiome.

Your gut microbiome—the community of bacteria that lives in your gut—plays a vital role in a number of functions, including your mood, the amount of energy you derive from your diet and, yes, your immune system. At the same time, your immune system and the gut work in a symbiotic relationship, moderating one another and working to support each other—an interaction that's underscored by the fact that, according to *Cellular and Molecular Immunology,* 70% to 80% of the body's immune cells are contained in the gut.

To build and maintain this healthy crosstalk, it's important to first think of your GI tract as a system as intricate as a rainforest, with a multifaceted system of life. It's been adapted to accommodate a wide range of microbes, and to upset its delicate balance may lead to a host of health problems, including an exaggerated response to an invader.

This internal ecological system is influenced by the way you live your life and the decisions you make on a daily basis. What you eat, how often you move, the quality of your sleep, your external environment, your emotions and moods, the medications you take, your social life—all can contribute to your gut health. While several factors can impact your gut health and influence a decreased or dysregulated immune system—including nutrient deficiency (such as a zinc deficiency, as seen in those with pyrrole disorder, as well as those who eat diets low in antioxidant-rich fruits and vegetables), stress, insulin resistance, food allergies and intolerances (which can create systemic inflammatory effects, impact the intestines, and contribute to irritable bowel syndrome), over-the-counter medications such as antacids and NSAIDs, toxin exposure (to, say, heavy metals, pesticides and prescription medication) and genetics—you can take your gut health into your own hands.

Given that it's your gut we're talking about, it makes sense that its health is to a large part dependent on your diet. In fact, the single most important factor for a strong microbiome is what you eat. A microbiome in equilibrium is full of bacteria that produce specific short-chain fatty acids that positively affect wellness. These include acetate, propionate and, especially, butyrate—highly biologically active compounds that promote gut health, blood sugar regulation, optimal blood fat levels, appetite control and immunity. This friendly flora needs nourishment, which can then have a huge impact in shifting the inflammatory cascade. *In addition to a healthy diet, rich in organic food, here are a few foods to nurture it right…*

GREEN TEA

EGCG—the chief catechin in green tea—has been linked to a variety of health benefits. Functioning as a powerful antioxidant, it not only protects cells from oxidative damage but also encourages gut health. A 2019 review of studies and trials published by *Nutrients* found that green tea consumption resulted in the reduction of *Firmicutes* (an unfriendly bacteria) and improved levels of *Bacteroidetes* (a friendly bacteria)—changes, the authors say, that could help prevent gut dysbiosis (microbial imbalance). Green tea can also inhibit NLRP3 inflammasome activity and increase Nrf2 (which decreases inflammation). What's more, a randomized control study out of Japan on 200 healthcare workers showed the incidence of influenza was lower in the group that took 378 mg of green tea catechins and 210 mg of the amino acid *L-theanine* per day. The amount of EGCG in each cup of tea depends on the quality of the tea. Some resources suggest 50 mg to 100 mg, and others as high as 180 mg.

POMEGRANATE

Also rich in antioxidants, pomegranate can have a positive impact on gut flora by acting as a prebiotic—compounds that help "good" bacteria flourish in the intestines. A 2015 study published in *Anaerobe* reveals that pomegranate extract and pomegranate juice increased the mean counts of *Bifidobacterium* and *Lactobacillus* (friendly bacteria) and inhibited unfriendly bacteria such as the *B. fragilis* group. Another study in *Anaerobe* found that pomegranate stimulates the growth of a bacteria known as *Akkermansia Muciniphila*—an intestinal bacteria superstar that supports microbiome health and offers protection from disease.

To boost your own intestinal health, you can drink eight ounces of pomegranate juice daily or take it as a supplement, 400 mg to 800 mg a day.

Note: Check with your doctor before making pomegranate a regular part of your diet. Pomegranate can lower blood pressure so if you are on a bp-lowering medication, your blood pressure could become too low if you drink a lot of pomegranate juice. Pomegranate may also interfere with some medications.

BROCCOLI SPROUTS

Broccoli sprouts—small, immature seedlings of the broccoli you typically eat—contain sulforaphane, a sulfur-rich compound, found in cruciferous vegetables, that has been shown to have immune enhancing benefits, and inhibit multiple inflammasomes that cause cytokine storms (one of which is the aforementioned multi-protein complex known as the NLRP3 inflammasome). Use them in lieu of lettuce or bean sprouts in a sandwich, on top of your avocado toast, in a salad, or as a soup topper. They have a spicy, almost radish-like, flavor so don't put them in your smoothie. And they are very easy to grow on a counter at home.

TURMERIC

One of the boons of turmeric—or, more specifically, the phytochemical curcumin that's found in it—is that it operates as an anti-inflammatory. Used in Ayurvedic medicine as a digestive healing agent, it began being recommended as treatment for acid reflux, flatulence and functional dyspepsia by the World Health Organization in 1999. What's more, it works synergistically with EGCG, vitamin C, and quercetin to stimulate the production of immune-boosting enzymes. To have more turmeric in your diet, enjoy eating curries, add it to smoothies, or make "golden milk."

WALNUTS

Eating a handful of walnuts per day—roughly 16 walnut halves—boosts the bacteria species that generates butyrate, thus changing the microbiome for the better. Other nuts that encourage a healthy microbiome include pecans, almonds, cashews, pistachios and hazelnuts.

FOODS RICH IN QUERCETIN

Quercetin is one of the most abundant antioxidants in many grains, fruits and vegetables (it also gives some of these their pigment) and naturally supports your ability to ward off free radical damage. It also increases gut microbial diversity, which protects your gut and immune health. While quercetin supplements are available, you can up your intake of it through the consumption of foods with a high quercetin content, such as apples, onions, grapes, broccoli, berries, cherries, citrus fruits and capers. Other options include tea (black and green), red wine, spinach, kale, buckwheat and olive oil.

PREBIOTIC AND PROBIOTIC FOODS

Prebiotics—a type of fiber the human body cannot digest—work as food for probiotics, microorganisms that help the body cultivate and maintain a healthy colony of bacteria. Prebiotics are present in many high-fiber foods, including Jerusalem artichokes, garlic, onions, leeks, barley, banana and flaxseeds. Foods rich in probiotics, meanwhile, include yogurt, kefir, miso, tempeh, Kombucha and fermented foods such as sauerkraut and kimchee.

Eat your way towards an effectual immune response? Absolutely.

Zinc and Licorice Root May Reduce Risk for COVID

Jacob Teitelbaum, MD, Hawaii-based holistic physician and author of numerous books including the upcoming, newly updated *Real Cause, Real Cure.* Vitality101.com

---

Zinc and glycyrrhizin (from licorice root) may reduce risk for coronavirus. In studies on 2003 SARS coronavirus, zinc killed the virus on contact. Sucking a zinc lozenge when in crowds may offer some protection. Drinking licorice tea each morning and taking vitamins A, C, D, E, zinc and elderberry (available in a combination called ViraPro) makes your body less hospitable to viruses—another line of defense.

Stay Healthy When You Fly

Philip M. Tierno, Jr., PhD, clinical professor of microbiology and pathology at New York University Langone Medical Center. He is author of *The Secret Life of Germs: Observations and Lessons from a Microbe Hunter.* Med. NYU.edu

---

Airline passengers spend hours stuck in a small space with fellow travelers, breathing the same air and touching the same surfaces—surfaces that might not get cleaned well or often. And their body's natural defenses against germs are compromised by the environmental conditions on planes. Beyond a pandemic and other germs, the shrinking airline seats, when combined with lack of movement, can lead to other serious health issues as well.

Luckily, there are ways to protect yourself, particularly on longer flights...

•**Stay hydrated.** You need moist mucous membranes to create a line of defense against germs that are inhaled. The air in airplane cabins is very dry—often only about 20% humidity or less. Healthful levels should be closer to 40%. Low humidity dries out the mucous membranes in passengers' noses and throats, limiting their ability to shield them from germs in the air they breathe. Drink four to eight ounces of fluid—preferably water—per hour. Avoid alcoholic beverages that can dehydrate the body.

Warning: Water is, of course, an excellent beverage for hydration—but consume bottled water, not water from the plane's bathroom tap, which can be contaminated with germs.

•**Turn your air vent on, but don't point it at your face.** In past decades, the standard advice was to leave the air vent above airline seats turned off—it blew air that could contain germs from passengers seated throughout the plane. That risk has been greatly reduced because commercial aircraft now have very effective air-filtration systems. In fact, breathing filtered air blowing from the vent above your seat could reduce your exposure to germs from a sick passenger seated near you. Still, filtration systems are not perfect, and this blowing air could further dry out your mucous membranes, so a prudent compromise is to turn your vent on but not aim its stream of air directly into your face.

•**Find the healthiest seat.** What's the healthiest seat on the plane? People often ask whether aisle seats or window seats are the better choice from a health perspective. The answer is, it's a trade-off—aisle seats make it easier to get up and move around, avoiding blood clot risk...but window seats mean that you have fewer passengers seated near you, decreasing the odds that you'll be near someone who is contagious.

Also: Politely ask a flight attendant if you can switch seats if someone near you on the plane is repeatedly sneezing or coughing. Passengers within three seats to the front or sides of someone who is contagious—or within one to two seats behind such a person—face much higher infection risks than passengers seated elsewhere on the plane.

•**Don't forget your mask.** Be sure to wear your mask, especially if you are seated near someone who is coughing or sneezing and you cannot switch seats, perhaps because the flight is full. At-risk or elderly passengers should wear a mask even if no one around them appears to be sick. Not all contagious people show obvious signs of an illness.

•**Get up and move every hour or two.** Stroll up the aisle and back or at least stand and stretch. Spending long hours stuck in a cramped airline seat isn't just uncomfortable…it can lead to a potentially fatal blood-clot condition called *deep vein thrombosis*—even in travelers who have no history of circulatory problems. If it isn't possible to move around because the "fasten seat belt" sign remains on, at least flex and stretch the muscles of your legs, feet and toes and do some shoulder rolls.

Note: Qantas, which plans to start running the world's longest flight—from Sydney to London

in 23 hours, 40 minutes—has created a video to help passengers benefit from easy-to-do inflight exercises. Go to YouTube.com and search "Qantas inflight exercises."

•**Wear eyeglasses rather than contact lenses.** The low humidity on airplanes can dry out your eyes, creating discomfort for contact lens wearers. If you must wear contacts on a flight, apply eyedrops periodically to keep your eyes moist.

•**Hand sanitizer and/or sanitizing wipes reminders.** Everyone should know by now to carry and use hand sanitizer during flights immediately before eating, drinking, removing contact lenses or doing anything else that involves touching your eyes or face on flights. Choose a product that contains at least 60% alcohol, and use a quarter-size drop for each hand cleaning—most people don't use enough. Also wipe down the seat-back tray table before using it—these are rarely cleaned by airlines and could be con-

---

Flying During COVID-19

Keep in mind that although airlines say they're deep cleaning, we really don't know how effectively. Also, it takes only one infected passenger to introduce germs to a "clean" cabin.

Helpful: The shorter the flight, the safer, as we've learned from norovirus and influenza studies, and flying nonstop limits the number of people you're exposed to.

Wear a mask on the plane and in the terminal. As you surely now know, being in close proximity to others is the key transmission risk, and a mask reduces exposure. Wearing a mask helps to keep you from touching your face. It must cover your nose and mouth, from just under your eyes to the bottom of your chin. Having a beard impairs proper fit…wear a neck gaiter, which covers from nose to neck.

Use hand sanitizer and/or wipes liberally. At this writing, the TSA allows passengers to bring up to 12 ounces of hand sanitizer aboard. Or bring a three-ounce bottle of 60% or higher rubbing alcohol and paper towels.

While everyone is afraid of breathing in the virus, most planes have good air-filtration systems. The greatest transmission risk is from someone shedding the virus in water droplets that linger on

surfaces that you then touch. Wipe down high-germ areas yourself, or use hand sanitizer after contact. Food trays and everything bathroom-related—the door latches (open and close), flush button, faucet handle—are the worst.

Put as much distance as possible between you and others. It's impossible to truly socially distance on a plane. The greatest probability of picking up an infection comes from people in the seats nearest you in all directions—on either side and one row in front and behind. When possible, create a perimeter around yourself even if that means changing your seat. An empty middle seat is better than no distance, so avoid planes with only two seats per side.

What you don't need to wipe: The virus doesn't survive well on most surfaces, so it's not necessary to wipe down purchases from airport shops or a soft suitcase after the flight. If you wipe down the tray, you don't need to wipe down your things that touch it, such as a book or computer.

Charles Peter Gerba, PhD, professor of microbiology and environmental science at the Mel and Enid Zuckerman College of Public Health of University of Arizona in Tucson and coauthor of The Germ Freak's Guide to Outwitting Colds and Flu.

taminated with germs from passengers on prior flights.

Washing your hands thoroughly with soap and water ordinarily is as effective as using hand sanitizers or sanitizing wipes, but hand washing can be problematic on commercial aircraft. It sometimes isn't possible to get to the bathroom to wash your hands immediately before eating or drinking—the food cart might block your path…the handles of airplane bathroom doors and soap dispensers are themselves often contaminated with germs…and sometimes there are germs in planes' tap-water reservoirs. Always wash your hands thoroughly as soon as you deplane.

Wipes Are Better Than Sprays

Charles Gerba, PhD, professor of microbiology and immunology and environmental science, University of Arizona, Tucson.

Wipes are better than sprays to kill germs on counters and other nonporous surfaces. You're more likely to let it dry naturally, giving it time to kill viruses. Make sure wipes contain *quaternary ammonium compounds* (quat), such as ones from Clorox and Lysol.

How to Kill the Coronavirus: When You're Home…When You're Out

Charles Gerba, PhD, a professor of microbiology and immunology and environmental science at University of Arizona College of Agriculture and Life Sciences, Tucson, Arizona. He is coauthor of *The Germ Freak's Guide to Outwitting Colds and Flu.*

It's hard not to get hysterical about the spread of the coronavirus. It's a novel virus—which means it's never been seen before—and the illness it causes, COVID-19, can be serious for people over 60 as well as those with underly-

ing health conditions, especially diabetes, heart disease and respiratory illnesses like asthma, bronchitis and emphysema.

Discovering how COVID-19 acts has become an ongoing process. We do know about other coronaviruses—including the one that causes SARS and the ones that cause many colds in the US every year—so we're presuming this coronavirus acts in similar ways. Based on these assumptions, there are things you can do to protect yourself from getting sick, both at home and when you're out and about.

AT HOME

Like the common cold and influenza virus, COVID-19 can survive very well in cool, dry temperatures—anywhere from a few hours to nine days, depending on the temperature and location.

COVID-19 enters your body when you touch a surface where the germ is living and then touch your nose, eyes or mouth. That's why not touching your face and washing your hands often is crucial. So is killing the virus to stop its spread. *Here's how…*

•**Clean high-traffic surfaces at least daily.** These include counters, desks, tabletops, phones, computer keyboards and mouse, tablets, television remote controls and your bedside table. You should also swab down the bathroom and kitchen sink, bathroom fixtures and the toilet. If someone in your house is sick with COVID-19, clean these areas two or three times a day.

•**Use a disinfectant wipe when you clean.** You want to concentrate on smooth, nonporous surfaces. The easiest way to clean these surfaces is to use a wipe that contains *quaternary ammonium compounds* (quat), which is found in most disinfecting wipes, such as from Clorox and Lysol. Why wipes? Because you are more likely to let the disinfectant dry naturally after you use one, which gives it time to kill the virus. Sure, you can use a quat-based spray on surfaces, but you have to wait about 10 minutes before you wipe it dry. Avoid white vinegar sprays for now because we don't know if it's effective against this virus.

•**Don't worry too much about soft surfaces.** Blankets, sheets, carpets, someone's jacket—it's harder for a virus to transfer to your fingers from these types of surfaces. Pillowcases could be a concern, although there is no data on this. You could change them nightly to be safe. Also, don't worry about mail and packages being contaminated even if the mail carrier is sick and doesn't know it yet. There is low transfer of virus from paper to the hands because paper is porous and absorbs a lot of the fluid the virus may be suspended in.

•**Use liquid soaps.** That way, when you and your family members wash hands, you're not contaminating each other.

•**Put a bottle of hand sanitizer next to entrances.** We have done studies on virus contamination of surfaces in homes, and once-a-day use of hand sanitizer seems to be enough to break the movement of viruses around the household. Place hand sanitizer near the front door, and ask everyone to use it when they come inside so no one brings viruses into the household. Even better, have everyone wash their hands thoroughly as soon as they come into the home. Don't rely on an air purifier to kill the virus. It won't unless it has a HEPA filter.

•**It is not necessary to shower as soon as you get home since it is largely your hands that spread the virus.** But if you are taking care of an ill person with coronavirus, change and wash your clothes every day.

WHEN YOU'RE OUT

It takes, on average, five days for people infected with COVID-19 to show symptoms, according to researchers from Johns Hopkins. So even if people aren't coughing and sneezing, they still could be passing on the virus. *Besides staying away from crowds and washing your hands as soon as you get home, here's how best to stay healthy...*

•**Always have a bottle of hand sanitizer in your purse or pocket.** Use one that contains 60% to 70% alcohol, and squirt it on your hands often—when you get off the bus, when you leave the grocery store, when you walk out of a public restroom. Keep one in your car, too.

•**Take extra care at the store.** Some areas that might contain more COVID-19, at least

based on studies done on viruses that cause colds—self-checkout counters and serving spoons at the prepared food stations. Apply hand sanitizer after using those. Consider going to the supermarket at off hours to minimize exposure to other people.

•**Swab down your car—especially if you've driven a sick person to the doctor or your children/grandchildren anywhere.** A car isn't a particularly germy place if you're the only person in it. But it can become a virus magnet once children or sick people go for a ride. Use disinfecting wipes to clean the often-touched areas—steering wheel, controls, armrests, door handles and the child/baby seat if there's one.

•**Don't go too crazy.** You don't have to wipe down the seat at the theater or on the train or in an Uber or taxicab—this virus isn't butt-borne. And you don't have to wear gloves so you don't touch the gas pump, door handles or elevator buttons with your bare hands. You could carry along tissues and use those, but honestly, if you squirt some hand sanitizer afterward and try not to touch your face you should be OK.

5 Smart Ways to Avoid Germs at the Gym

Bryan Combs, PhD, CRNP, a nurse practitioner and assistant professor of nursing at the University of Alabama at Birmingham School of Nursing. His research has been published in *Orthopedic Nursing, Workplace Health and Safety* and other leading professional journals.

Hopefully as you read this, after massive closures due to the coronavirus, gyms and fitness centers are open and in full swing to meet your workout needs. A trip to the gym is supposed to improve your health. So why do so many people get sick after hitting the treadmill, pumping some iron or sweating their way through spin class?

No matter how clean your gym looks, there's a good chance that it is crawling with microbes ranging from garden-variety cold and flu viruses to the infamous fungi that lead to athlete's foot and a host of bacteria such as *staphylococ-*

cus (more commonly known as "staph") and *Escherichia coli* (E. Coli).

Interestingly, many people assume that winter is the worst time of year for germy gyms—and certain pathogens, such as the flu virus, are more likely to be hanging around during that time. But the truth is, gyms are a hotbed of icky microbes year-round.

That doesn't mean you should sacrifice the health benefits of regularly working out at your local gym or fitness center. Just be sure to follow these five steps to avoid picking up a nasty bug from the germiest places at the gym.

STEP #1: Wipe down gym equipment before using it. Whether it's an elliptical machine, stationary bicycle, weight machine or free weights, never assume that it was cleaned by the previous user. Any piece of gym equipment that a person can touch could be teeming with germs. Don't believe it?

Consider this: When researchers took 288 samples at 16 fitness facilities in Ohio, *S. aureus* bacteria, which causes everything from skin infections to pneumonia, were found in the greatest concentrations on the following equipment—half of treadmill handles…56% of weight plates…and 63% or medicine balls, according to a 2019 study published in *BMC Infectious Diseases.*

What to do: To protect yourself, always use a disinfectant spray or towelette to clean any piece of exercise equipment before you touch it. And, of course, be a sport and do that for the next person.

Helpful: If the gym doesn't keep a disinfectant spray or wipes on hand, bring along a travel-sized antibacterial hand sanitizer to apply to your hands between machines and/or a time or two during your workout.

STEP #2: Beware of gym towels. When your face is dripping with sweat, it's handy to grab one of those towels that your gym may have on hand for a quick dry-off. Think twice before doing this. You probably assume that those towels are germ-free because they are freshly laundered, but that may not be the case.

While the towels have been washed, a lot of gyms use the same container to carry dirty towels to the washing area and to bring clean towels back, so they can become contaminated again.

What to do: To be safe, bring your own clean towel…and make sure you wash it after each workout.

STEP #3: Don't go barefoot. By now, everyone knows that you need to wear flip-flops or some other waterproof shoes in the shower. But don't get careless and walk barefoot in the locker rooms either. Both are ideal places to pick up athlete's foot or even a methicillin-resistant *Staphylococcus aureus* (MRSA) infection, which can spread by skin contact.

What to do: Wear shoes in the shower—and the locker room. You can buy a pair of shower shoes for less than $20 online and in stores.

STEP #4: Watch that water bottle. Staying hydrated is good for you, but an unwashed water bottle can make you sick. That's because it's common for people to use the same water bottle each time they go to the gym. But how often do they wash the outside, which may be covered with bacteria or viruses? Most likely, not very often.

What to do: Wash the outside of your water bottle with dish soap and hot water after every workout. It's also a good idea to rinse the inside with hot water—just as you would any drinking glass.

STEP #5: Don't forget about your gym bag. Surprisingly, your own gym bag may carry the most bacteria.

Here's why: Your gym bag does double duty, carrying your clean clothes to the gym and your dirty, smelly ones back home. It probably also holds your sweaty shoes. But do you ever clean your gym bag? Probably not.

What to do: To prevent the spread of germs, opt for a plastic or vinyl gym bag and clean the inside and outside with a disinfectant spray after each use, if possible, or at least a few times a week if you're a frequent gym-goer. As an alternative, choose a cloth bag that you can wash in hot water and bleach at least once a week and then dry in a hot drier.

Flu Mystery Solved

Proceedings of the National Academy of Sciences.

Why is the flu so easily transmitted during winter? There have been many theories, but research now says that low humidity plays a key role because of its effects on immunity. In lab studies performed on mice, low humidity impaired the animals' ability to repair viral damage.

Pneumonia Rx Danger

Valerie Vaughn, MD, MSc, is an assistant professor at VA Ann Arbor Healthcare System and University of Michigan Medical School. UofMHealth.org

Two-thirds of pneumonia patients receive antibiotics for longer than necessary when discharged from hospitals. The median prescription was two days longer than needed. Excessive antibiotic use increases the risk for antibiotic resistance, infections and—in the case of fluoroquinolones—torn tendons, ruptured arteries and suicidal thoughts. If an antibiotic prescription following hospitalization for pneumonia extends more than five days total (seven days for those with severe issues beyond pneumonia), ask why.

Power Soup That Helps Boost Immunity

Jackie Newgent, RDN, CDN, a registered dietitian, classically trained chef and author of several cookbooks, including *The Clean & Simple Diabetes Cookbook*. Check out her plant-based recipes on her blog at JackieNewgent.com.

If there's ever been a time when you need a well-functioning immune system, it's now. And the first place to start strengthening your immune system is with the foods you eat. Immune-boosting foods protect us in several ways—they provide antioxidants and reduce inflammation in the body…they stimulate the

Don't Touch That Pen!

At the hospital or a doctor's office, use your own pen—not theirs—to fill in forms. Writing implements in medical settings harbor vast amounts of germs.

Miryam Z. Wahrman, PhD, professor of biology at William Paterson University, Wayne, New Jersey, and author of *The Hand Book: Surviving in a Germ-Filled World*.

immune system to do its job…and they help to fight infection. We asked Jackie Newgent, RDN, CDN, a nutritionist and classically trained chef known for creating delicious healthy dishes, to come up with a list of 10 of her favorite foods that help boost immunity. Her list includes a bit of everything—from spices and protein-packed picks to vegetables and even tea.

Best of all: These foods can be eaten separately…or together in a delicious soup that helps boost immunity. The recipe is on page 198.

10 IMMUNE-BOOSTING FOODS

Find out how these 10 super-germ-fighting foods do their job…

•**Lentils** provide a significant amount of iron. Getting iron from the food you eat can help your body fight fatigue.

•**Garlic and onion** both contain compounds called *allyl sulfides*, which work to protect immune function.

•**Mushrooms** contain a naturally occurring compound called *lentinan*, which stimulates immune function. They also contain a significant amount of zinc, a nutrient that also can help the immune system. Studies suggest that the white button mushroom, in particular, can help the body fight viruses.

•**Spinach** is an amazing source of folate. This nutrient can help increase the body's ability to fight infection.

•**Sweet potatoes** are rich in beta-carotene, a carotenoid that has a positive effect on immune cell function.

•**Tomatoes** get their red pigment from the phytonutrient *lycopene*. Regular consumption of tomatoes has been associated with enhanced immunity due to lycopene's role in immune cell function.

•**Yogurt** that contains probiotics from live friendly bacteria helps to improve your body's immune response—and protect you from infection. When choosing yogurt, read the label carefully. Look for brands that ideally contain at least two probiotic types and no added sugars, including high-fructose corn syrup.

•**Green tea** is loaded with flavonoids that have powerful antioxidant and antiviral properties. When regularly consumed, green tea may help protect against the flu.

•**Cinnamon** is a warming spice, so called because it seems to warm our bodies by playing a role in promoting circulation. Cinnamon's antioxidant and anti-inflammatory properties help stimulate the immune system.

AMAZING IMMUNITY-BOOSTING SOUP

1 Tablespoon olive oil or avocado oil

1 large onion, chopped

2 large garlic cloves, finely chopped

½ teaspoon ground cumin

½ teaspoon ground cinnamon

4 cups reduced-sodium vegetable broth

¾ cup dry brown or green lentils

4 ounces cremini, shiitake or white button mushrooms, stemmed and sliced

1 (15-ounce) can diced tomatoes

1 medium garnet yam or sweet potato, scrubbed, unpeeled and diced

1 cup freshly brewed green tea, unsweetened

1 (5-ounce) package fresh baby spinach

Sea salt and freshly ground black pepper to taste

⅓ cup reduced-fat plain Greek yogurt and/or 6 lemon wedges (optional)

In a large saucepan, heat the oil over medium-high heat. Add the chopped onion, and cook until lightly browned, about eight minutes, stirring occasionally. Add the garlic, cumin and cinnamon, and cook one minute longer, stirring constantly. Add the broth and lentils. When the liquid boils, reduce the heat, cover and simmer for 25 minutes.

Add the mushrooms, tomatoes, diced yam and tea. Cook until the lentils are soft and the yam just holds its shape, about 12 minutes.

Stir the baby spinach into the soup by the handful. Cover and heat for five minutes. Add seasoning as desired.

To serve, divide the soup among six wide, shallow bowls. Add a dollop of Greek yogurt to each bowl and/or serve with lemon wedges, if desired. Makes six servings.

A New Use for CBD?

American Society for Microbiology annual meeting

Cannabidiol (CBD), derived from cannabis (aka marijuana or hemp), is growing in popularity as a natural remedy for pain, insomnia, anxiety and other health problems.

Latest discovery: CBD kills S. aureus and other dangerous bacteria—and appears to be as effective as high-powered antibiotics.

Plants and Superbugs

Keck School of Medicine, University of Southern California.

About one-fifth of antibiotic-resistant infections are linked to agriculture—including the consumption of plant foods. Foodborne organisms can "silently" colonize the intestine and eventually emerge to cause a future illness. This finding may lead to new treatments for superbugs.

Hand Sanitizer at the Hospital

The New York Times.

Hospital hand sanitizers are used less often than they should be because they cannot be placed close to patients. Fire marshals require sanitizer dispensers to be removed altogether or located far from patients' bedsides because hand sanitizers contain at least 60% alcohol and are flammable. Fire regulations also limit how much hand sanitizer can be kept on site.

Result: Sanitizer dispensers usually are in hallways—but greater use of sanitizers closer to patients could be more effective at germ control. In one study, 50% more hand sanitizer was used when the product was hung over patients' beds on a trapeze-bar construct.

Tiny But Deadly

Roundup of experts on mosquito-borne disease, reported in *Nature*.

Mosquitoes are humans' deadliest enemies. The diseases they carry may have killed almost half the 108 billion human beings who have ever lived.

The Natural Way to Boost Your Immune System When the Grandkids Come to Visit

Jamison Starbuck, ND, naturopathic physician in family practice in Missoula, Montana, and producer of *Dr. Starbuck's Health Tips for Kids*, a weekly program on Montana Public Radio, MTPR.org.

Not long ago, my patient Kathy guiltily admitted that she sometimes dreads visits from her grandchildren—when the kids leave, her husband is exhausted and she ends up in bed, sick with a cold or bad sore throat. Kathy's situation is not unusual. Parents, grandparents and all adults who share close quarters, hugs and kisses and frequent meals with little ones often find that their immune systems are unable to defend against the onslaught of contagious ailments that kids carry around.

Here's what I suggest to help my patients strengthen their immune systems...*

• **Don't forget the basics of healthy eating and hydration.** When you're busy with child-care, it's easy to fill up on quick "kid" snacks and forgo healthy meals...and many grandparents and parents forget to hydrate sufficiently. Make sure to nourish yourself (and your little ones) with healthy food, such as plenty of fruits and vegetables, lean meat, beans and whole grains, and to hydrate well—water is always best. Aim to drink half your body weight in ounces daily.

• **Take antioxidants daily.** A common regimen: 1,000 mg of vitamin C...400 international units (IU) of vitamin E...and 10,000 IU of vitamin A. *Note:* It's beneficial to take these antioxidants all the time, not just when around young kids.

Additional help: The week before your grandkids come to visit, or at the first sign of a child getting ill, start taking an immune-boosting herbal tincture. I particularly like a combined formula of astragalus, ligusticum, lomatium and elder. However, if you can't find a combo formula, taking just two or three of the four herbs is beneficial. Take 60 drops of a combined tincture in two ounces of water, twice daily, in between meals. Continue to take the tincture throughout the child's visit, or his/her illness, and for three days afterward.

• **Get good sleep!** This can be hard to do with the excitement of visitors or when the kids are sick. A safe, non–habit-forming natural sleep aid is the amino acid L-tryptophan. You may already know that tryptophan is abundant in turkey and thought to be responsible for that sleepy feeling after the Thanksgiving meal. Tryptophan promotes the production of serotonin, a neurotransmitter that facilitates relaxation. Take 500 mg of L-tryptophan at bedtime, with water, away from food.

• **Manage your stress.** Caring for kids can be fulfilling and lots of fun, but it can also cause impatience, confusion, irritability and self-criticism. This emotional stress takes a toll on the immune system. Another amino acid, *gamma-aminobu-*

*Before taking any supplement or herbal remedy, check with your doctor.

tyric acid (GABA), can help manage these strong emotions. Take 200 mg of GABA up to four times a day, as needed, for emotional stress.

Kathy followed my plan and six months later happily reported back that she was no longer getting sick after her grandkids came to stay. She had convinced her husband to do the protocol as well, and except for the very messy house after the kids depart, they both now thoroughly look forward to visits with the grandchildren!

Measles Does Long-Term Damage to the Immune System

Stephen Elledge, PhD, geneticist, Harvard Medical School, Boston, and coauthor of a study published in *Science*.

Measles eliminates up to 73% of children's protective antibodies, deleting the immune system's "memory" of other diseases. Children who have measles are more vulnerable to other infections long after measles is gone.

HPV Vaccine Is Important for Boys as Well as Girls

Maura Gillison, MD, PhD, professor of medicine, department of cancer medicine, The University of Texas MD Anderson Cancer Center, Houston, and leader of a study published in *JAMA*.

Cancer caused by the human papillomavirus is wrongly thought of as only a female issue. But of the 34,800 HPV-caused cancer cases in the US every year, 40% are in men. HPV is sexually transmitted, usually through oral sex. In men, the cancer that HPV most commonly causes is of the mouth and throat. But the vaccine against HPV, Gardasil, is not approved to prevent mouth or throat cancer—only cervical cancer—so it is generally only given to girls. Also, insurance may not cover an unapproved use. It takes decades between an HPV infec-

tion and the time cancer develops, so early vaccination is a good idea.

The Search for Flu Strains Continues

The Ohio State University College of Veterinary Medicine

Far-flung flu research! Scientists travel to county fairs each year, where they swab the snouts of pigs and look for new—and dangerous—strains of flu. The 2009 flu pandemic began in pigs and eventually infected 50 million and caused 12,000 human deaths.

Why You Need a Tetanus Shot

Mark K. Slifka, PhD, professor of microbiology and immunology, Oregon Health & Science University, Beaverton.

Tetanus is a serious bacterial infection that can be life-threatening if not treated promptly. The bacteria that cause tetanus are typically transmitted via soil, dust or manure. Rusty nails are widely thought to cause tetanus, but rust itself does not necessarily carry the bacteria—any sharp object that's rusty could have been exposed to dirt, dust or manure that contains the bacteria that cause tetanus.

In the US, the current recommendation by the Advisory Committee on Immunization Practices is for adults to be revaccinated for tetanus every 10 years throughout adulthood. In other countries, such as the UK, there is no recommendation for adult booster vaccination against tetanus once a person has completed his/her childhood vaccination series.

If you don't remember when you got your last tetanus shot (or if you don't know whether you got the full childhood series), you should get a booster. A booster dose may be given when someone is exposed to the bacteria to help prevent severe disease, but the vaccine works best

Common Flu-Shot Side Effects

Soreness or aching in your arm usually lasts a day and indicates that your immune system is responding properly to the shot. Redness, pain or swelling at the injection site may last a few days—this too shows that your immune system has been activated. Low-grade fever is possible but uncommon—if the fever is above 101°F, you are probably sick with a virus different from the flu virus. Nausea, headaches or fatigue occasionally occur.

Caution: Severe allergic reactions to flu shots or their components are rare but do occur. Anyone who develops breathing trouble, wheezing, hives, high fever, swelling around the eyes or lips, or a fast heartbeat should get to a doctor or emergency room quickly.

Centers for Disease Control and Prevention, Atlanta.

when given before exposure to allow time for protective levels of antibodies to build up.

Even though tetanus is rare in the US, the majority of reported illnesses occur in people who didn't receive the full childhood vaccination regimen or didn't complete their booster shots in adulthood. Side effects from the shot are rare but may include fever and/or swelling at the injection site. If you have questions about your vaccination history, consult your doctor.

Syphilis and Gonorrhea Are at Epidemic Levels

Sexually Transmitted Disease Surveillance Report by the US Centers for Disease Control and Prevention, Atlanta.

Until recently, these sexually transmitted diseases were declining in the US, with syphilis nearly eliminated. But both are increasing significantly. Gonorrhea cases rose 5% in 2018 over the previous year (latest data available) to more than 580,000...and syphilis increased 13.3%, to 115,000 cases. Combined cases of gonorrhea, syphilis and chlamydia—the most common STD, with 1.7 million cases reported—reached an all-time US high in 2018.

Do Adults Need a Measles Shot?

William Schaffner, MD, professor of preventive medicine and infectious diseases, Vanderbilt University Medical Center, Nashville.

The recent spate of measles cases—the worst outbreak in 25 years—has generated a great deal of concern.

The good news is that most adults are at low risk for measles, and few cases have spread into the general population. The majority of recent cases have occurred in unvaccinated children in certain close-knit communities with some adults in those communities getting the illness.

Most unvaccinated people will become ill if they come in contact with someone who is infected. But for people born in 1957 or earlier, it's highly likely that they had measles as a child, and once you've had the disease, you're immune to getting it again.

That said, some adults are at higher risk for measles—namely those living in a community with a measles outbreak, health-care workers, college students living in close quarters and those planning international travel. If you're in any of these categories—and don't remember whether you had measles as a child—check your records to be sure that you got two doses of the measles, mumps, rubella (MMR) vaccine.

If you're not sure if you got two doses of the MMR vaccine or had measles as a child, there's no harm in getting vaccinated.

Exceptions: The vaccine is not recommended for pregnant women and adults who have a weakened immune system, a bleeding disorder or recently received a blood transfusion. A blood test also can confirm whether you have immunity to measles.

Where Germs Hide in Your Home

FamilyHandyman.com

Sheets are a breeding ground for microscopic dust mites—wash sheets in hot water weekly, and keep humidity below 50%. *Showerheads* may contain bacteria that can cause lung infections—clean heads by submerging them overnight in vinegar if the manufacturer says that will not harm the finish. *Refrigerators* can have mold and bacteria growing in them—wipe up spills immediately, clean regularly with hot soapy water, and throw out spoiled food at least weekly. *Hand towels* may hold germs for hours after use—avoid sharing them, and change and wash them regularly. *Remote controls* are covered with germs—disinfect them weekly with antibacterial wipes. *Vacuum cleaners* may contain bacteria, molds and allergens—clean them regularly and consider wearing a mask while vacuuming.

Protect Yourself from Germs in Public Bathrooms

Philip M. Tierno, Jr., PhD, clinical professor of microbiology and pathology at NYU Langone Health in New York City. He is author of *The Secret Life of Germs.* Med. NYU.edu

Public bathrooms can be a hotbed of viruses and bacteria. *My advice…*

•**Don't fret so much about the toilet seat.** Unless there's noticeable liquid or a smear of something gross on the seat, it is less contaminated than most people fear. That's because there's usually a low germ count on smooth-surfaced toilet seats and you have a protective skin barrier.

•**Flush with your shoe.** The flush handle is often contaminated, so flush with your shoe instead of your hand. If balance is a problem for you, at least use toilet paper to press the handle, then drop it quickly into the bowl.

•**Use paper towels.** The soap dispenser, faucet handle and door handle are often contaminated. Use a paper towel instead of your bare hand.

•**Avoid electric hand dryers.** Research shows that these machines can actually spread bacteria into the air and onto your hands.

•**Count to 30.** Even if your hands get contaminated, it's not a problem as long as you wash them with soap and water before touching your eyes, nose or mouth or a break in the skin (the conduits of entry into your body). With soap and warm water, vigorously rub your hands, including the tops and under your fingernails, for 30 seconds. Use the same paper towel you dry your hands with to open the door.

Good idea: Consider carrying your own paper towel in a pocket or bag in case the bathroom doesn't have any.

Say Goodbye to Toenail Fungus

Douglas F. Tumen, DPM, a board-certified foot surgeon and fellow of the American College of Foot and Ankle Surgeons. He is author of *Ask the Foot Doctor: Real-Life Answers to Enjoy Happy, Healthy, Pain-Free Feet.* AskTheFootDoctor.com

Most people know the telltale signs of toenail fungus, but few are aware of the best ways to get rid of this wily infection.

The condition is more common as we age, with about half of adults over age 70 dealing with this unsightly problem.

Onychomycosis (the medical term for nail fungus) is notoriously difficult to treat—some people spend years, or even decades, trying to eradicate their thick, brittle and crumbly toenails that may have turned yellow or brown.

But some therapies are more effective than others. In fact, new research shows that even particularly stubborn toenail fungus can now be eliminated with few risks for side effects.

HOW THE BATTLE BEGINS

The environment inside your shoes is ideal for fungus—warm, humid and dark. What's more, the hard nail structure makes it difficult for topical drugs to penetrate effectively.

Your feet encounter fungus every day—in the shower (be it public or in your home)…in your gym locker room…at nail salons…or when going through airport security if you're barefoot when you pull off your shoes. These are common ways to contract athlete's foot.

Toenail fungus, however, more often results from repeated nail injuries, such as your toes hitting the inside of your shoes when walking or running…or banging your toe into a chair or other furniture. Such injuries weaken the nail bed, allowing fungus to invade the toenail. Long toenails and snug shoes make the toenails vulnerable to these injuries, so proper nail care, including keeping your toenails trimmed, and proper shoe fit are crucial.

Important: A fungal infection can spread from one toenail to another, and early treatment helps minimize this. People with diabetes, poor circulation or compromised immunity should seek medical advice for toenail fungus.

To give yourself the best odds of vanquishing toenail fungus, here are five options that you may not know about—use one or more of these methods…

TREATMENT #1: **Vicks VapoRub.** Dabbed onto the affected toenail once or twice daily, this over-the-counter (OTC) topical cough suppressant often reduces—and sometimes cures—fungus in five to 16 months. It's one of VapoRub's "inactive" ingredients—*thymol*, a derivative of thyme used for its scent—that helps fight fungus. Other ingredients, including camphor, eucalyptus and menthol (all cough suppressants), may help combat fungus, too. You can apply it at night and then go to bed with or without socks.

Scientific evidence: When 18 adults with toenail fungus applied Vicks VapoRub daily for 48 weeks, the condition improved or was eliminated in 15 of the study participants, according to research published in *Journal of the American Board of Family Medicine.*

Avoid Athlete's Foot

Forgot your flip-flops and worried about the fungus you might pick up walking barefoot on the locker room floor? Use hand sanitizer to clean your feet before putting your shoes back on.

Jeffrey Benabio, MD, FAAD, dermatologist and physician director of Health Care Transformation at Kaiser Permanente, San Diego.

TREATMENT #2: **Nail file and OTC topical antifungal.** For an early-stage fungus called white superficial *onychomycosis*, topical medication applied to freshly trimmed nails may help. This fungus appears as tiny (a couple of millimeters in diameter) circular or oblong spots. Because it rests on top of the nail bed, rather than inside or underneath the nail, this infection may respond well to topical treatments.

What to do: File the nail as low as possible using a single-use emery board. This will remove some of the fungus-infected nail and deprive the remaining fungus of its preferred food source—the nail itself.

Caution: Never dig under the nail with instruments. Doing so can loosen the nail from the nail bed, making it easier for fungus to enter.

Next, apply an OTC topical antifungal product containing *tolnaftate, ciclopirox* or one of the -azole medications (*clotrimazole, miconazole* or *ketoconazole*) daily. Although OTC antifungals marketed for athlete's foot, such as Lotrimin AF (which contains clotrimazole), have only been FDA-approved for use on skin, they can be safely used off-label for onychomycosis.

Important: While the fungal-infected nail grows out, avoid nail polish for at least a few months. Conventional nail polishes act like paint, trapping and essentially protecting lingering fungus. In fact, many patients first notice white superficial onychomycosis at the end of the summer when they stop getting regular pedicures and there's no polish hiding the spots.

If you do wear nail polish, choose a nontoxic formula that is free from chemicals such as formaldehyde and toluene. These versions are more "breathable" than traditional nail polishes, so they're less apt to trap fungus underneath. For added protection, try a product (such as daniPro) that contains antifungal compounds to help prevent toenail fungus. Men, or women who wish to avoid color, can use a clear version.

TREATMENT #3: Lasers. With the power to vaporize and disable toenail fungus, lasers are one of the more effective treatments. As the nail grows, healthy nail should begin emerging from the base, indicating that the fungus is being killed. Lasers are painless, require no aftercare and improve the majority of cases. Laser treatment for toenail fungus, which is performed by a podiatrist, is typically administered once a month for at least three months.

Note: Laser therapy for onychomycosis is FDA-approved, but is not covered by insurance because it's considered a cosmetic treatment. In some cases, the treatment may be covered if it's medically necessary—for instance, if you have diabetes or are immuno-compromised. Ask your insurer. The fee varies widely—a course of treatment may cost up to $1,000.

TREATMENT #4: Oral antifungals. For patients whose onychomycosis is stubborn and affects more than half of the nail plate, oral antifungals may be the most effective option. For years, the standard protocol called for 250 mg of Lamisil, a costly prescription antifungal, once a day for 90 days. The treatment is effective in about 60% of cases, but side effects can include gastrointestinal upset, headache and liver toxicity. Liver damage occurs in less than 1% of patients who use the drug but is potentially fatal.

A new, safer option: A less expensive generic version of Lamisil, terbinafine hydrochloride, is now widely available and can be prescribed via an equally effective, more liver-friendly "pulse dosing regimen"—four cycles of 500 mg (two pills) daily for seven days each month (a total of 56 pills over four months). Pulse therapy was as effective at treating onychomycosis as the conventional daily regimen with the brand-name medication (typically one pill daily for three months), according to a 2019 study published in *Journal of Fungi*.

Note: Most insurers only cover terbinafine, the generic medication, and not the brand-name version.

TREATMENT #5: Sanitized shoes. The fungus in your toenail is most likely living in your shoes. That's why it's smart to invest in an ultraviolet (UV) light shoe sanitizer. The Steri-Shoe Essential, for example, is a small device that you place in your shoes (closed-toed or even sandals) and plug in so that UV light can kill the fungi that can lead to toenail fungus. This product, which has the American Podiatric Medical Association Seal of Acceptance, sanitizes shoes and turns itself off in 45 minutes. It's available online for $99.95. Even though it's unlikely that socks will spread fungi when doing laundry, it's best to wash socks in hot water and use bleach to be safe.

A Fishy Solution?

Oregon State University

With the ongoing threats posed by antibiotic resistance, the search for new antibiotics is urgent.

Recent finding: The slimy mucus that acts as a protective coating for fish may contain infection-fighting components that could lead to the discovery of new antibiotics.

Bonus: One compound that was identified from the mucous coating inhibited the growth of human cancer cells.

Petting Zoo Precautions

Howard Smith, MD, a pediatric ear, nose and throat physician and former radio talk show host, broadcasts the weekly podcast "Dr. Howard Smith On Call." DrHoward Smith.com

Petting zoos can spread antibiotic-resistant germs. A recent Israeli study of 228 petting zoo animals found that 12% carried strains of bacteria that are resistant to antibiotics and capable of infecting humans. Children who cannot yet be trusted to keep their hands out of their mouths should not directly touch the animals or go to petting zoos. Everyone else should wash their hands vigorously and repeatedly after touching these animals.

Dangerous Mice

mBio

Watch out for Big Apple mice! In research conducted on 416 New York City mice, the ubiquitous pests were found to carry bacteria, including Salmonella and E. coli, that cause gastrointestinal diseases in humans. Some of the bacteria appear to be resistant to common fluoroquinolone antibiotics, such as Cipro and Levaquin.

The Truth About Fecal Transplants

Henning Gerke, MD, gastroenterologist, University of Iowa Health Care, and clinical professor of internal medicine, gastroenterology and hepatology, University of Iowa, Carver College of Medicine, Iowa City.

Admittedly, a fecal transplant—putting someone else's poop into your body—sounds unpleasant. However, it may be the only way to cure some very serious gastrointestinal conditions that resist conventional treatment. And the procedure is not really as gross as what you're probably imagining.

The medical name for the procedure is fecal microbiota transplantation (or FMT)—and the serious condition it most commonly treats is C. difficile (C. diff), a bacterial infection that sickens half a million Americans and kills up to 30,000 each year. In fact, both the Infectious Diseases Society of America and The Society for Healthcare Epidemiology of America have recently added FMT to their official guidelines for treating C. diff.

AN ANCIENT THERAPY MADE MODERN

The concept of curing illness with donor fecal matter dates back to 4th-century China, when a cruder version of the procedure (which truly was gross—it involved making a soup!) was used to treat severe food poisoning and diarrhea. Today's procedure administers FMT via colonoscopy, enema or a tube run through the nose and into the stomach. (An oral capsule is being tested in clinical trials.) The procedure is simple and usually performed outpatient. In most cases, the patient leaves the hospital the same day and C. diff symptoms ease within days.

The fecal matter used in FMT comes from either a local donor (someone you know or the hospital's donor program) or from a national nonprofit stool bank called OpenBiome. In all cases, donors are screened first for illnesses, the same as for blood donors. With a local donor, medical staff mixes the stool with saline (often in a basic kitchen blender) to prepare for a transplant. OpenBiome stool donations are filtered and homogenized, then sealed and kept frozen.

The risk for side effects is low—for instance, abdominal discomfort or a mild fever. FMT has become so accepted as a treatment for C. diff that 97% of Americans live within two hours of a facility that performs the procedure, according to OpenBiome.

HOW FMT WORKS

The main culprit behind C. diff and many other gastrointestinal upsets is a disruption of the gut microbiome. This can be caused by medical conditions, such as a compromised immune system, diabetes or obesity...or from taking certain drugs, such as antibiotics. FMT transplants gut organisms from a healthy donor into a sick patient's gut, repopulating the disrupted gut and helping to restore the natural balance. Numerous studies show FMT to be about 70% to 90%—or more—effective for treating recurrent C. diff infections. (If you're wondering why probiotics don't help, they contain only a few strains of microorganisms, not the wide, diverse spectrum contained in the stool of a healthy donor.)

C. diff bacteria actually are present in a normal, healthy gut in small numbers. But when antibiotics—even a single course—kill off healthy gut bacteria while they're killing the pathogens that made you sick, C. diff can take over, triggering severe diarrhea. Ironically, the standard first line of treatment for C. diff is more antibiotics, which explains why recurrent C. diff is a common problem. Especially vulnerable are children, people over age 65 and those who have a compromised immune system.

THE FMT FRONTIER

While the effectiveness of FMT has only been established for treating C. diff—which is the only FDA-approved use outside of research—the procedure shows promise for other conditions. Because your gut microbiome is critical to your whole immune system and your general health, scientists are studying how FMT might also treat irritable bowel syndrome (IBS), Crohn's disease, diabetes, obesity, peanut allergies and melanoma.

The National Institutes of Health is currently funding a large study that is being conducted by the Fecal Microbiota Transplantation National Registry under the guidance of the American Gastroenterological Association's Center for Gut Microbiome Research and Education.

The study plans to track about 4,000 FMT patients for a decade after their transplants. The researchers will be gathering data on FMT's effectiveness for C. diff and other illnesses, including information on the short- and long-term effects. Currently, more than 20 hospitals, medical centers and medical schools across the country are participating—a number that's expected to grow to 75.

Meanwhile, you can search for a doctor who performs FMT by going to OpenBiome.org.

Credit Cards Are as Germy as Cash

Timothy E. Riedel, PhD, assistant professor of practice, College of Natural Sciences at The University of Texas at Austin. CNS.UTexas.edu/fri

---

Recent study: Germs found on credit cards included *Staphylococcus aureus*, the cause of staph infections…and *Salmonella enterica*, a source of food poisoning. Consumers tend to imagine, incorrectly, that their cards are cleaner than cash because they don't pass through as many hands. Periodically use alcohol wipes to disinfect cards. Wash your hands or use hand sanitizer between handling cards and eating.

Superbugs in Cosmetics

Amreen Bashir, PhD, lecturer in biomedical sciences at Aston University in Birmingham, England, and lead researcher of the study of used makeup published in *Journal of Applied Microbiology.*

Ninety percent of cosmetics were found to have superbugs ranging from staph to E. coli. Makeup sponges carried the most bacteria—more than mascara, eyeliner and lipsticks—because they're rarely washed, even after being dropped on a bathroom floor. Protect yourself by washing them with soap and hot water weekly and discarding sponges every two months.

Bat Bites and Scratches Can Be Easily Overlooked

Data from Centers for Disease Control and Prevention, Atlanta, reported in *University of California, Berkeley Wellness Letter.*

Bat bites and scratches can be hard to see and easy to overlook. Some people have been bitten while asleep without knowing it. If you suspect that you may have had a bat bite…or wake up and find a bat in your room…or have a close encounter with a bat behaving oddly—such as being unable to fly or being active during daytime—see your doctor to discuss whether you should get treated for possible rabies exposure. Bats are the leading cause of the disease in the US. Of 89 cases reported between 1960 and 2018, 70% were caused by bats.

CHAPTER 12

Medical News Alerts

The Oxygen Factor

You've probably never thought about it this way, but whether or not you develop a disease like heart disease, cancer, stroke or chronic obstructive pulmonary disease (COPD) depends, in large part, on how the cells of your body respond to oxygen. Because these diseases cause about two-thirds of all the deaths in the US, understanding these cell reactions is a big deal…in fact, it's big enough to win a Nobel Prize.

How the journey began: The story of this groundbreaking discovery began in 1995 when researchers at Johns Hopkins University, led by Gregg L. Semenza, MD, PhD, identified a protein that controls how cells respond to low levels of oxygen (hypoxia). Twenty-four years later, Dr. Semenza was awarded the 2019 Nobel Prize in Physiology or Medicine for his seminal work on this protein, which was dubbed hypoxia inducible factor-1 (HIF-1).

A MASTER REGULATOR OF OXYGEN

What is HIF-1? Simply put, it is a type of protein that binds to part of your DNA, allowing it to turn on or off genes that control cell functions. As such, HIF-1 is the so-called "master regulator" for genes that regulate your cellular response to oxygen. This is important because the low levels of oxygen that occur with hypoxia can be deadly to cells.

Think of it this way: The human body has about 100 trillion cells that need a steady supply of oxygen. Imagine if, say, FedEx had to make 100 trillion deliveries 24 hours a day…every day. At the cellular level, that is the scope of the body's oxygen supply challenge.

To protect cells, HIF-1 turns on genes that increase oxygen in several ways. For example, HIF-1 can increase the production of red blood

Gregg L. Semenza, MD, PhD, professor of genetic medicine, pediatrics, radiation oncology and molecular radiation sciences, biological chemistry, medicine and oncology at Johns Hopkins University School of Medicine in Baltimore. Dr. Semenza is director of the Vascular Biology Program at Johns Hopkins' Institute for Cell Engineering and the recipient of the 2019 Nobel Prize in Physiology or Medicine.

cells, which carry oxygen to cells, by triggering production of a hormone called *erythropoietin* (EPO). EPO is made in your kidneys, but it triggers production of red blood cells in your bone marrow.

HIF-1 also can increase oxygen by promoting the growth of new blood vessels to deliver oxygen to the body's tissues—a process known as *angiogenesis*. This occurs when HIF-1 activates a protein called *vascular endothelial growth factor* (VEGF).

In the presence of hypoxia, HIF-1 triggers glycolysis, a process that breaks down glucose to promote the production of cellular energy.

HOW DOES HIF-1 AFFECT DISEASE?

When it comes to the effects of HIF-1, there's good news and bad news. By increasing oxygen-carrying red blood cells…creating new blood vessels…and activating glycolysis, HIF-1 can help prevent the cell damage that results from diseases caused by decreased blood supply, such as anemia, heart attack, stroke and diabetes.

On the other hand, HIF-1 can worsen such diseases as cancer, COPD and certain eye diseases of the retina. *Here's how that happens with…*

•**Cancer.** With a developing malignancy, cells divide very rapidly, which uses up lots of oxygen and causes hypoxia. HIF-1 can be activated by hypoxia in cancer cells to provide more oxygen and increase their blood supply. In cancers that grow quickly and spread (metastasize), HIF-1 is more active (overexpressed), research shows.

•**COPD.** With COPD, HIF-1 is required for the constriction of pulmonary blood vessels in response to hypoxia. This constriction makes it more difficult for the heart to pump blood to the lungs, which can lead to heart failure.

•**Eye disease.** Blood flow into and out of the retina (the thin layer of sensory tissue that lines the back of the eye) can be impaired due to a condition such as diabetes. To compensate for the lack of oxygen, HIF-1 kicks into high gear, triggering new blood vessel growth, which gradually covers the retina, leading to ischemic retinopathy, a major cause of blindness among people with diabetes.

HIF-1 TREATMENTS

Depending on the disease, either increasing or blocking HIF-1 activity could be beneficial. Treatments that increase HIF-1 activity are called HIF-1 inducers, while those that block HIF-1 are called HIF-1 inhibitors. With studies now under way in animals and humans, such treatments are close to becoming a reality.

For example, an HIF-1 inducer is being studied to treat anemia due to chronic kidney disease, which causes your kidneys to stop making the hormone EPO. The reduced EPO production inhibits the production of red blood cells, leading to anemia. To treat this anemia, researchers have developed a man-made (recombinant) form of EPO. However, the major drawback of recombinant EPO is that it must be injected, whereas HIF-inducers are administered as pills that can be taken by mouth.

Final-stage human studies show that an oral HIF-1 inducer medication, called a small-molecule drug, is a more natural and effective way to increase EPO and reverse anemia. One of the HIF-inducers (*roxadustat*) has been approved for use in China and Japan. There are large clinical trials under way in the US, the results of which will determine whether the medication gets FDA approval. The decision will probably be made within a year or so.

Meanwhile, an HIF-2 (a closely related protein) inhibitor drug is in clinical trials for the treatment of kidney cancer. So far, the drug has only been tested in a phase 1 trial, which tests drug safety, not drug efficacy. However, the results are promising.

THE FUTURE FOR HIF-1

In the next 10 years, several FDA-approved treatments should become available for diseases using HIF-1 inducers and inhibitors. In addition to those discussed earlier, treatments for conditions including heart attack, stroke, COPD, wounds, diabetes and even spinal cord injury are hoped for in the future.

Latest development: HIF-1 gene therapy—by promoting blood vessel growth in the legs, for example—might be useful for the treatment of localized disease, such as limb ischemia, a narrowing or blockage of an artery that significantly reduces blood flow.

Noise Pollution Harms More Than Your Hearing

Richard L. Neitzel, PhD, associate chair and associate professor of environmental health sciences and global public health at University of Michigan School of Public Health in Ann Arbor. He is a certified industrial hygienist (CIH) and Fellow of the American Industrial Hygiene Association (FAIHA). His research has been published in professional journals including *Environmental Science & Technology, Noise & Health* and *International Journal of Audiology.*

Screeching sirens, thunderous jackhammers and other earsplitting noises are known to harm a person's hearing—or even mental health. But these aren't the only dangers.

A growing body of evidence shows that "noise pollution" is worsening with each passing year...and potentially harming our overall health in the process. The impact of noise is comparable to air pollution, according to the World Health Organization. But unlike smog and diesel exhaust, noise pollution receives scant attention by the media. What's more, people are often unaware when noise pollution is wreaking its insidious damage.

What you need to know about the growing threat of noise pollution...

WHAT'S THE PROBLEM?

Noise (aka "unwanted sound") can come from just about anywhere. It can be the drone of cars on a nearby road...your neighbor's barking dog...or the TV in the next room. And it doesn't take much to cause harm.

What most people don't realize: While very loud noises—such as fireworks at close range or a jet plane takeoff—pose obvious threats to your hearing, damage often begins at more modest levels, such as that produced by a leaf blower or the music you listen to in your car or with earbuds.

As with many environmental toxins, impact depends on three things—intensity, duration and frequency. What determines adverse effects, experts believe, is the average noise exposure over time.

If you live in a city, harmful levels of noise are likely to be your constant companion. But even if you live in the suburbs or a rural area, you're also at increased risk if you have a lengthy commute, which is likely to include loud traffic sounds, or a noisy work environment.

DAMAGE YOU MIGHT NOT EXPECT

As scientists continue to dig into the negative impacts of noise pollution, evidence is mounting for a wide range of health problems. *For example...*

•**Hearing.** Some researchers believe that much of what is generally considered a natural age-related decline in hearing (presbycusis) may actually reflect the cumulative impact of noise.

•**Cardiovascular disease.** There's strong evidence linking noise pollution and cardiovascular disease. Rates of heart attack, heart failure, high blood pressure and stroke increase with higher levels of noise.

For example, a research review published in 2018 in *Journal of the American College of Cardiology* noted that road traffic and aircraft noise increased risk for coronary heart disease by 6% for every 10 decibels (dBA), starting as low as 50 dBA.

The actual culprit here is stress. Noise activates the autonomic nervous system—the body's "fight or flight response"—triggering the release of hormones (such as cortisol) that put the cardiovascular system into chronic overdrive. Excess stress hormones also promote generalized inflammation, which is linked to heart disease.

Note: Noise at night carries special risk. So-called "microarousals"—periods during which noise arouses the nervous system, but not quite enough to cause a person to wake up or remember the event—are linked to heart disease. The normal restorative drop in blood pressure at night fails to occur when sleep is fragmented.

•**Cognitive function.** Noise also appears to impair cognitive function, with working memory and attention especially affected, according to a study published in *Noise & Health.*

•**Diabetes.** Even though the evidence is thus far inconclusive, the stress of noise pollution may disrupt proper endocrine function, raising risk for diabetes, a study published in *Environmental Health Perspectives* has found.

•**Breast cancer.** Preliminary research has identified a link between aircraft noise and an increased risk for certain types of breast cancer—perhaps due, in part, to sleep disruptions, according to a study published in 2017 in *Scandinavian Journal of Work, Environment & Health.*

TO PROTECT YOURSELF

The first step in minimizing noise-related health risks is to recognize that these harms to your overall health do exist. *Here are simple steps you can take...*

•**Create some distance.** When waiting to cross a busy street or catch a train, stand back from the curb or train tracks—a few feet farther from noise makes a substantial difference in its intensity.

•**Avoid the noise.** Avoiding noisy areas or ensuring that you take regular breaks from noise in a quiet area reduces your exposure and gives your ears a chance to recover.

•**Consider hearing protection.** If you will be exposed to a noisy situation or event, whether recreational or occupational, consider hearing protection. There are earplugs and earmuffs that dial down decibels without shutting sound out altogether. Noise-canceling headphones are useful for steady low-frequency sounds, such as background noise on a train or plane.

•**Use caution when listening to music.** For many people, music is their biggest source of noise exposure. Don't deprive yourself of music's stress-reducing benefits, but be prudent. If you use a personal listening device, invest in high-end earbuds or headphones that block out external noise and allow you to lower the volume.

Because amplified concerts can be extremely noisy, wearing hearing protection is a good idea, particularly if you're close to the speakers.

Rule of thumb: If you're having to raise your voice to talk to someone at arm's length, it's probably too loud. If you have to shout, it's definitely too loud.

•**Cut noise levels at home.** To reduce noise pollution at home, start with obvious steps such as not blasting the TV. Consider features such as double-paned windows to mute street noise

Push "Print" for a New Heart...or Ear

Organ printer. Scientists at Tel Aviv University used human cells as bio-ink to create the world's first complete heart, with blood vessels and other structures. Within 10 years, 3-D "organ printers" might be available at major hospitals.

Advanced Science

Cartilage structure creator. 3-D printing can use wood cellulose to create anatomically correct structures that are seeded with cartilage cells. This approach could be used to create ears or other cartilage structures (such as joint tissue) for implantation.

Empa (Swiss Federal Laboratories for Materials Science and Technology)

and the clamor of lawn mowers and other landscaping equipment. Additional insulation, rugs and carpeting can help, as well as keeping the windows closed and using air-conditioning.

Be especially mindful of the bedroom. White-noise machines won't reduce overall sound levels, and can even raise them, but the addition of some white noise will make brief noise intrusions less stress-provoking, which may prevent sleep-disturbing arousals. Sleeping with foam earplugs, which are comfortable, can also help.

Helpful: If you're looking for a new home, check the noise levels by entering the address on the website HowLoud.com, which provides a soundscore rating. There's also a free sound-level app at CDC.gov/niosh/topics/noise/app.html. Alternatively, you can find sound-level meters online for $20 to $40.

Important: Even if you're so accustomed to a particular noise that you don't really "hear" it anymore, it's entirely possible that the noise doesn't bother you any longer because you've already lost some hearing! Remember that it's the total exposure that counts.

Fix for a Broken Heart?

Nature Communications

An experimental glue could replace stitches for heart repairs. When tested in pigs with a punctured left ventricle, the powerful, UV light–activated glue formed chemical bonds with proteins in the tissues and stopped bleeding in less than 30 seconds.

Bonus: The glue was absorbed by the body over time.

What You Don't Know Is Harming Your Kidneys

Joseph Vassalotti, MD, chief medical officer of the National Kidney Foundation, Kidney.org, and associate clinical professor of medicine in the division of nephrology at Icahn School of Medicine at Mount Sinai in New York City. His research has been published in peer-reviewed journals such as *American Journal of Nephrology, Kidney International* and *American Journal of Kidney Diseases*.

The early stages of chronic kidney disease (CKD) cause no symptoms. In fact, 90% of people with the condition don't know they have it. But even if your kidneys are still healthy—so far—you could be doing things that harm them without realizing it.

Kidneys are critical to the health of the whole body. They filter waste, balance body fluids, maintain blood pressure, control the production of red blood cells and regulate electrolytes and minerals, such as potassium, sodium and magnesium. When kidney health declines, waste builds up and causes health issues—including high blood pressure, anemia and metabolic bone disease (such as osteoporosis). The final stage is kidney failure and the need for regular dialysis or a kidney transplant.

THE GREATEST DANGER

More than 10% of Americans—30 million adults—have CKD, which is the ninth-leading cause of death in the US, according to the CDC. One factor that drives the prevalence of this disease is that people who are at risk often don't realize it...so they're less likely to get tested... take necessary precautions to protect their kidneys from further damage...and/or take steps to reverse early stages of damage.

People with diabetes and high blood pressure are at especially high risk. Together, these two conditions are responsible for two-thirds of CKD. Other risk factors include age (being 60 or older)...having a family history of kidney failure...being of non-Caucasian descent (African-American, Hispanic, Asian, Pacific Islander and/or Native American)...obesity...lupus...and cancer.

If you have risk factors for CKD, you should be tested with a Kidney Profile annually. The profile combines a urine albumin-to-creatinine ratio (ACR) test and an estimated glomerular filtration rate (eGFR) blood test.

THE THREAT FROM THE DRUGSTORE

Healthy kidneys are able to filter out medications and supplements without harm to the kidneys themselves. However, drugs and supplements can cause kidney damage or other side effects. *If you take any of these worst offenders, check with your clinician and be sure to get an annual Kidney Profile...*

•**Nonsteroidal anti-inflammatory drugs (NSAIDs).** The kidney danger from long-term use of NSAIDs, such as *ibuprofen* (Advil, Motrin) and *naproxen* (Aleve), is well-known, but few people realize how easy it is to do harm. A recent large study published in *JAMA Network Open* that looked at nearly 800,000 active young and middle-aged adults found that using eight or more doses a month put them at a 20% higher risk for kidney damage compared with not taking any NSAIDs.

•**Proton pump inhibitors (PPIs).** Heartburn/reflux/GERD drugs such as *omeprazole* (Prilosec), *esomeprazole* (Nexium) and *lansoprazole* (Prevacid) pose a risk to the kidneys if taken long-term. A recent study published in *Scientific Reports* found that compared with people who took other antacids, those who took PPIs (including over-the-counter versions) were 28.4% more likely to develop CKD.

•**Herbal and dietary supplements.** Since supplements are not regulated in the US, there is no guarantee that ingredients and amounts listed on a supplement label are what is actually in the bottle. Even if the label is accurate, "natural" herbs and supplements can be toxic to the kidneys, especially in large amounts.

For instance, kidney injuries have been reported from using the herbs Chinese yew extract, St. John's wort and wormwood. Talk to your doctor about the health risks of any herbal and/or dietary supplements you take—ideally, before you use them.

•**Prescription medications.** Patients who know they have CKD with decreased kidney function should make sure all their doctors are aware of this. Dosages for some drugs may need to be adjusted for these patients—and some medications, such as *metformin* (Glucophage), used to treat diabetes, and the muscle relaxant *baclofen* (Lioresal), may need to be avoided. But people who don't know that they have CKD are in danger of getting harmful dosages of certain drugs, including beta-blockers used to treat high blood pressure…antimicrobials…antifungals…and insulin.

KIDNEY-COMPROMISING LIFESTYLE

Lifestyle factors also can damage kidneys…

•**Insomnia.** Chronic insomnia has been associated with kidney damage. One study of more than one million veterans found that insomniacs were 2.4 times more likely to develop kidney failure than those who slept normally. Poor sleep is linked to high blood pressure and vascular disease, which may in turn lead to kidney disease. People who already have CKD also are at higher risk for sleep disorders, such as sleep apnea and restless legs syndrome.

•**Too much protein.** Low-carb diets that emphasize fat and protein, such as Keto or Paleo, may jeopardize the health of people at risk for CKD—particularly if they heavily consume processed red meats. White meat, fish and dairy protein do not seem to carry the same risk. Vegetable proteins may actually be protective. The research as to whether excessive amounts of protein also are harmful for people who aren't at increased risk for CKD is not conclusive.

•**Processed foods and phosphorus.** Our bodies need some phosphorus for strong bones, and healthy kidneys are able to remove any excess so that toxic amounts don't build up in the body. However, not all phosphorus is the same.

Organic phosphorus occurs naturally in many protein-rich animal and plant foods and is only up to 60% absorbed by the body. There is little danger of consuming too much plant-based phosphorus, as long as the kidneys are healthy. *Inorganic* phosphorus is an additive used to improve the shelf life and/or color of processed foods, such as processed cheese and sodas. Inorganic phosphorus is more than 90% absorbed…and too much can easily accumulate in the body. Excessive phosphorus throws off the body's delicate calcium balance. It can lead to calcium being drawn from the bones and dangerous deposits of calcium accumulating in blood vessels, the lungs, the eyes and the heart. Because our diet is so heavily processed, most of us get up to twice the recommended dietary allowance of 700 mg/day for adults. Check the ingredients list before buying packaged foods—phosphorus additives have "phos" in the name. Or better yet, stick to whole, fresh foods.

•**Air pollution.** A major study of almost 2.5 million veterans published in *Journal of the American Society of Nephrology* estimated that air pollution causes nearly 45,000 new cases of CKD in the US each year. Other research compared county levels of air pollution with the incidence of CKD among one million Medicare patients. The researchers found that diagnoses of CKD were highest in counties that had the highest levels of air pollution. Air pollution as a cause of CKD is being studied further. But for the time being, it makes sense to avoid or limit exposure as much as possible.

SHOULD YOU WORRY ABOUT ANTIPERSPIRANTS?

You may have noticed an FDA warning for people with kidney disease on labels of antiperspirants. Antiperspirants contain small amounts of aluminum, which temporarily plug sweat ducts to reduce perspiration. Excessive amounts of aluminum can be toxic. However, the amount of aluminum that is absorbed by the skin from antiperspirants is tiny—especially compared with the amount of aluminum people are exposed to naturally from water and soil.

Recommended: If you have kidney disease, ask your doctor if you should stick with plain deodorants that don't contain aluminum.

---

9 Ways to Love Your Liver

Robert S. Brown, Jr., MD, MPH, the Gladys and Roland Harriman Professor of Medicine and clinical chief in the division of gastroenterology and hepatology in the department of medicine at Weill Cornell Medical College, New York City, and a member of the National Medical Advisory Committee for the American Liver Foundation. LiverFoundation.org

---

You probably give your liver little thought, but your body's largest internal organ is a multitasking miracle, filtering toxins, working with your immune system to fight off infection and storing and releasing nutrients from food so that your body can access and use them to function.

If you don't protect and nurture your liver—or worse, out-and-out ignore it—it can get overtaxed, and the spillover affects your entire body. Liver disease is on the rise—30 million Americans suffer from some sort of liver disease that can, if untreated, lead to scarring (cirrhosis), organ failure or even death. The problem is most people don't know it, because liver disease is silent.

The good news is that loving your liver isn't complicated. It benefits from many of the same healthy habits you already know to do (but maybe aren't yet doing) for your heart and your body as whole. *Here, nine easy ways to love your liver…*

1. Brew a pot of coffee. Aside from coffee's ability to help you get up and go in the morning, it has many health benefits, including boosting liver health. A study at Southampton, University, UK, of 430,000 people found that consumption of two cups of coffee a day was related to a 44% lower risk for liver cirrhosis.

Note: The benefit isn't related to the caffeine, so you can enjoy decaf if you would rather. Coffee beans contain hundreds of antioxidants and other compounds that offer protection from liver disease and cancer.

Tip: Green tea is another source of antioxidants that are good for the liver, though it is not as well-studied as coffee.

2. Eat oatmeal for breakfast. Your digestive tract loves all fiber, of course, but you can show your liver extra TLC with foods that help move toxins through the body and out of your system. That lightens the load your liver needs to process. If you don't like oatmeal, other top fiber sources are oat bran, barley, flaxseed, beans, apples and citrus fruits.

Also: If you replace starches and simple carbs with these high-fiber foods, you'll eat fewer calories and feel less hungry.

3. Avoid high-fructose corn syrup. If you make only one change to your diet, eliminate all sugar-sweetened beverages, especially those with high-fructose corn syrup (HFCS). As you probably know, HFCS has been associated with a greater risk for obesity, diabetes and heart disease, but you may not be aware that HFCS has a direct impact on your liver. It raises your risk of developing non-alcoholic fatty liver disease (NAFLD), a very common disorder affecting nearly one in three people. In human trials, consuming HFCS was found to be more likely to contribute to NAFLD than dietary fat. NAFLD can lead to liver damage and the more serious condition nonalcoholic steatohepatitis and ultimately cirrhosis. Also, HFCS fails to activate the body's normal signal to stop eating when full— your appetite isn't satisfied, so you continue to eat, putting even more stress on your liver.

While there has been a push in recent years to remove HFCS from foods and beverages, read all labels carefully because it is still hidden in many packaged products such as ketchup and salad dressing.

4. Lose weight. Carrying extra weight is toxic to your liver. NAFLD occurs in about 15% of nonobese patients but its prevalence increases along with your body mass index (BMI). Obese (BMI of 30.0 to 39.9) and extremely obese (BMI of 40 or more) patients have a prevalence of 65% and 85%, respectively.

Livers don't need fancy or quick weight-loss diets. A healthy, balanced eating plan that you can stick with for life, such as the heart-healthy Mediterranean diet, is the best way to lose weight and support your liver. Focus on good fats, such as olive oil, nuts, fish and avocado, and more vegetables than animal protein.

5. Add strength-training to get your liver in fighting shape. While better muscle tone is the obvious benefit of strength training, having more muscle mass boosts health in many ways that you can't see, including reducing fat in the liver. Though the exact mechanism isn't yet known, a three-month study at Tel Aviv Medical Center found that three strength-training sessions a week led to reduced fat in the liver. Another study found that doing just push-ups and squats, three sets of 10 reps of each exercise, three times a week over six months lowered markers for liver disease.

6. Know your liquor limits. You think you know how much is "too much," but safe alcohol limits are probably lower than you realize—just one drink a day for women…two for men. One drink means 12 ounces of beer (5% alcohol content), five ounces of wine (12%) or 1.5 ounces of hard liquor (40%). Getting one generous pour, ordering beer by the pint or sharing a full bottle of wine with a friend can put you well over that limit. That's fine for special occasions, but steady drinking damages your liver even if you don't have an alcohol-use disorder, also known as alcoholism. The number of deaths from cirrhosis is on the rise across the country, especially among adults ages 25 to 34.

Important: Saving up during the workweek for a Saturday night splurge is not a safe plan and does not keep you within the week's alcohol limits—overindulging is always toxic to the liver.

7. Limit your liver's exposure to acetaminophen. Most people think of *acetaminophen* (Tylenol) as safe, but it's often overused. In fact, overdoses account for about 50,000 emergency room visits, 25,000 hospitalizations and nearly 500 deaths a year, half of them unintentional. A total of 12 regular-strength, 325-milligram (mg) pills per day is considered safe. Beyond that, the risk increases. At 25 regular-strength pills a day, it's toxic.

Important: To avoid getting a double dose by mistake, always read a medication's ingredients list because acetaminophen is in many other over-the-counter remedies such as cold medicines.

8. Boost liver health with CoQ10, an enzyme that helps generate energy in your cells, and n-acetylcysteine (NAC), a powerful antioxidant. Both are found in many foods, such as spinach, legumes and certain fish—but it may be hard to get enough in your diet. That's where supplements can help. Studies have found that 600 mg of NAC twice a day improved liver function. Between 100 mg and 300 mg a day of CoQ10, also known for heart health, did this as well. Ask your doctor or nutritionist if either or both of these may be helpful to you.

9. Have your liver enzyme levels checked. Your blood pressure and cholesterol are taken by your doctor at every doctor's visit, but you probably have no idea about your liver enzyme levels. Liver enzymes are the proteins needed for the liver to do its work. They're also markers of liver health. When the liver has to work harder than normal or is damaged, higher levels of enzymes show up in your blood. Unfortunately, the basic blood tests done at wellness visits may not include checking liver enzyme levels. For that you need what's called a comprehensive metabolic blood test. An elevated number could be the only early warning sign of liver problems.

Important: Some general practitioners might not think that mildly elevated enzymes, such as *alanine aminotransferase* (ALT), warrant investigation, but if your enzymes are at all high, you should be checked to see if fatty liver disease or another condition is the cause.

Slimy Creepy-Crawler Provides Adhesives

Study by researchers at University of Pennsylvania, Philadelphia, published in *Proceedings of the National Academy of Sciences.*

Snail slime may lead to better adhesives. Snails have a slimy moisture layer called an epiphragm that hardens to protect their bodies and lets them cement themselves in place—and then loosens when the snail wants to move again. This reversible adhesive has now been duplicated in the lab. Researchers hope to use this to develop adhesives that can be quickly released when needed.

Liver Transplant: Living Donors Are Saving Lives...

Koji Hashimoto, MD, PhD, director of living donor liver transplantation and pediatric liver transplantation at Cleveland Clinic. His research has been published in *Annals of Surgery, Liver Transplantation* and other leading medical journals.

Deciding to have major surgery is never easy. So imagine how tough the decision might be if the surgery meant giving up a piece of the largest organ in your body, entirely for the benefit of another person—someone whose life might well be saved by your generosity.

The quandary is real for increasing numbers of Americans. That's because doctors are urging more and more people in need of liver transplants to seek out living donors, just as many kidney transplant patients have done for years.

Faced with uncertain odds of getting a timely transplant the old-fashioned way—by waiting for an organ from a deceased donor—patients whose livers are failing due to life-threatening conditions, such as cirrhosis, viral hepatitis and primary liver cancer, are reaching out to family, friends, faith communities and sometimes even strangers on social media.

What's at stake: About 14,000 Americans each year need a new liver, but only about 8,200 get one. Many remaining patients become too ill to qualify for a transplant or die waiting.

Living donation is possible because the liver is the only human organ that can regenerate. That means the person who gives up part of his/her healthy liver will have most of the organ's original size again within two months—and so will the recipient.

The procedure, developed over the past three decades, has continued to evolve over the years and now offers improved surgical techniques and postoperative care. As a result, living liver donations work at least as well as a transplant from a deceased donor with one-year survival often exceeding 90%. And it often means patients get their transplants at earlier stages in their illnesses. But that does not mean the decision to donate is simple.

WHO CAN DONATE A LIVER?

Most transplant centers will accept donors between the ages of 18 and 55 or 60. Older adults have increased surgical risks, and younger people are not considered mature enough to give informed consent.

Most living liver donations are "directed"—meaning you offer to donate to a particular patient who has reached out for potential donors among family, friends or strangers. The baseline for consideration is whether you have a blood type that matches or is compatible with the blood type of the patient.

If you think you'd like to be considered as a living liver donor, you can start the process by calling the patient's transplant center. During the initial phone call, a staff member will ask a few questions about your overall health and your reasons for considering donation. If you and the transplant team agree that you might be a good candidate, you will go to the transplant center for a couple of days of tests and interviews.

You can expect a thorough examination of your physical health, including blood draws... tests of your heart and lungs...scans of your liver...and a psychological evaluation to ensure that you understand the risks and that there has been no coercion to participate in a living liver donation. Some people, including those who are significantly overweight and at risk for fatty liver disease, may be asked to undergo a liver biopsy.

If you have certain health problems, including bleeding or clotting disorders or a history of alcoholism or drug addiction, you won't be able to donate. But some common conditions, such as mild high blood pressure that is well-controlled with medication, will not disqualify you.

If the transplant team believes you are a good candidate, a separate donor advocate team, including a physician, social worker, bioethicist, coordinator and psychiatrist, will review the decision with your interests in mind.

Important: If you are accepted, you can change your mind at any point. The final decision is always yours.

WHAT WILL I NEED TO DO TO PREPARE?

If you are accepted and decide to donate, you usually will have a few weeks to get ready—though in some cases, a patient is in such desperate need that surgery is scheduled within a couple of days. If you do have a waiting period, the transplant team will encourage you to limit or avoid alcohol, which is hard on the liver…eat a healthful diet…and avoid putting on weight, which can lead to fat buildup in the liver.

You also will want to use this time to talk to your family and, if need be, your employer about the support you will need after the surgery.

WHAT HAPPENS DURING THE SURGERY?

You and the recipient will show up for surgery on the same day, in adjoining operating rooms. You will be put under general anesthesia, so you won't feel any pain. During an operation that can last about six hours, surgeons will remove a portion of your liver—15% to 70% of the volume, depending on the needs of the recipient. Children need the smallest amount of tissue.

At some transplant centers, all donor surgeries are done with a large abdominal incision, shaped like a hockey stick that extends across half the belly and up the chest. Elsewhere, some surgeries are now done with smaller laparoscopic incisions, reducing postsurgical pain and recovery time.

WHAT ARE THE RISKS?

The donor faces a risk for death of about one in 500, according to the best available data. That's comparable to the risk faced by anyone having major abdominal surgery. Other risks include wound infection, hernias, excess bleeding and leakage of bile, a digestive fluid made by the liver. A leak can temporarily cause pain, nausea and vomiting. The rate for a major complication, such as a bile leak, incisional hernia or liver failure, varies by transplant center, but typically is below 10%.

WHAT'S THE RECOVERY LIKE?

Most donors need to stay in the hospital for five to six days after the surgery, but you may be able to leave sooner after a laparoscopic procedure. If you live far from the transplant center, you may be asked to stay nearby for another week or two to be monitored by your caregiver for fever, shortness of breath or other symptoms that might indicate a complication. Recovery can take time due to the fatigue and pain caused by a large incision, which is commonly used. If you have a desk job, you may be able to return to work in two months or less…someone with a physically demanding job might need three months after conventional surgery.

While no long-term health risks have been found, you will be asked to return to the transplant center for periodic checkups and to continue yearly physicals with your primary care physician at home.

WHAT ABOUT COSTS?

The recipient's insurance will cover the cost of your surgery and medical care related to any complications from the donation, but not the cost of travel, lodging and time off from work. You should talk with your employer to determine whether your time off can be covered by vacation, sick time or disability pay.

Help with travel, lodging and meals away from home is available to some donors through certain charities or the National Living Donor Assistance Center (888-870-5002 or Living DonorAssistance.org). While a donor cannot benefit financially from the donation, the recipient and his/her family may be able to help you with some related expenses as well. A transplant center social worker will walk you through the help that is available.

Life-Saving Smart Tattoos

Angewandte Chemie International Edition

"Smart tattoos" will soon be able to monitor your health.

New lab discovery: Chemical sensors embedded in tattoo ink could be used to detect changes in glucose, albumin and other important biomarkers.

"Magic Mushrooms"—the Promise and the Risks

Albert Garcia-Romeu, PhD, instructor in the Behavioral Pharmacology Research Unit of Johns Hopkins University School of Medicine, Baltimore. HopkinsPsychedelic.org

Many people were surprised when Denver and Oakland decriminalized "magic mushrooms," which contain the naturally occurring hallucinogen *psilocybin*. But mushrooms containing *psilocybin* have been used sacramentally and recreationally for hundreds of years. They have not been shown to be chemically addictive, and preliminary studies suggest that they could be useful for treating anxiety, depression and addiction to alcohol and tobacco.

Example: In a 2016 Johns Hopkins University study, two doses of psilocybin given five weeks apart significantly decreased anxiety and depression in cancer patients—and for six months afterward.

Even though laws have changed locally, it will be years before mushrooms are approved for use in medical treatments in the US. *Until then, they likely would be obtained from unregulated suppliers, which creates possible risks…*

•**Psilocybin can trigger psychotic episodes in people predisposed to certain psychiatric disorders.** In controlled settings, medical personnel would screen for these disorders.

•**Psilocybin's hallucinogenic effects could cause unintentionally dangerous behavior,** such as walking into traffic. Effects can last for four to six hours after consumption. In a medical setting, patients would be closely monitored.

•**Magic mushrooms can look a lot like other wild mushrooms that contain dangerous toxins**—a supplier could provide the wrong ones.

•**Very rarely, some people could experience long-lasting perceptual disturbances.**

The wisest option is to not use magic mushrooms medically for now. Or seek out approved clinical trials at ClinicalTrials.gov. The underground marketplace is uncontrolled. The data on regular usage and interactions with other drugs and conditions are lacking. They show promise and generally are nontoxic, but more research is needed.

Supplement for Space Travel?

Frontiers in Physiology

Resveratrol, an antioxidant found in red wine and blueberries, may prevent muscle loss during space travel. Animals given resveratrol and subjected to Mars-like gravity (which is just 40% of the Earth's) experienced almost total protection.

Could a Fitness Tracker Save Your Life?

James E. Ip, MD, associate professor of clinical medicine and director of cardiac pacing and implantable devices at Weill Cornell Medicine's division of cardiology in New York City. He is author of the articles "Evaluation of Cardiac Rhythm Abnormalities from Wearable Devices" and "Wearable Devices for Cardiac Rhythm Diagnosis and Management," both recently published in *JAMA*.

If you are among the millions of Americans who wear a wrist device that counts your steps, you probably already know that many of these fitness trackers also can monitor your sleep patterns, nudge you to get up and move when you sit too much and estimate how many calories you burn in a day.

But did you know that some of the newer devices are being credited with saving lives? Consider these recent press reports…

•**A 73-year-old Connecticut woman with unexplained shortness of breath noticed that her device showed a higher-than-usual heart rate**—and it kept getting higher over a period of a few days. She went to a hospital, and it turned out she had life-threatening blood clots in her lungs.

•**A 34-year-old Utah man noticed his device was showing a much lower-than-**

normal heart rate. At his wife's insistence, he went to a hospital, where he learned he had dangerous blockages in two coronary arteries.

•**A 42-year-old man who had a seizure was taken to a New Jersey emergency room,** where he was found to have a rapid, irregular heartbeat known as atrial fibrillation (A-fib). The condition can lead to stroke or heart failure. Because he was wearing a fitness device, doctors asked to see his heart rate recordings, which allowed them to time the onset of his abnormal heartbeats and choose the best treatment.

The people in all of these examples happened to be using Fitbit devices, but the data that alerted them and their doctors to their health risks are available on many devices.

The key feature in most of the devices: A sensor, called a photoplethysmogram (PPG), that sits against the wrist and uses light-emitting diodes (LEDs) to continuously detect blood volume changes that can be translated into a heart rate—the number of times your heart beats in a minute.

For a healthy adult who is sitting quietly and not under any unusual stress, the normal "resting" rate is 60 to 100 beats per minute. In general, younger, fitter people have lower resting heart rates.

While consumer fitness devices are not perfect heart rate monitors, they can give you a good estimate of your resting rate and your rate during exercise. When you work out, you want your heart rate to rise. How much your heart rate should increase depends on your age, fitness level and goals. A rule of thumb is that moderate-to-intense exercise should get you to 50% to 85% of your maximum heart rate, which you can calculate by subtracting your age from 220.

Here's what you don't want: A spiking heart rate when you are sitting still or a heart rate that stays sluggish even when you get moving.

What a fast or slow heart rate could mean: A fast heart rate can be caused by a number of conditions ranging from anxiety or dehydration to infection or an actual heart rhythm problem. A slow beat can signal anything from heart damage to sleep apnea to an underactive thyroid.

With most popular devices, you can see your current heart rate on your wrist and check your heart rate history—going back hours, days or weeks—on an app or a website.

At least one device, the Apple Watch, has an additional optional feature—you can set it to send you an alert if a rapid heartbeat develops at a time when the device senses you are not moving much. The watch also can send you alerts for slow heartbeats. The latest version has two more features approved by the FDA—a notification for irregular heartbeats that could signal A-fib and an app that lets you take a brief electrocardiogram (ECG)—a test of your heart's electrical activity. If results look abnormal, the device will urge you to seek medical care.

Some wearable devices, including the Apple Watch, also can detect hard falls. If the wearer seems unresponsive, it can even be set to make automatic calls to 911 or other emergency contacts.

People who may want to consider using a fitness tracker include those who have a personal or family history of cardiac problems…and those who have a medical condition such as high blood pressure or diabetes.

Important: If you have one of these devices, take the time to read through online user guides before deciding whether to turn on the various alerts.

And don't forget the cost. The latest Apple Watch will set you back $400 or more, while other smartwatches and trackers with heart rate detection start at under $100 and go up to around $350. In addition to Fitbit, popular brands include Garmin, Polar and Samsung. *Other considerations…*

•**None of these devices or features is a substitute for medical advice.** If you see something worrisome or confusing, you should always check with your health-care provider.

•**The risk for false alarms is real.** A preliminary report from a study conducted for Apple said that 16% of watch wearers who got a notice about irregular heartbeats were not actually experiencing A-fib. Doctors expect accuracy rates to vary among consumers, with young and healthy users most likely to get false alarms.

●**Risks and benefits remain unclear.** There's no study showing that wearing one of these devices leads to better medical care or outcomes. Even what seems like an obvious benefit—early detection of A-fib—comes with risks. For example, many people diagnosed with the condition are prescribed a blood thinner, which increases bleeding risks. The risks of taking the drug must be balanced against the potential benefit of preventing stroke.

●**Your doctor may not be sure how to interpret data from these devices.** Because medical systems have not yet developed best practices for incorporating the information produced by wearable devices into the patient's medical record, doctors typically handle this issue on a case-by-case basis.

However, there's reason to think wearable devices that monitor our health will only become more common and useful. Paired with data from other connected devices—such as weight scales, blood pressure monitors and blood glucose monitors—they will produce a torrent of data. Consumers and medical providers will have to work through how best to use it all.

In the meantime, if you decide to wear a fitness tracker, speak to your doctor about the data you should be collecting and how to best use it to help protect your health.

You're Eating Plastic!

Review of 26 studies analyzing the prevalence of microplastics by researchers at University of Victoria, British Columbia, Canada, published in *Environmental Science & Technology.*

Americans eat 70,000 microplastic particles every year. Microplastics are tiny, often microscopic, bits of plastic from food and water containers and the breakdown of larger plastic products in the environment. The health effects of microplastic consumption are unknown.

Light Up Your Insides
Frontiers in Microbiology

Recent discovery: Brief exposures to the UVB light in sunshine increase microbial diversity in the gut. The intestinal organisms, along with increased vitamin D, may protect against multiple sclerosis and other inflammatory diseases.

Vitiligo: Treatments Are Available for This Mysterious Skin Disorder

John E. Harris, MD, PhD, director of the Vitiligo Clinic and Research Center at University of Massachusetts Medical School in Worcester, UMassMed.edu/vitiligo. He has published textbook chapters on vitiligo and research in *Science Translational Medicine, Journal of the American Academy of Dermatology* and elsewhere. Dr. Harris serves on a number of advisory boards and committees, including the Vitiligo Research Foundation and American Academy of Dermatology.

Michael Jackson may be the most famous person ever to have vitiligo, but he's definitely not alone. The autoimmune disorder, in which the body attacks cells that give skin its pigment, affects roughly one out of every 100 people in the world—regardless of race or gender.

In the US, it's estimated that up to five million people have this condition. Even though vitiligo ("vittle-eye-go") occurs most commonly before age 30, it can develop at any age. People with certain other autoimmune disorders, such as the thyroid condition known as Hashimoto's disease and type 1 diabetes, are at greater risk.

Good news: While vitiligo is still incurable, recent scientific advances are uncovering important facts about the condition that are leading to more—and better—treatment options than ever before. *What you need to know...*

In a person with vitiligo, pigmentation can be lost anywhere on the body, but common areas include the face, neck, scalp, hands and arms. Sometimes vitiligo affects the armpits, mouth and genitals.

Vitiligo is highly individualized. One person might lose all pigment in his/her body over the course of a lifetime, while another develops a single white patch later in life. For some, the condition remains stable for decades, until something triggers the immune system and it spreads again. Triggers can include a bout of severe stress…a cut or burn…or environmental exposure to certain chemicals, including phenols found in permanent hair dyes and some detergents.

The most common risk factor for vitiligo seems to be genetic. Up to 25% of people with vitiligo also have a relative with the disorder. The more genes you have in common with a person affected by vitiligo, the greater your risk.

Having another autoimmune disorder also increases risk. When researchers looked at nearly 1,100 people with vitiligo, close to 20% had another autoimmune disease, such as alopecia, inflammatory bowel disease, lupus or Sjögren's syndrome, according to research published in *Journal of the American Academy of Dermatology.*

TREATMENT OPTIONS

At this time, there are no FDA-approved medical treatments to reverse vitiligo—but that could be changing as promising new treatments are now in clinical trials (see below). In the meantime, people with vitiligo are prescribed treatments "off label," meaning that the medication was originally intended for another condition. Most insurers cover these treatments for people with vitiligo, but check first. *Current treatment options…*

•**Prescription topical steroids** can help restore the pigmentation in smaller areas of the body. The cream provides moderate improvement, and side effects may include stretch marks and thinning of the skin.

Note: When a person's vitiligo is rapidly expanding, a low-dose oral steroid is sometimes used until the disease has stabilized.

•**Topical tacrolimus** is a newer treatment that can be applied to parts of the body that are more sensitive to the side effects of long-term use of steroid cream, such as the face, genitals, breasts and underarms.

•**Narrow-band UVB phototherapy** is recommended when depigmented areas are too extensive (typically more than 5% of the body) for topical treatment alone. In most cases, it requires two to three visits per week with each treatment lasting only about one to four minutes. However, the treatment may take up to a year to be effective and must be continued indefinitely to maintain results.

Note: This type of phototherapy uses UV radiation that does not increase risk for skin cancer.

What happens: This treatment is administered in a booth in which the patient stands with the affected areas of the body exposed to UVB light. UV goggles are worn to protect the eyes. The treatment usually is covered by insurance and is offered at dermatologists' offices throughout the US.

Note: A laser therapy, similar to narrow-band UVB phototherapy, is highly effective on small areas of the skin. Brand names include XTRAC and Pharos.

•**"Bleaching" therapy,** *monobenzone* (Benoquin), is a topical "depigmenting" cream that can be used if a person has extensive vitiligo (covering more than 80% of the body). With this treatment, skin is permanently lightened in unaffected areas of the body so that the spots caused by vitiligo are no longer noticeable. The treatment may take one to two years to complete. Side effects may include burning, itching and redness of the treated skin.

•**JAK inhibitors** are drugs that are already on the market to treat conditions such as rheumatoid arthritis and bone marrow disease. The drugs, *tofacitinib* (Xeljanz) and *ruxolitinib* (Jakafi), can be used both orally and topically. These medications block the cellular pathway that fuels vitiligo. While FDA approval specifically for vitiligo has not yet been finalized, this treatment is in clinical trials and shows tremendous promise. Until then, the medications can be prescribed off-label.

LIVING WITH VITILIGO

Because vitiligo is so visible, it impacts a person's self-esteem and quality of life. Strangers may stare or make rude comments. Up to one-third of people with vitiligo experience symptoms

Artificial Intelligence to the Rescue!

AI determines dangerous nodules. Up to 67% of Americans have thyroid nodules, and the vast majority are benign—but sometimes the cancer risk is unclear based on traditional ultrasound imaging and/or a fine-needle biopsy.

In development: Ultrasound software that uses artificial intelligence (AI) to more accurately distinguish between high- and low-risk nodules.

JAMA Otolaryngology—Head & Neck Surgery

AI predicts cancer symptoms. Using an AI algorithm based on symptoms reported by cancer patients during their treatment, doctors may be able to identify those who are at risk for future problems with depression, anxiety and disturbed sleep. With more study, AI may be able to improve these patients' quality of life.

University of Surrey

of depression. Because melanocytes are found not just in skin but also in the eyes and ears, vitiligo can, in rare cases, affect those areas, too. Hearing loss can occur if the immune system attacks the melanocytes in the inner ear.

One step should be followed at all times—wearing sunscreen. Patches of skin without pigment burn easily. Skin damage also can trigger an autoimmune response that may lead to more vitiligo, so take particular care with cuts and burns. For the same reason, people with vitiligo may not want to get tattoos, especially if the disease is actively spreading or existing spots are getting larger. Makeup can be helpful.

Good brands: Dermablend and Cover FX.

Support groups for individuals with vitiligo are a good resource for coping with the psychological effects of the disorder. To find such a group, consult the website of Vitiligo Friends, VITFriends.org, a nonprofit dedicated to enhancing the quality of life for people with vitiligo. Global Vitiligo Foundation, GlobalVitiligoFound ation.org, is another good resource.

High-Tech Toilets Can Monitor Health

NBCNews.com

Japanese hospitals use them to look for abnormalities in urine flow that could indicate bladder or prostate disease. Toilets under development for home use could examine residents' waste for signs of infections, diabetes, kidney disease and some forms of cancer, as well as detect a spreading disease before it becomes an epidemic.

New Treatment for Crohns?

Gastroenterology

Immune cells from Crohn's patients contain less of a gut-specific protein found in the cells of healthy patients.

Recent finding: Infusions of modified cells that produce more of the protein may reduce cramps, diarrhea and other symptoms.

Next step: Clinical trials.

New Ulcer Treatment Guidelines Help Dodge Antibiotic Resistance

Carlo A. Fallone, MD, associate professor of medicine, McGill University, Montreal, Canada, and lead author of a study titled "Reconciliation of Recent Helicobacter pylori Treatment Guidelines in a Time of Increasing Resistance to Antibiotics," published in *Gastroenterology*.

For decades, a week or so of antibiotic therapy has been prescribed to successfully treat the cause of stomach ulcers. Alarmingly, though, the *Helicobacter pylori* (H. pylori) bacterium that causes ulcers is becoming resistant to the antibiotics.

Good news: New guidelines show how to kill H. pylori in an era of increasing antibiotic resistance.

Since the 1990s, standard care for ulcers caused by H. pylori has been a treatment called triple therapy: Seven to 10 days of two different antibiotics—*clarithromycin* (Biaxin) and *metronidazole* (Flagyl) or *amoxicillin*—plus a proton pump inhibitor (PPI) antacid, such as *esomeprazole* (Nexium) or *omeprazole* (Prilosec). Initially, triple therapy was 90% effective against H. pylori. Now the bacterium is becoming resistant to the antibiotics, especially to *clarithromycin* and to *levofloxacin*, which is sometimes substituted for clarithromycin. To make matters worse, if one round of triple therapy doesn't eradicate the H. pylori, doctors frequently prescribe additional rounds, exposing patients to more antibiotics.

ERADICATING H. PYLORI SAFELY

To address what has become a worldwide concern, three expert groups—the European Helicobacter and Microbiota Study Group, the American College of Gastroenterology and the Canadian Association of Gastroenterology—separately developed their own guidelines for safer ways to treat H. pylori. Researchers from these three groups and from McGill University reviewed all three sets of recommendations and came up with a new set of guidelines that incorporates the key points from all three. *Here is what they are…*

First-line therapy: Instead of triple therapy, patients who have been diagnosed with H. pylori ulcers should start by taking *bismuth quadruple therapy* for 14 days—bismuth, two different antibiotics (*metronidazole* and *tetracycline*) four times daily plus a PPI antacid twice daily. Bismuth is a natural element and has been safely used since ancient times as a remedy for heartburn. It is, in fact, the main ingredient in Pepto-Bismol (which is sometimes the bismuth used in the therapy). Research shows that when given along with metronidazole, tetracycline and a PPI, it significantly inhibits H. pylori.

Second-line therapies: If the first treatment is not effective, the following can be tried…

- For patients who have not previously been treated with *metronidazole* (for instance, because they were treated with triple therapy using amoxicillin instead), bismuth quadruple therapy for 14 days should be used. For patients who were treated with metronidazole but not with bismuth (because they were treated with a non-bismuth quadruple therapy), bismuth quadruple therapy can be used—preferably with levofloxacin substituted for metronidazole if the patient is not resistant to that antibiotic.

- If metronidazole is ruled out because of previous use, triple therapy substituting levofloxacin for clarithromycin (as long as the patient is not resistant to levofloxacin) should be given for 14 days.

And if those therapies fail to kill off H. pylori…

- High-dose amoxicillin plus a PPI for 14 days.

- As a "last resort," triple therapy substituting *rifabutin* (another antibiotic often used to treat tuberculosis) for clarithromycin for 10 days can be used. This therapy is reserved only for patients for whom multiple previous attempts have failed because of the potential for serious adverse side effects, such as bone marrow suppression.

The new guidelines do not generally recommend probiotics during H. pylori treatment. Patients on ulcer therapies often take these to help reduce side effects from the medications, but evidence so far is weak for any benefit from probiotics—both for preventing side effects and for helping to treat the H. pylori. More research is needed to determine if specific strains of probiotics might help in still undetermined ways, and if so, how much to take.

CLARITHROMYCIN CAUTION

The new guidelines don't completely rule out triple therapy, but they advise that it should be limited to patients living in areas where local H. pylori resistance to clarithromycin is low (less than 15%). Since that is hard to know in the US—few people get the endoscopic testing to verify H. pylori, and unlike Europe, we don't keep local resistance registries in this country—most US patients should stick to bismuth-quadruple first-line therapy.

Note: The guidelines stipulate that triple therapy should be avoided for patients who have already had clarithromycin or other macrolide antibiotics, which include *erythromycin* and *azithromycin.*

GOING FORWARD

As stool-based molecular tests become more advanced, it may become easier and cheaper to routinely test for antibiotic susceptibility to determine the best medication combination for each patient. If such testing were to become routine, it would also make it easier for regions to maintain a database of local rates of resistance to specific antibiotics—which would be invaluably helpful in global efforts to address antibiotic resistance. Another treatment option that may become more widely available is a more powerful and longer-lasting antacid called *vonoprazan*, a *potassium-competitive acid blocker* (PCAB), that is now being used in Japan. Clinical trials have shown that when used in triple therapy, it is more effective than PPIs against H. pylori.

H. pylori infection is a common infection mainly acquired in childhood, although the likelihood of having it increases with age. The bacterium is found in about 20% of 40-year-olds and 50% of people over age 60. However, why only some people with the infection develop stomach ulcers while most do not is not known. H. pylori also causes more than 80% of stomach cancer cases, the third most common cause of cancer deaths worldwide.

The symptoms to watch for include gnawing or burning stomach pain that may last for minutes or hours...tends to be worse in the morning or on an empty stomach...and may be relieved by eating or taking an antacid. Diagnosis usually starts with a blood or breath test to determine if you have H. pylori.

If it turns out that you do have stomach ulcers, discuss these new guidelines with your doctor. Even if you don't have ulcer symptoms, if you are at high risk for stomach cancer—for instance because of family history—it's a good idea to be tested for H. pylori and treated if you have the bacterium.

You Can Help Scientists Beat COVID-19

Louis Dron, MSc, director at Cytel, a research organization headquartered in Waltham, Massachusetts. Cytel. com

Patient-volunteers for clinical trials have been key in the fight against COVID-19. Sponsored by the Bill and Melinda Gates Foundation and Fast Grants, my company, Cytel, is tracking more than 2,000 COVID-related clinical trials worldwide, 422 of them in the US, of which 194 are actively recruiting. They'll need more than 175,000 participants to complete all of this research. *Here's what you need to know if you want to get involved...*

•**Why participate?** Volunteering allows everyday people to join the front lines in the battle against coronavirus. If the trial therapy works, you'll be among the first to be treated with it, ahead of regulatory and manufacturing delays.

•**What's being studied?** Trials are under way to better understand risk factors and disease behavior, as well as effectiveness of drug therapies and vaccines.

•**Is it safe?** Many therapies being studied have been used extensively in other contexts, so they have well-known safety profiles...other therapies are new. No treatment is without potential side effects and interactions with other medications, which can vary from person to person. Medically trained staff will explain the safety of each trial and risk factors. Participants can withdraw consent at any time.

•**Do you need to have tested positive for COVID-19?** No. Trials exist for healthy individuals without risk factors for infection...for people who test negative but are at high risk for exposure...for patients with mild disease...and for hospitalized and critical patients.

•**How do you get involved?** The sites below allow you to search for trials in your area. Or ask your health-care provider what's available. Read the materials to decide whether any trial is right for you.

Covid-Trials.org, Cytel's global compilation of ongoing COVID trials.

Better Healing with Self-Repair

No more dental fillings? A calcium/phosphate gel appears to trigger self-repair in tooth enamel. The gel stimulates the growth of new enamel that closely resembles the original—and may bond to tooth surfaces better than porcelain and other materials.

Science Advances

Hard-working molecules... Synthetic molecules known as TrAPs (traction force-activated payloads) activate the body's natural repair mechanisms and could improve tissue repair after bone fractures and other injuries.

Advanced Materials

ClinicalTrials.gov, a searchable registry covering almost all USA trials.

ResearchMatch.org, an initiative endorsed by the NIH.

CenterWatch.com, a repository of ongoing COVID trials.

Speech Improvement with Facial Transplants

Face Transplant Program, NYU Langone Health

Facial transplant surgery—in which donor tissues are used to replace facial nerves, muscles and bones—may improve speech after severe facial traumas, according to a new case study. To date, more than 40 facial transplants have been done worldwide.

HIV Drug Could Possibly Work on Alzheimer's

Nature.

Lamivudine, a drug used to treat HIV/AIDS, has been shown in animal studies to reduce inflammation in as little as two weeks.

Implication: The medication could be used to treat age-related inflammatory diseases, including Alzheimer's disease, macular degeneration and other age-related disorders.

Next step: Human trials.

Canine Cancer Sniffers Make the Grade

The Journal of the American Osteopathic Association

Canine cancer sniffers make the grade!

Recent finding: After just eight weeks of training, cancer-sniffing beagles were able to distinguish lung cancer–positive blood samples from healthy controls with 97% accuracy.

Next step: Canines will be tested for their ability to detect other types of cancer by using patients' breath—with the ultimate goal of developing an over-the-counter screening device.

CHAPTER 13

Medication Smarts

The Truth About Generic Drugs: They May Not Be as Safe as You Think...

Every year, doctors in the US write nearly six billion prescriptions—and nine out of 10 are filled with a generic drug, which the FDA says, "works in the same way and provides the same clinical benefit as its brand-name version."

As a pharmacologist and lifetime advocate for consumer health, I've been one of the biggest champions of generic drugs for more than 25 years. They can cost much less than brand-name drugs. And the FDA assures us that their stringent oversight guarantees generics are as effective and safe as brand-name products. Along with most doctors and pharmacists, I believed the FDA. But no more.

From carcinogenic contaminants...to an increased incidence of side effects...and/or even poor efficacy, there can be problems with ge-

neric drugs, ranging from blood pressure and antiseizure drugs to heartburn medications and antidepressants.

WHAT CAN GO WRONG WITH GENERICS

There are three main reasons why generic drugs may not be as effective and safe as the FDA promises—possibly because generic drugs have thinner profit margins, with less money available for quality control. The issues are...

•**Instant release vs. timed-release.** Decades ago, most prescription drugs were instant release—the active ingredient was immediately released into the bloodstream. To maintain an effective level of medicine in the blood, you had to take pills two or three times a day. But in the 1980s and 90s, companies began to market timed-release or extended-release formulations,

Joe Graedon, MS, a pharmacologist and cofounder with his wife, Terry Graedon, PhD, of The People's Pharmacy, PeoplesPharmacy.com, which educates consumers about the use of medications and natural remedies. He is an adjunct assistant professor at University of North Carolina Eshelman School of Pharmacy and coauthor of numerous books, including *Top Screwups Doctors Make and How to Avoid Them*.

225

allowing for a once-daily dose. Today, most popular drugs are available in a timed-release form.

A hidden threat: The approval process the FDA uses for generic drugs is still based on the decades-old concept of instant release. If a generic drug reaches a "maximal concentration" in the bloodstream that is similar to its equivalent brand-name drug, the FDA approves it. But the hour-by-hour level of the drug in the blood may be quite different from the brand-name drug, possibly reducing effectiveness and increasing side effects.

•**Foreign manufacturing.** About 80% of drug ingredients—the active pharmaceutical ingredients (APIs)—are now made in foreign countries, including India, China, Thailand, Turkey, Brazil, Mexico, Bangladesh, Slovakia and others. Many pills are also manufactured abroad.

Unfortunately, FDA oversight of the foreign production of APIs and pills is inadequate. In the US, for example, the FDA makes unannounced inspections of drug manufacturers. Abroad, the FDA usually schedules its visits, allowing companies to prepare in advance. This contrasting oversight has led to products with inadequate levels of the active compound, contamination and falsification of testing data.

•**Transportation.** The FDA has stringent temperature and humidity guidelines for the transportation of drugs (generic and brand-name versions) to ensure that they stay intact. But the FDA exercises little oversight of those guidelines. For example, what happens if an API is manufactured in China…goes to India to be formulated into pills, which travel by container ship to Houston…then get shipped to a wholesaler or distributor in San Diego or Phoenix…and are finally distributed to pharmacies? No one knows the consequences of this odyssey.

HOW TO PROTECT YOURSELF

It's difficult to figure out if a generic drug you're taking could harm your health. Complicating matters is the fact that there are no specific categories of generics that are worse than others. Problems have been found in many classes of generic drugs.

Case in point: Some of the worst offenders are foreign-manufactured angiotensin II receptor blockers (ARBs). There have been repeated reports of these popular medications, such as *losartan, irbesartan* and *valsartan*, typically used for high blood pressure and heart failure, being contaminated with carcinogens (nitrosamines). The FDA has now recalled untold numbers of these pills and has published a list of ARBs it considers safe. To see the list, go to FDA.gov and search "ARB Drug Products."

To minimize potential harm…

•**Assume nothing.** Don't assume that your generic drug is flawed—but don't assume that it's perfect either. Because of the failure of the FDA to protect us from harmful generic drugs, you need to personally evaluate the safety and effectiveness of your generic drug.

•**Ask for lab results.** You and your physician need to monitor your health with all of the data that is available. With that in mind, make sure your physician supplies you with all lab results so you can track any changes.

Example: HbA1c, a measure of long-term blood sugar levels—if it rises but you haven't made any changes in your diet or lifestyle, your generic diabetes drug may not be working.

•**Keep records.** Once you have your lab results, be sure to record them so you can closely track the effectiveness of the drug. If those numbers stay steady, it's likely the medicine is working. If they change significantly after you start a generic substitution or get a refill, tell your doctor immediately. You may need to revert to the brand-name drug or a different generic manufacturer.

Smart ideas: If you revert to the brand-name drug, consider buying from a Canadian online pharmacy, which will have lower prices. (You will most likely have to pay out of pocket, but the drug may be covered by a private insurer if you submit a receipt.)

Important: To make sure it's a reliable pharmacy, visit the website PharmacyChecker.com.

If you switch generics, ask your pharmacist for an "authorized generic drug"—a type of generic that is identical to the original brand-name drug. (The authorized version is often made by the same manufacturer that makes the brand-name version.)

Example: Pfizer makes Viagra, and a Pfizer subsidiary makes its authorized generic, sildenafil.

•**Monitor symptoms.** Some conditions aren't measured in numbers.

Examples: You're taking a generic prostate drug for urinary symptoms, but you still have to get up several times a night to urinate—a sign the drug isn't working. Or you switch to a generic pain reliever, and your arthritis pain comes roaring back. In both cases, the generic drug is the likely culprit.

•**Challenge and rechallenge.** This is a time-honored way to assess your reaction to medication. If generic drug X causes a headache, going back on the brand name should solve the problem. To confirm that the problem lies with the generic, take the same one you used before to see if the symptom reappears. If it does, it's highly likely the generic is at fault.

•**Find out the manufacturer.** There may be dozens of different companies making your generic medicine. Ask the pharmacist to always put the name of the generic manufacturer on your prescription bottle. If a generic drug from a particular manufacturer works, stick with it… and ask your pharmacy to keep it on hand or order it just for you—not all drugstore chains, however, will be able to fulfill this request.

•**Seek allies.** If you decide not to use the generic, ask your doctor and/or pharmacist to go to bat for you if your insurance company balks at paying for the brand name. (If your doctor or pharmacist insists that all generic drugs are identical to their brand-name counterparts, ask him/her to read this article.)

Helpful: To find out the latest on recalled drugs, sign up for recall alerts at FDA.gov/safety/recalls.

Has Your Medication Supply Been Affected by the Coronavirus Pandemic?

Jack E. Fincham, PhD, RPh, emeritus professor of public health and pharmacy, and dean emeritus, The University of Kansas School of Pharmacy in Lawrence. He is also a faculty member of the Osher Lifelong Learning Institute, The University of Arizona in Tucson.

As the tumultuous effects of the new coronavirus pandemic are being felt worldwide, hand-washing and social distancing aren't the only steps you should be following to stay safe. You also should check your supply of the medications you regularly take.

Here's why: Close to 90% of active drug ingredients for generic medications are manufactured in China, which has been significantly impacted by the illness caused by the new coronavirus (COVID-19).

To complete the entire manufacturing process, most of the medications that get dispensed by your pharmacy have to travel along an international supply chain that also includes India and other countries. For brand-name medications in the US, it's been estimated that 70% are manufactured in foreign countries.

The FDA has been monitoring the drug-supply chain, but the increasing international spread of the new coronavirus recently caused the federal agency to suspend inspections of drugs overseas (possibly through the end of 2020), which could threaten the quality of those manufactured products. That includes temporarily pulling inspectors out of China, which is the largest source of drug ingredients for aspirin, ibuprofen (Motrin) and penicillin.

If you are taking a drug that can't be interrupted, it is wise to plan for the possibility of a drug shortage.

ARE YOU AT RISK?

Other things besides the recent COVID-19 pandemic have contributed to drug shortages. For example, natural disasters, such as the hurricane that struck Puerto Rico in 2017, have triggered shortfalls of certain medications. Shortages also have occurred when drug products are abruptly discontinued.

Medication shortages are most likely to affect older, lower-priced drugs that don't provide significant financial gain for manufacturers, such as the fluoroquinolone antibiotic *gemifloxacin* (Factive).

There are shortages for the following medications (at press time)…

•**Cardiovascular drugs, such as *diltiazem* (Cardizem)**

•**Antiviral drug *letermovir* (Prevymis) injection,** used in bone-marrow transplant patients

•**Immunosuppressive drug *tacrolimus* (Prograf)**

•**Liquid *nystatin* (Mycostatin),** an antifungal medication used to treat yeast infections in the mouth or stomach.

Other medications, such as certain injectables and anti-epileptic and antipsychotic drugs, also are in short supply. People who take any of these drugs are more vulnerable if new shortages occur due to the COVID-19 outbreak. For a list of current drug shortages, check the FDA website, AccessData.FDA.Gov/Scripts/DrugShortages/.

Older antibiotics, such as penicillin, also are susceptible to shortages. Antibiotics, of course, are not used to treat viral infections, but secondary bacterial infections can occur with such illnesses and require antibiotic treatment.

You also need to be alert to possible shortages if you take a drug that causes side effects if the medication is stopped suddenly. These include prescription pain medicines, certain antidepressants and some blood pressure medications, such as the beta-blocker *bisoprolol* (Zebeta) and the angiotensin II receptor blockers *irbesartan* (Avapro) and *losartan* (Cozaar).

If you take medication for one or more of the following conditions, it's important that you maintain an adequate supply of the drug to control the condition…

•**Lung conditions,** such as chronic obstructive pulmonary disease (COPD) or asthma

•**High blood pressure**
•**Heart disease**
•**Cancer**
•**Diabetes**
•**Seizures**
•**AIDS**
•**Autoimmune diseases,** such as rheumatoid arthritis, lupus or multiple sclerosis
•**Depression**
•**Thyroid disease**

WHAT TO DO?

Start by talking to your doctor. Especially if you're taking medication for one of the conditions listed earlier, ask your doctor to write a prescription for a 90-day supply. Most insurance companies and drug plan providers are already easing up on restrictions for 90-day supplies.

If you run into problems, ask your doctor's office for help or consult your pharmacist for advice. If the larger refill you're requesting doesn't coincide with your refill date, your doctor can call your prescription drug plan provider and explain why the medication is essential for your health. With the doctor's prescription and advocacy on your behalf, the provider may be more apt to approve the larger refill.

You should also ask your doctor if there are alternative medications that you can take if you have difficulty getting your regular medication. For example, if you take a beta-blocker, there may be other medications in the same class of drugs that are available and will have the same effect.

If you still have trouble getting or paying for a 90-day supply, an online pharmacy might be able to provide your medication.

Important: To ensure that you are using a reputable online pharmacy, consult the website of the National Association of Boards of Pharmacy (nabp.pharmacy/programs/dotpharmacy, click on the "Pharmacy Verified Websites" list).

For information on online Canadian pharmacies, consult the website of the National Association of Pharmacy Regulatory Authorities (napra.ca/online-pharmacies). Ask your doctor to fax a written 90-day prescription and have the medication sent to you.

REMEMBER OTC MEDICATIONS

While you're reviewing your prescription-drug supply, also make sure to have some commonly used over-the-counter (OTC) medications on hand. It may be best to buy these now. *Here are OTC medications that are useful for everyone to have in their medicine cabinets…*

•**Analgesics,** such as *acetaminophen* (Tylenol), *ibuprofen* (Motrin) and/or *naproxen* (Aleve)

•**Lubricating eyedrops,** such as Systane

•**Oral antihistamine medicine for allergies and colds,** such as *cetirizine* (Zyrtec) and *loratadine* (Claritin)

•***Guaifenesin* (Mucinex) for bronchial congestion**

Helpful: Look for liquid versions of any oral medications that might be needed for children or adults with swallowing difficulties. Plus, get disinfectant wipes, which are needed for certain medical treatments.

Also: Find out if your pharmacy or other pharmacies in your area will deliver or mail medicines in case you get quarantined at home. Although hand sanitizers may be in short supply, you can make your own by mixing isopropyl alcohol (at least 91%) with aloe vera gel. Use a ratio of one-third aloe vera and two-thirds alcohol.

BE VIGILANT…BUT DON'T PANIC

While it's prudent to seek a 90-day supply of medications, it's important to avoid stockpiling drugs, as we have seen with people hoarding face masks, hand sanitizers and toilet paper. This can turn a potential shortage of any product—including medications—into an actual shortage.

With the COVID-19 outbreak subsiding in China and the massive quarantines that slowed their workforces being loosened, production of drug ingredients has resumed there. But other countries along the production chain may still have problems, especially India, so don't panic…but do plan ahead.

Some Drugs Cause Loss of Smell

Alan Hirsch, MD, neurological director of The Smell & Taste Treatment and Research Foundation in Chicago.

Some drugs cause loss of smell, including *atorvastatin* (Lipitor) and other statins… ACE inhibitor *captopril* (Capoten)…*azithromycin* (Zithromax) and other antibiotics…and antidepressants such as *amitriptyline* (Elavil) and *fluoxetine* (Prozac). These drugs may affect taste or smell receptors by causing dry mouth, which diminishes smell. If you've noticed this, ask your doctor about a lower dose or a different drug.

Choking Alert

Nearly 4,000 people (most over age 65) reported problems swallowing dietary supplement pills during a 10-year period, according to a report from the FDA. Three deaths also were reported.

Self-defense: Swallow supplements with plenty of water…or ask your pharmacist or doctor if your supplement can be cut into pieces, or if there is a liquid, powder or chewable form.

Cecile Punzalan, MD, MPH, medical officer, Center for Food Safety and Applied Nutrition, FDA, College Park, Maryland.

Many Grandparents Do Not Secure Medicines Properly

Preeti Malani, MD, director, National Poll on Healthy Aging, Institute for Healthcare Policy and Innovation, University of Michigan, Ann Arbor.

More than 80% of grandparents say that they keep their medicines in the same easy-to-access place when young grandchildren visit. This heightens the risk for accidental poisoning of children—especially since nearly one-third of grandparents report keeping their medicines in easy-to-open containers instead of childproof ones.

Don't Die from Your Heartburn Medication

Ziyad Al-Aly, MD, director, Clinical Epidemiology Center, VA St. Louis Health Care System.

People who took a proton pump inhibitor (PPI), such as *omeprazole* (Prilosec) or *lansoprazole* (Prevacid), for more than 90 days were 17% more likely to die than those who took an H2 blocker, such as *cimetidine* (Tagamet) or *ranitidine* (Zantac), for the same amount of time, according to a 10-year study of nearly 160,000 participants.

Important: 80% of the PPI prescriptions were at the low-dose level found in over-the-counter formulations.

Heart Drugs May Increase Risk of Falls

Frederik Dalgaard, MD, is a cardiovascular researcher at Herlev and Gentofte Hospital, Hellerup, Denmark, and leader of a study published in *Journal of the American Geriatrics Society.*

Taking A-fib drugs may increase risk for falls and fainting in older patients.

Latest finding: *Amiodarone* (Nexterone and Pacerone) was associated with fainting and falls in older people with A-fib, in part because it can lead to bradycardia (slow heartbeat). Use precautions—such as rising from a seated position slowly—especially in the first two weeks after starting the medication.

Other A-fib drug previously linked to falls: *Digoxin* (Lanoxin).

Beware This Blood Thinner

Derjung M. Tarn, MD, PhD, associate professor of family medicine, David Geffen School of Medicine, University of California, Los Angeles.

One-third of people taking an anticoagulant, such as *apixaban* (Eliquis), to prevent stroke also take one or more over-the-counter drugs or supplements that when taken with an anticoagulant can cause dangerous internal bleeding, according to a survey of nearly 800 men and women.

Examples: Painkillers such as aspirin, *ibuprofen* (Advil) and *acetaminophen* (Tylenol)…and dietary supplements, including fish oil, as well as turmeric, ginger and other herbs and herbal teas.

If you take an anticoagulant: Ask your doctor which drugs and supplements to avoid.

The Lowdown on Laxatives

Joshua Levitt, ND, naturopathic physician and medical director at Whole Health Natural Family Medicine, Hamden, Connecticut. He is a clinical preceptor for Yale School of Medicine and author of *The 21-Day Revival, The Science-Based Truth About CBD* and *The Honey Phenomenon.*

If you're 60 or older, chances are one in three that you have occasional or chronic constipation. For people under age 60, the odds are one in six, and women of all ages are 50% more likely to have constipation than men.

But not all constipation is created equal. It occurs for several reasons, and different causes call for different treatments. Use the wrong treatment, and your problem may only get worse. *Naturopathic physician Joshua Levitt, ND, explains what you need to know…*

CHRONIC CONSTIPATION

An aging colon is a major culprit when it comes to chronic constipation. Reduced muscle function in the large intestine makes defecation more difficult. The smooth muscles in the wall of the colon become weaker, impairing peristalsis, the automatic muscular contractions that propel stool through the bowel.

Other causes: You may not be getting as much exercise as you used to. Less physical activity results in less intestinal motility—the movement of the stool. Or your diet may be low in fiber. You need roughage from fruits, vegetables, beans, grains, nuts and seeds to add bulk to your stool.

Growing problem: Chronic constipation is a side effect of certain medications.

Worst offenders: Pain relievers such as opioids and nonsteroidal anti-inflammatory drugs (NSAIDs)...antidepressants...and proton pump inhibitors for heartburn.

Note: There also are a number of diseases that cause constipation, including Parkinson's and hypothyroidism. If you have disease-caused chronic constipation, see your doctor.

THE RIGHT LAXATIVE FOR CHRONIC CONSTIPATION

It's important to understand your unique type so that you can choose the laxative that will work best for you. *At the most basic level, there are two types of chronic constipation...*

•**Spastic.** This is characterized by pellets or thin ribbons of stool that require you to strain to pass them. This happens because of a tense bowel—the smooth muscles of the colon are overly tight.

•**Atonic.** This is characterized by large, hardened stools that accumulate in the bowel. It happens in people who have been constipated for a while—they have trouble squeezing out the stool due to an atonic, or flaccid, bowel.

What to do...

For spastic constipation: There are osmotic or softening laxatives, some with magnesium, such as Phillips Milk of Magnesia, and some using other compounds, such as *polyethylene glycol* (MiraLAX).* So-called "stool softeners" usually are osmotic laxatives, such as *docusate* (Colace, Surfak). They work by drawing water into the bowel, softening stool.

*Check with your doctor before taking any supplement—especially if you have a chronic medical condition or take medication.

But my favorite osmotic laxative—because it's the most effective due to higher absorbability and better muscle relaxation—is magnesium citrate, a nutritional supplement taken as a powder, pill, capsule or liquid. To find your tolerance level, start with a dose of 300 milligrams (mg) of magnesium citrate, taken with dinner, to hopefully produce a morning bowel movement. Because magnesium requires digestive acid and digestive enzymes for absorption, it's best taken with a meal. Take the 300-mg dose for three days. If it doesn't produce results, increase the dose to 450 mg. Continue to increase the dose by 150 mg every third day until you produce a laxative effect. If you get to the point of watery diarrhea, cut back to the previous dose. Magnesium citrate can be taken on an ongoing basis as long as it's 150 mg below your tolerance level. I suggest Magnesium Citrate by Vital Nutrients or Natural Calm by Natural Vitality.

Another option for spastic constipation is enteric-coated peppermint oil. Peppermint is an antispasmodic, making it ideal for spastic constipation.

My advice: I favor Mentharil from Integrative Therapeutics. Take one capsule (0.2 milliliters of enteric-coated peppermint oil) at bedtime. If that doesn't work, take two the next night. If that doesn't work, take three the next night. If it still isn't working, it's not the right laxative for you.

Note: For mild constipation, a cup of peppermint tea is a great option.

For atonic constipation: While there are many fiber-rich (bulking) laxatives—*wheat dextrin* (Benefiber), *methylcellulose* (Citrucel), *calcium polycarbophil* (FiberCon) and *psyllium* (Metamucil)—the most effective "laxative" is simply high-fiber food.

Try a daily breakfast of one-half cup of oatmeal, a tablespoon of ground flaxseed, a handful of slivered almonds or walnuts and a sprinkling of berries. Throughout the rest of the day, eat five servings of fruits and vegetables and plenty of beans, legumes, whole grains and/or nuts and seeds.

Alternative: Add ground flaxseed to a smoothie. The optimal dose is two tablespoons—but don't start at that level because it can produce increased gas. Instead, start with one-half tablespoon for three days, increasing it to one tablespoon on day four…to one-and-a-half tablespoons on day seven…and to two tablespoons on day 10.

•**Stimulant laxatives.** Popular stimulant laxatives include *bisacodyl* (Dulcolax) and *sennosides*, the active ingredient in the herb senna (Senokot, Ex-Lax). These over-the-counter products work by stimulating the bowel to contract and expel stool—but I suggest trying a gentler, natural alternative with fewer side effects first. Drink one-half cup of senna tea daily. Try Traditional Medicinals Smooth Move senna tea.

FOR OCCASIONAL CONSTIPATION

If you want quick relief from a bout of constipation that is not chronic, try this protocol, which helps prevent rectal tears caused by passing stool that has accumulated in the colon over several days.

Day 1:

1: Drink one cup of prune juice, and eat three to four prunes (dried plums). Prunes contain naturally occurring *sorbitol*, which works like an osmotic laxative.

2: Take magnesium citrate—from 300 mg to 500 mg.

Day 2: If bowels have not moved…
Continue the steps above and…

3: Drink one cup of senna tea. Steep two bags for five minutes.

4: Take an aloe vera extract, which "greases" the bowels, helping stool move. Try one 450-mg capsule of Super Aloe from Ortho Molecular Products.

Caution: If there is an abrupt change in bowel movements…you're constipated for more than a week…constipation is accompanied by severe abdominal pain…or you see blood in your stool—see your doctor.

Green Tea Strengthens an Antibiotic

Journal of Medical Microbiology

A chemical compound found abundantly in green tea, known as EGCG, appears to make drug-resistant bacteria more susceptible to the antibiotic *aztreonam* (Azactam). The drug is commonly used for respiratory/bloodstream infections.

Daily Aspirin Not Right for Everyone

Robert Eckel, MD, is professor of medicine at University of Colorado School of Medicine in Aurora, Colorado, and past president of the American Heart Association. UCDenver.edu

---

Most people should not take a daily aspirin for heart health, says Robert Eckel, MD. Daily low-dose aspirin was long-considered an effective way to reduce the odds of blood clots that could lead to heart attacks and strokes, but recent research suggests that the benefits are outweighed by the risks for dangerous internal bleeding.

Keep Everything Moving

The following good habits help to prevent constipation…

•**Go when you need to go.** Delaying defecation stretches the bowel, creating and worsening atonic constipation. When your body is telling you it's time to go—go.

•**Use a toilet footstool.** The optimal position for effortless defecation is squatting, not sitting. A way to mimic this pose is to use a footstool in front of your toilet, which raises your knees, creating a squat-like position that helps open the rectum. (Squatty Potty is a popular brand.)

•**Don't sit around.** To prevent constipation and for general health, the pelvic floor should be toned and tight. Unfortunately, sitting too long on the toilet relaxes the pelvic floor—stretching layers of muscle and tissue like a hammock. If defecation isn't happening, come back later. If you're finished, don't hang around.

—Joshua Levitt

Exception: Daily low-dose aspirin is generally beneficial for someone who already has experienced heart attacks or thrombotic strokes.

Medicines That Cause Night Sweats

Sharon Orrange, MD, associate professor of clinical medicine in the division of geriatric, hospitalist and general internal medicine, Keck School of Medicine, University of Southern California, Los Angeles.

Pain relievers such as *acetaminophen*, aspirin and *ibuprofen*...tricyclic as well as SSRI antidepressants...migraine medications including *frovatriptan* (Frova) and *eletriptan* (Relpax)...and diabetes medications such as insulin, *glipizide* (Glucotrol) and *pioglitazone* (Actos) can cause overstimulation of sweat glands. (For more information about night sweats, see page 14 in chapter 1, "Aging Well.")

Opioids After Surgery? Not so Fast

Michael Kim, DO, clinical assistant professor of anesthesiology at Keck School of Medicine, University of Southern California in Los Angeles. Dr. Kim is the collaborative team leader for the Enhanced Recovery After Surgery program at Keck Medicine of USC.

Unless you live in a bubble, you know that the US is in the throes of an opioid crisis.

Even though doctors have begun to recognize that opioid use after surgery may play a part in the opioid crisis, more than two million Americans still begin to use and abuse opioids following surgery every year.

Now: Many medical centers have adopted a program known as Enhanced Recovery After Surgery (ERAS). ERAS involves a range of measures to provide a better surgery experience for the patient, resulting in shorter hospitals stays, a reduction in complications and readmissions, and greater patient satisfaction. It also is curbing or eliminating opioid use for surgical procedures. Hospitals using an ERAS protocol are seeing opioid use drastically decline.

THE BASICS OF ERAS

Although the specific ERAS plan differs depending on the type of surgical procedure and the individual patient's needs, there are some basic principles. *Five key steps of ERAS...*

PREADMISSION

If your surgery is not an emergency, your pain-management plan should start before your procedure. For example, before surgery, you will talk to your surgeon and also get a pre-op anesthesia consultation with the anesthesiologist. At this time, your medication needs will be assessed. Knowing what to expect—and working with your team on a pain-management plan—reduces a lot of the anxiety and fear that contribute to pain after surgery.

Before surgery, you'll likely be asked to stop smoking and drinking alcohol. Tobacco and alcohol use generally does not affect the type of drugs that are administered during surgery, but eliminating both may reduce complications from anesthesia. A few weeks before, you also may be started on an exercise plan (such as daily walking) and/or a healthful diet to prepare your body for the stress of surgery.

Several days before surgery, you may be started on a nonopioid pain medication, such as over-the-counter *acetaminophen* (Tylenol), a nonsteroidal anti-inflammatory such as *celecoxib* (Celebrex) or the nerve-pain drug *gabapentin* (Gralise). This allows the medication to saturate your tissues before surgery and reduces the pain and inflammation reaction during surgery.

PREOPERATION

Previously, it was common to have nothing to eat or drink after midnight the day before surgery. This was done to prevent any potential risk for aspiration (unintended inhalation of liquid or solid material into the trachea and lungs). An ERAS protocol recognizes that this level of fasting is not necessary. It can cause your body to use up valuable proteins, fats and nutrients that it needs to undergo surgery.

You may be able to have a light diet of a few crackers up to six hours before surgery and drink clear liquids, such as water or apple juice, up to two hours prior to surgery. In addition, you may be instructed to drink a high-carbohydrate drink the day before surgery and another three to four hours before surgery.

DURING SURGERY

A lot can be done during surgery to reduce your pain afterward. Your anesthesiologist may use nonopioid pain medication, such as acetaminophen, celecoxib or gabapentin, just prior to surgery and give you medications to prevent nausea and vomiting when you wake up.

You also may get a nerve block just before the procedure begins to reduce pain when you wake up. The anesthesiologist or surgeon will give the nerve block at the beginning or after the surgery, and its effects can last from hours to a few days. Your anesthesiologist will constantly check your fluid levels, blood glucose and body temperature. Preventing cold stress during surgery reduces the surgical stress.

AFTER SURGERY

An ERAS plan kicks into high gear following surgery. *It typically includes the following promptly after surgery…*

•**Mobilization.** This can mean sitting in a chair instead of lying in bed and getting up to walk as soon as you can, even if you use a walker. If you can walk, you will be encouraged to go as far as comfortably possible at least twice on the first day after surgery.

•**Nutrition.** Depending on your surgery, you may be given clear fluids to drink within two hours after surgery. If you can't drink, you may get fluids through an IV. Many patients can have a full diet the day after surgery.

•**Removal of tubes and drains.** If you have IV tubes, a Foley catheter, a surgical drain or a nasogastric tube, your surgical care team will try to get these out as soon as possible (usually 24 to 48 hours after surgery) to reduce the risk for infection. Some may go home with a drain, based on their procedure.

•**Pain management.** For medication, opioids are no longer the first choice. Other options include acetaminophen, an over-the-counter or prescription-strength nonsteroidal anti-inflammatory drug or gabapentin.

In many cases, these non-narcotic options may be as effective as an opioid. Opioids, if needed, may be used for "breakthrough" pain (a pain flare-up that occurs despite the regular use of pain medication). You may also be given a local anesthesia patch to wear.

RECOVERY AT HOME

Your discharge instructions will depend on the type of surgery you have, but opioids will not be an automatic part of the plan. A non-narcotic pain reliever will be the first choice.

If you need an opioid for breakthrough pain, you will be prescribed the lowest effective dose for a shorter amount of time. For example, instead of a 10-day prescription, you may get a three-to-five-day prescription. Your ERAS plan will include follow-up phone calls from the nurse or the nurse practitioner to see how you are doing and how you are handling any pain.

If you are scheduled for surgery: Ask your surgeon if your hospital has an ERAS program. To learn more about ERAS, go to the website of the ERAS Society USA, ERASUSA.org.

How Does CBD Treat Pain Versus Opioids… and Is It Addictive?

Diana Martins-Welch, MD, assistant professor of medicine at the Donald and Barbara Zucker School of Medicine at Hofstra/Northwell in Lake Success, New York. Board-certified in internal medicine and hospice and palliative care, she is a member of the Association of Cannabis Specialists, which is dedicated to providing best clinical practices for the use of cannabis medicine.

Cannabidiol (CBD) is a chemical found in the cannabis plant and is different from tetrahydrocannabinol (THC), the substance that produces the marijuana "high." We don't yet fully understand how CBD works to relieve pain, but studies show that it is an anti-inflammatory agent. Many painful conditions, such as arthritis and lupus, are inflammation-driven.

Opioid drugs, such as *fentanyl* (Duragesic) and *oxycodone* (Oxycontin), work on different pain receptors in the brain and also release dopamine, the "feel-good" brain chemical that creates a powerful sense of well-being. CBD does not produce an excessive release of dopamine, as opioids do. While pain can diminish drastically with opioids, these drugs can also cause people to feel sleepy, dizzy or "cloudy." CBD's analgesic effect does not result in mental cloudiness.

We don't know why some people become addicted to opioids, while others do not, but a genetic component may affect how the body responds to them. CBD is not thought to be addictive because there isn't a surge of dopamine, so the brain's reward system isn't stimulated, as occurs with opioids. Therefore, there's no craving for CBD, as some people might experience with opioids.

Important: Before trying CBD, be sure to check with your doctor if you have a chronic medical condition or take any medication or supplement.

Sleeping Pills May Block Threats

Frontiers in Behavioral Neuroscience

People who take sleeping pills, such as the benzodiazepine *triazolam* (Halcion), can sleep so soundly that a fire alarm won't wake them.

In the works: A new class of sleeping pills that allows patients to wake up long enough to detect threats.

Medical Cannabis for Autism

Study by researchers at Ben-Gurion University of the Negev and Soroka University Medical Center, both in Beersheba, Israel, published in *Nature*.

Medical cannabis relieves autism symptoms. In a study of 188 child patients formally diagnosed with autism spectrum disorders—average age of 13—use of cannabis oil containing 30% nonpsychoactive CBD and 1.5% psychoactive THC resulted in nearly 80%

reporting moderate or significant symptom improvement within a month. Fourteen percent said cannabis did not help symptoms, and 6% reported side effects including sleepiness, restlessness, reflux or lack of appetite. After six months, with 155 patients remaining in the study, about 85% reported moderate or significant improvement in symptoms…67% said that their quality of life had improved…and more than 63% reported a more positive mood.

Beware This "Safe" Opioid

Molly Jeffery, PhD, scientific director of research, Division of Emergency Medicine, Mayo Clinic, Rochester, Minnesota.

Tramadol (Ultram), long considered to be less addictive than *hydrocodone/acetaminophen* (Vicodin) or *oxycodone* (OxyContin), may be just as risky. When researchers reviewed almost 450,000 records of surgery patients, those who had been prescribed tramadol were more likely than those given other opioids to refill their prescriptions long past when their surgical pain should have ended.

If you're prescribed an opioid after surgery: Ask your doctor if an alternative over-the-counter or prescription drug will relieve your pain.

What to Do About Weight Gain If You Take Prednisone for Back Pain

David Sherer, MD, a retired anesthesiologist who now focuses on patient education, writing and patient advocacy. He is author of the blog "What Your Doctor Isn't Telling You" at BottomLineInc.com.

Prednisone is a powerful prescription steroid drug with lots of possible side effects, including weight gain. Used as an anti-inflammatory for back pain or immune suppressant, prednisone is also commonly prescribed for such conditions as arthritis, ulcer-ative colitis, psoriasis, lupus, asthma and other breathing disorders.

Like other steroids, prednisone also can cause high blood pressure, headache, nausea, muscle weakness, anxiety and sleep problems. When used long term (typically for more than three months), the drug increases risk for infections, bone loss, cataracts and elevated blood sugar.

Weight gain can contribute to back pain. To keep back pain at bay, a good rule of thumb is to stay within about 10 pounds of your ideal body weight. If you are sedentary, getting up to walk for a few minutes every hour will help.

In addition to weight-loss strategies, talk to your doctor about seeing a physical therapist who can suggest pain-relieving exercises such as stretching. Swimming, yoga and/or massage therapy also can help. Over-the-counter (OTC) topicals, such as capsaicin or arnica, are worth considering as well. Some people report that CBD formulations relieve their pain.

If those steps don't work, ask your doctor about an OTC nonsteroidal anti-inflammatory drug (NSAID), such as *naproxen* (Aleve).

Note: NSAIDs also can cause side effects, such as ulcers and even kidney damage or heart prob-lems. Some people get relief from *acetamino-phen* (Tylenol), but liver damage can occur if the dosage exceeds the recommended maximum daily dose. Ask your doctor to identify the saf-est medication for you.

Painkiller Danger

mBio

In a recent lab study, mice infected with *C. difficile*, a dangerous bacterial infection that causes severe diarrhea, had shorter sur-vival times if they received a nonsteroidal anti-inflammatory drug (NSAID) called *indometha-cin* prior to the infection.

Theory: NSAIDs disrupt the immune system and reduce intestinal defenses. More study is needed to determine if humans are similarly affected.

CHAPTER 14

Men's Health

Myths About Male Sexuality

Do men crave sex more than women? Are they always in the mood? Do men really enjoy the "chase"? The honest answers may surprise both genders.

In the movies, men always initiate sex—and like being in charge. Real life doesn't necessarily match that mystique. Male sexuality is far more complicated, and these myths not only hold couples back from finding deeper intimacy and connection, they can damage their sex lives with inappropriate expectations. When a man doesn't want sex, his female partner often feels alarmed. (He's supposed to want this, so there must be something wrong with me or our relationship.) And he may worry that his lagging interest is a sign that he's not masculine enough.

These are the most common misconceptions about men and sex—and the reassuring truths behind them that will help both of you connect in a more open way...

***MYTH #1:* Men are always in the mood for sex.** We have been taught that men have higher sex drives than women have. On the flip side, we're all familiar with the stereotype of a wife saying, "Not tonight, honey. I have a headache."

Reality: Research on men between the ages of 30 and 60 found that the guys were no more likely than their female partners to be the one with higher desire. While some research shows that 15% of men have had "problematic sexual desire" over the past six months, the percentage of men who have episodes of low desire is probably higher than that, according to my research. Ideally partners have a similar level of sexual interest, but when there is a discrepancy,

Sarah Hunter Murray, PhD, sex researcher and relationship therapist in private practice in Winnipeg, Manitoba. She is author of *Not Always in the Mood: The New Science of Men, Sex, and Relationships.* SarahHunterMurray.com it's just as common for the female as the male to be in the mood.

Problem: Because we believe the myth, women often squash down their desire, thinking, *I really shouldn't want sex more than he does.* They don't feel that it's their place to initiate it. A woman also may see his lack of interest as a sign that she's not attractive to him. Meanwhile, he may feel embarrassed or confused by his lack of desire. They're both left wondering, *Is there something wrong with us?*

New way of thinking: There's so much variability in sexual drive that there really is no "normal." Understanding that men have many of the same issues that women have—they're stressed, they're tired, they don't feel attractive—helps both partners feel understood. A man's desire at any given moment is not a marker of his partner's level of attractiveness. Your desires won't always be perfectly synced—leave a little space for each other to not be in the mood sometimes. Consider simply cuddling, since you don't need an orgasm to have intimacy. If "not tonight" starts becoming a pattern, try saying in a loving way, "I've noticed I've been in the mood a few times, and you haven't been. Is anything going on there?"

MYTH #2: Men's desire is driven solely by a woman's physical appearance. You've probably heard that male arousal starts with physical cues, such as seeing his wife's legs when she is wearing a short skirt.

Reality: When I ask men how important physical appearance is, they say, "Yes, I like it when she shows off her body, but if I'm not feeling emotionally connected to her, if we're not on the same page, then that isn't enough to do it for me." They feel most turned on when their relationship is running smoothly.

Problem: Believing the myth that all men want women with a 36-24-36 body completely ignores the depth of a man's sexuality. Women sometimes worry when they put on weight or get older that their partners will no longer be attracted to them.

New way of thinking: Yes, looks matter to some degree, but men have different views of beauty and are, in reality, most drawn to a woman's confidence and her ability to let him know,

I want to connect with you sexually. Again and again, I have heard men talking about their sexual desire for partners who had a physical disability or who had put on weight after having children or who were in their 50s or older. It was her comfort in her own skin and willingness to share her body with him that was the real turn-on.

MYTH #3: Men are selfish in bed. The common stereotype is that a guy is looking out for only his own sexual needs—it's mainly about him climaxing and then rolling over and going to sleep.

Reality: Men want so much more than one-sided gratification. Men repeatedly told me how important their partners' sexual pleasure was to them. If she was acquiescing to sex—consenting but not really excited about it—that was a major turnoff. They would say, "I don't want to be having sex with somebody who isn't super-excited to be having sex with me." Bringing a woman pleasure and providing an orgasm feed into his feelings of masculinity. Men see their mate's enjoyment as a sign that they are on the same page. Pleasing her in the bedroom helps him feel connected to her outside the bedroom, too.

Problem: If a woman believes this myth—that he is looking only for his own sexual needs to be met—she might feel dismissive of him, thinking, *This is only for you. What's the point?*

New way of thinking: Recognize that he might want sex because he is longing to feel closer and that he truly wants to make you happy. This, in turn, will make you feel more receptive, which can lead to greater intimacy.

MYTH #4: Men like to be in charge in the bedroom. Society tells us that men should be the ones to initiate sex. Some of this goes back to college, when men tend to get socially rewarded for having sexual partners, while women are taught to be gatekeepers. ("Good girls don't have sex.") So a man still may feel pressure to pursue and make the first move.

Reality: Research tells us that men are getting tired of that standard. They feel enormous pressure to be the ones who make the first move, and they long for their partners to initiate, too. Why? It makes them feel good. It makes them feel wanted. And it makes them feel that some of that responsibility to take charge in the bedroom is off their shoulders. Also, it makes them feel vulnerable to always initiate sex and deal with the fear of rejection.

New way of thinking: While you may not be used to making the first move, it can be really empowering to step into a more assertive role. It's a mind-set of, *Hey I want closeness—so why not reach out instead of sitting passively waiting to see if he reads my signals?* Nonsexual overtures can be a good place to start—rubbing his shoulders or giving a little foot massage.

MYTH #5: **When men don't want it, something serious must be going on.**

Reality: The reasons that men might not be in the mood are the same as the ones that women report. It's been a long day. They're stressed. They're tired. We all have reasons to say no to sex that have nothing to do with our partners, and we need to be understanding about that.

Problem: While we're used to talking about what happens to a woman's sexuality after having kids, we don't discuss that a man's desire can take a nosedive, too. Research shows that dads today are more involved in their children's lives. They're changing diapers at night...they're coaching the hockey team...and they're feeling worn out and not always up for romance.

New way of thinking: Both sexes need time to recharge in order to be receptive to sex. It's essential to find pockets of time both separately and together. Allow for transition time after work—a little time to change clothes or read the mail. Ease into together time. Don't feel pressured to schedule special events—just going to bed at the same time can help you feel more in sync.

MYTH #6: **Men are confident and don't need compliments.** Have you noticed that women get complimented on their appearance much more than men do? They hear, "Your dress is so cute" or "I love your haircut." Men? Not so much.

Reality: Over the course of my research, I learned something startling—men wish they had this sort of attention from women. They want to be looked at by their partners. They want to be able to say, "Yes, I have been working out!" It's important to their desire, and it's something that rarely gets talked about because it goes against that norm.

New way of thinking: How can a woman make her partner feel noticed? Giving him compliments such as, "I love how that shirt brings out your eyes," shows that you appreciate him in a physical way. Nonverbal cues (a peck on the cheek or a pat on the bum) also send him the reassuring message that he still does it for you.

Eat Nuts for Better Sex

Albert Salas-Huetos, PhD, postdoctoral researcher, University of Utah School of Medicine, Salt Lake City.

In a study of 83 men, eating just two ounces of an almond, walnut and hazelnut mixture (about 45 nuts) a day improved sexual desire and orgasm quality, even though they ate an otherwise unhealthy diet.

Theory: The nuts are rich in the amino acid arginine, a precursor of nitric oxide, which increases circulation by relaxing and widening blood vessels.

Important: There are about 320 calories in two ounces of nuts, so you may need to cut daily calories elsewhere.

Prostate Biopsy: Avoid This Hidden Danger

Michael Liss, MD, principal investigator at SWOG (formerly Southwest Oncology Group) and medical director for clinical research, University of Texas Health Science Center, San Antonio.

More than one million US men get prostate biopsies every year. The procedure is simple—but, unfortunately, it is increasingly being followed by complications that can be serious...and even life-threatening. *What you need to know...*

INFECTION RISK IS RISING

While a prostate biopsy is an easy procedure, it has a high potential for infection. That's because prostate tissue samples are taken by needle punctures made through the rectum. *E. coli* bacteria are part of the natural environment of the rectum and can easily attach to the biopsy needles and infect the prostate, causing serious infection.

For this reason, prostate biopsy patients are given the antibiotic *ciprofloxacin* (Cipro) prophylactically to protect against prostate infections—and for years that worked. Now, however, with the rise of antibiotic resistance, about 10% to 20% of people have Cipro-resistant E. coli bacteria in their rectums, increasing risk for prostate infection from biopsy fourfold.

Some urologists try to reduce infection risk by cleaning biopsy needles after each needle puncture (typically 12 or more for each biopsy), cleaning the rectal area with a disinfectant before the procedure and/or giving extra antibiotics. Studies have not confirmed the effectiveness of these strategies.

REDUCING INFECTION RISK

Avoiding prostate infection from biopsies is challenging but not impossible. *These strategies are showing effectiveness…*

•**Determine if rectal *E. coli* are Cipro-resistant by doing a rectal swab culture several days before the biopsy.** If that is the case, a different antibiotic—for instance, an injection of a broad-spectrum antibiotic—can be given about one hour before the biopsy to kill off the E. coli bacteria. (Adding antibiotics also carries risk, including more antibiotic resistance and antibiotic-associated diarrhea.)

You may want to consider having a rectal swab if you are at high risk for Cipro-resistance. Risk factors include…

•Use of any antibiotic, including Cipro, in the last six months.

•Recent travel outside the country.

•An infection after a prior prostate biopsy.

•Working in the medical field and being exposed to resistant bacteria.

However, Cipro-resistance isn't the only thing that raises risk for prostate biopsy infections.

Men are also at higher risk if they have diabetes…take steroids…are undergoing chemotherapy…and/or have a recent history of prostatitis or urinary tract infection.

•**Take a safer route to the biopsy.** A procedure called *transperineal prostate biopsy* takes prostate tissue samples through the skin between the anus and scrotum (perineum). Transperineal prostate biopsy has a lower infection rate (less than 1% compared with 5% to 7%) than traditional prostate biopsy, but is not routinely performed. It is usually done in an operating room under general anesthesia and has a higher rate of temporary urinary retention (inability to urinate) after the procedure. It is also much more expensive than traditional prostate biopsy and may or may not be covered by insurance.

POST-BIOPSY SYMPTOMS

Alert your doctor immediately to any signs of infection. Infections can quickly become severe and may require a hospital stay and intravenous antibiotics. Symptoms to look for include chills, fever and urine that burns or is difficult to pass. The American Urological Association recommends that patients with fever post-biopsy be assessed for sepsis, a potentially life-threatening blood infection, and not be given a fluoroquinolone antibiotic, such as Cipro or *levofloxacin* (Levaquin), or *trimethoprim-sulfamethoxazole* (Bactrim), all of which are likely to be ineffective because of antibiotic resistance.

If you're scheduled for a prostate biopsy, ask your urologist about his/her infection rate and what he does to lower risk.

Prostate Cancer Treatment Linked to Dementia

Ravishankar Jayadevappa, PhD, research associate professor of geriatrics, Perelman School of Medicine, University of Pennsylvania, Philadelphia.

When more than 154,000 men with localized or advanced prostate cancer were tracked for an average of eight years, 13% of those who received *androgen deprivation therapy* (ADT) within two years of their diagnosis developed Alzheimer's disease compared with 9% who did not get the treatment. The prevalence of other forms of dementia was even greater—22% among those who got ADT versus 16% who did not. ADT can be life-saving in men with advanced prostate cancer, but those with localized prostate cancer must carefully weigh the long-term risks and benefits.

Mushrooms Fight Prostate Cancer

Men who ate about one-quarter cup of mushrooms three or more times a week had a 17% lower risk for prostate cancer, compared with those who ate them less than once a week, according to a study that followed more than 36,000 men for up to 24 years.

Theory: Mushrooms, including shiitake, oyster, maitake and white button, help protect against the inflammation that contributes to the development of prostate cancer.

Shu Zhang, PhD, assistant professor of epidemiology, Tohoku University School of Public Health, Sendai, Japan.

"Man Up" and Take Control of Your Health

David Sherer, MD, retired anesthesiologist who now focuses on patient education, writing and patient advocacy. He is author of the blog "What Your Doctor Isn't Telling You" at BottomLineInc.com.

Men tend to be very stubborn about taking care of themselves. Articles put out by *The Huffington Post* and The American Heart Association have focused on the reasons why this is so.

The former publication has pointed out that men die earlier than women. Part of this may be due to men taking more risks than women, as well as smoking and drinking to excess more

than women. Men's relative social isolation and more dangerous jobs also put them at risk for earlier death. Given all this, why would men avoid the doctor? *The Huffington Post's major reasons...*

- **Too busy to go.**
- **Fear of finding out bad news.**
- **Discomfort of examination (prostate, rectal, etc.).**
- **The doctor's "personal" questions.**
- **Getting weighed!**

Do visits to the doctor really save lives? You bet! Blood pressure screening, blood sugar tests and skin and testicular examinations are but a few of the easy interventions that can prevent or help treat diseases before they have gone too far. Lifestyle changes, medical and surgical therapies, as well as psychiatric counseling can literally save lives. But symptoms have to be heard and signs of disease have to be seen to be recognized and treated, and the only way that gets done is to visit the doctor. There is no substitute (short of telemedicine if that's an option) for a face-to-face visit with the physician. So why is this still an issue?

Well, men appear to have no shortage of dumb reasons. "I don't want to ask for directions." "I don't want to show that I have no knowledge of a particular topic." These are typical foolish sentiments that Dr. Glenn Good, an expert on masculinity and the psychology of men at the University of Florida, highlighted in a statement to *The Huffington Post*. The American Heart Association expanded on this issue, exploring other birdbrained but genuine excuses for not taking proper medical care of oneself. *These include...*

- **"I don't have a doctor."**
- **"I don't have insurance."**
- **"I don't have time."**
- **"I don't want to spend the money."**
- **"I'd rather tough it out."**

So men are still playing the stoic Marlboro Man of decades ago. Along with this machismo BS, the lame justifications listed above may seem silly and trivial, but they stand up to scrutiny. Indeed, men will say and do just about anything to avoid the doctor's office. What is a spouse, girlfriend, friend or other loved one to do to combat this foolish and boneheaded behavior? *I have a few suggestions…*

1. Show your loved one this blog post and read to him how lives have been saved and countless suffering (physical, emotional AND financial) has been averted by a simple visit to the doctor.

2. Get on the web and research "Why Men Avoid the Doctor" and show your XY chromosomal friend the potential disasters of not going.

3. Play on his conscience. If he won't do it for himself, at least he can do it for his life-partner, his children, his friends, coworkers and community.

4. Tell him that hypertension, diabetes, prostate cancer, colon cancer and cardio-vascular diseases are relatively common in Western-society men and that these conditions can often be cured or effectively treated if recognized early.

5. "Scare him straight." Tell him about someone you know who avoided the doctor only to learn that a condition had gone too far or, worse yet, caused an unexpected death to occur in a guy who appeared to be "healthy as a horse."

Most men, I believe, when pushed will listen to reason. But there will still be some guys out there who, despite your best efforts, will resist. At that point, radical measures may be needed. You might have your doctor call your loved one (if the doc is willing) to stress the importance of a physical. You might have a friend (preferably male), clergy member, trusted relative or grown child work him over as well. You can also play the "don't you want to dance at 'fill in the blank's' wedding?" (Insert child or grandchild's name there.)

It's going to take a cultural shift for men to "man-up" and take control of their health. I fear it is an uphill battle, but one well worth fighting.

Men: It's time to drop the macho act and drop your pants for the doctor. It's the right thing to do!

Peyronie's Disease: Men Can Now Overcome This Nightmare

Peter J. Stahl, MD, director of Male Reproductive and Sexual Medicine at NewYork-Presbyterian Hospital/Columbia University Medical Center and assistant professor of urology at Columbia University College of Physicians and Surgeons, both in New York City.

What if there were a disease that caused a man's penis to shrink and bend… and it led to painful erections that could make sex impossible?

Sadly, for up to 10% of men ages 40 to 70, this nightmare—a condition called Peyronie's disease—is a reality. If you haven't heard of it, that's because many men who are affected never talk about it or seek help.

Even though a host of treatments for this disease have been recommended over the years, few have offered much relief. Now there are new and better options available, so it's time for men with Peyronie's to finally seek help.

What you need to know…

PEYRONIE'S DISEASE: NEW ANSWERS

Peyronie's disease was first described by a French surgeon named Francois Gigot de la Peyronie in 1743. While the cause has long been a mystery, over the years, some medical experts have blamed Peyronie's on vigorous or acrobatic sex that injures the penis and causes scar tissue. However, many men who develop Peyronie's have no history of injury.

Now researchers believe there is a genetic cause. Peyronie's is related to other diseases that cause thickening of connective tissue such as Dupuytren's contracture, a hand deformity that makes it difficult or impossible to straighten one or more fingers.

SIGNS AND SYMPTOMS

Peyronie's sneaks up on men, starting as a hard lump (called a plaque) that forms under the skin in the shaft of the penis. Most of the time, the plaque is on top of the shaft.

The disease occurs in two phases. During the acute phase, the lump is painful and gets progressively bigger and harder. The plaque may cause the penis to shrink or to bend. The resulting change in the shape of the penis is typically noticeable only during erections, which can be very painful. In some cases, it becomes impossible to have an erection hard enough or straight enough for sexual intercourse. The acute phase typically lasts from as few as three months to as many as 18 months.

During the chronic phase, the plaque stops growing. Pain with an erection stops, but the deformity is permanent without treatment. Other symptoms are anxiety and depression, reported by more than 70% of affected men. Intercourse is still possible except when there's severe deformity. Ejaculation is not affected. But for many men who have erectile dysfunction (ED) with Peyronie's, it's the psychological trauma that causes ED, not the disease.

TREATMENTS TO AVOID

For years, men were told to use a topical cream that was rubbed into the area of the plaque and absorbed through the skin. Today, we know that topical treatments are not effective for Peyronie's.

Many oral treatments have been used that don't work or may be too hard to take. Vitamin E…a vitamin B antioxidant called Potaba…the cancer drug *tamoxifen* (Soltamox)…and the amino acid derivative supplement carnitine have been shown to be no better than a placebo. The drawbacks of these treatments are numerous. For example, Potaba requires 24 pills a day for three to six months. The gout medication *colchicine* (Colcrys) is sometimes helpful to reduce pain, but it has no impact on penile deformity and can cause severe upset stomach.

Injecting the penis with *interferon*, a protein used to treat hepatitis and some cancers, is an effective treatment that may slow the rate of plaque growth, but it makes men feel like they have a bad case of the flu.

Vacuum devices have also been tried, but there is no evidence that they help.

BEST TREATMENT OPTIONS

The best treatment for Peyronie's involves shared decision-making between doctor and patient. The goal is to find treatment with the least risk that will get a man's penis hard enough and straight enough for sex. It does not need to be perfect. Men who notice symptoms of Peyronie's, such as those described earlier, should be sure to discuss them with their doctor. *Effective treatment options include…*

•**Oral medication.** One oral drug that may help during the acute phase is *pentoxifylline* (Pentoxil), which is typically used to improve blood circulation. Studies show about a 40% chance of improvement after six months with low risk for side effects.

Other oral drugs to try during the acute phase include ED drugs, such as *sildenafil* (Viagra) or *vardenafil* (Levitra), and pain medicine, usually nonsteroidal anti-inflammatory drugs (NSAIDs), including *ibuprofen* (Motrin) or *naproxen* (Aleve). These drugs help control symptoms, such as ED and pain, that often occur during the acute phase.

•**Penile injection with *verapamil* (Verelan)**—a drug typically prescribed for high blood pressure or chest pain—has been used to treat Peyronie's for years. Studies show that it slows plaque progression during the acute phase. You need injections every two weeks for up to six months. Your doctor will numb your penis first with lidocaine. The treatment has only minor side effects, such as penile bruising and temporary nausea.

None of the treatments described above are approved to treat Peyronie's. They are used "off label," meaning that they are FDA-approved for other uses. Off-label treatments are sometimes covered by insurers. Check with your insurance provider.

Latest treatment options include…

•*Collagenase clostridium histolyticum* **(Xiaflex)** is the first drug to receive FDA approval for the treatment of Peyronie's disease. It improves the condition by breaking down connective tissue. Studies show, on average, a 34% improvement in penile curvature when eight injections are given over 32 weeks. There is some risk of bruising or swelling and, in rare cases, risk of rupturing one of the erection chambers of the penis, which could require urgent surgical repair. This treatment is approved only for chronic disease in men with at least a 30-degree curvature deformity.

•**RestoreX,** a new painless traction device, may also be worth a try. When men used the device 30 to 90 minutes a day for three months, 77% experienced about a 30% reduction in curvature and 94% achieved increased length of 1.6 cm, according to research published in *The Journal of Urology.*

WHEN SURGERY IS NEEDED

Many men get adequate relief from the treatments described above. If not, there are relatively safe and effective surgical options.

•**Plication surgery** involves simply straightening the penis by placing sutures or using other reconstructive techniques to shorten the side of the penis opposite the plaque. It is considered a "preferred and reliable technique," according to research published in *Translational Andrology and Urology.* The downside of penile plication is that it shortens the penis by 1 cm to 2 cm in most cases.

•**Grafting surgery** involves excising the penile plaque and inserting a graft into the penis to lengthen the affected side. While this sounds preferable to most men at first, grafting surgery involves risks for penile sensory loss and ED that can be very impairing. It is generally reserved for patients with excellent erectile function and moderate-to-severe penile deformities.

•**Penile implant** is appropriate for men who have both Peyronie's and severe ED. This procedure, which involves the placement of an inflatable penile prosthesis, is considered the gold standard for men with both conditions, notes a study in *Current Urology Reports.*

A TEAM EFFORT

Peyronie's disease can be a major quality-of-life issue, not only for men but also for their sexual partners. It helps to get your partner involved in treatment decisions and discuss other ways to maintain intimacy while treatment is under way.

Also: Don't ignore the psychological aspects. Working with a mental health counselor for psychological support or seeking couples therapy can be a key element of treatment.

Finding the right specialist is also important. Ideally, look for a urologist with subspecialty training in sexual health. Ask your doctor for a referral, or to find this type of specialist near you, consult the website of the Sexual Medicine Society of North America, SexHealthMatters. org, and click "resources."

Breast Cancer in Men Is Rising

Xiao-Ou Shu, MD, PhD, Ingram Professor of Cancer Research, Vanderbilt University Medical Center, Nashville, and leader of an analysis of data on 16,025 men diagnosed with breast cancer, published in JAMA Oncology.

Men with breast cancer have poorer outcomes than women with the disease. Breast cancer is rare in men but the incidence of the disease is rising. Procedures and drugs to treat it have almost all been tested only on women. Male breast cancer patients usually are older when diagnosed and more likely to have advanced disease. Therefore, at three and five years after diagnosis, they have lower survival rates than women after the same time periods. The Food and Drug Administration is asking drug companies to include men in future breast cancer studies.

Be Careful When Removing Nose Hairs

Nose hairs protect nostrils from harmful environmental particles. Getting rid of the hairs reduces immunity and makes you more subject to infections. Plucking nose hairs or anything else that removes the hair follicle (such as waxing) raises infection risk.

Safest: Invest in a good trimmer and keep nose hairs short and comfortable, but do not remove them entirely.

Roundup of experts on nose hairs, reported at Your-SkinOnline.com.

The Best PET Scan

Geo Espinosa, ND, LAc, a naturopathic doctor, licensed acupuncturist and certified functional medicine practitioner in private practice, and clinical assistant professor and holistic clinician in urology, New York University Langone Medical Center, New York City. He is recognized as an authority in holistic urology and men's health and is author of *Thrive, Don't Only Survive!* DrGeo.com

Prostate cancer recurs up to 40% of the time within 10 years after initial treatment. But until recently, there has not been a test that could detect a recurrence before the cancer is already at an advanced stage...and harder to treat.

Good news: A new kind of scan finds prostate cancer recurrence months or even years before other tests can.

Treatment lowers levels of *prostate specific antigen* (PSA)—a protein produced by prostate cells—to zero or nearly zero. Rising levels of PSA are the classic sign that prostate cancer has recurred. Doctors then order tests to see whether the recurrence is local (in the prostate) or has spread (metastasized).

Until now, tests available—such as a bone scan or *positron emission tomography* (PET) scan—have been able to detect recurrence only when the growing cancer has caused PSA levels to rise to at least 10 nanograms per milliliter (ng/mL) to 30 ng/mL or even higher. At that point, the cancer is much harder to treat and outcomes are poorer.

Now a new kind of PET scan can detect recurrence at much earlier stages than any other test currently available—with tremendous lifesaving potential. But first, some background on PET scans.

HOW A PET SCAN WORKS

All PET scans involve injection of a radioactive tracer, followed by a *computed tomography* (CT) scan of the patient's whole body. Depending on the type of PET, tracers include a radioactive drug that gravitates to damaged cells in bones...a sugar (*fluorodeoxyglucose/* FDG) that is absorbed by glucose molecules in cells...or a radioactive form of the vitamin-like nutrient choline, called Choline C 11, that is also absorbed by cells, similar to FDG.

The different tracers all work on the same principle—that cancer cells multiply more rapidly than normal cells and don't undergo normal cell death, so more of the tracer ends up in the cancer cells, which makes those cells "light up" on a scan. *However, there are also differences...*

•**A bone scan can detect cancer in bones when PSA is as low as 10 ng/mL** but is not able to detect cancer metastasis in other parts of the body.

•**An FDG PET can detect cancer recurrence in other parts of the body,** but only once the cancer has spread beyond the prostate...and cannot reliably differentiate between cancer and prostate gland enlargement.

•**Choline C 11 PET can detect cancer when PSA is as low as 2 ng/mL,** but the scan is not widely available. The radioactive choline has a very short shelf life...can be made only in specialized facilities...and must be administered within minutes of being produced.

A NEW AND BETTER PET

Recently, the FDA approved a new type of PET scan called Axumin. Axumin PET uses an amino acid antibody that binds to PSA proteins in blood. Prostate cancer cells "eat up" this amino acid more quickly than other tracers—cutting the time for the tracer to circulate through the patient's body—and the cancer cells that the tracer attaches to are at a very early stage. Axumin PET can detect prostate cancer when PSA produced by the cancer cells is as low as 1 ng/mL.

Studies show that Axumin PET scan is more successful at finding early recurrence than Choline C 11.

Plus: Axumin PET is covered by Medicare and is available at many US prostate cancer "centers of excellence" treatment centers, which are typically found at academic institutions. Search online for one near you and ask if it offers Axumin PET scan.

BOTTOM LINE

PSA should be undetectable after surgery or very low after radiation treatment. Men whose PSA starts to rise—especially rapidly—should consider asking their doctors about Axumin PET. It could be a lifesaver.

Low T Treatment Risk

Christel Renoux, MD, PhD, is assistant professor of neurology and neurosurgery at McGill University, Montreal, Canada, and coauthor of a study of 15,401 men age 45 and older, published in *The American Journal of Medicine.*

Testosterone replacement therapy (TRT) could put your cardiovascular health at risk. An almost five-year study of men with low testosterone levels found that TRT users had greater risk for stroke, transient ischemic attack and heart attack, especially during the first two years of use. TRT is increasingly being prescribed to aging men, but there's limited evidence about the long-term benefits. Proceed with caution.

Osteoporosis: What Men Need to Know

Robert R. Recker, MD, professor of medicine and director of the Osteoporosis Research Center at Creighton University School of Medicine in Omaha. His research has been widely published in leading medical journals, including *Journal of Bone and Mineral Research, Osteoporosis International* and *Bone.*

Osteoporosis wouldn't appear on most people's list of diseases that affect men. But it should. Men over age 50 are more likely to break a bone due to osteoporosis than they are to develop prostate cancer.

Other eye-opening facts: About two million American men already have this bone-weakening disease, and at least another 12 million have no idea that they are at increased risk for it.

All told, about one man in five will experience an osteoporosis-related fracture during his lifetime—and when this occurs, the consequences are even more dire than for a woman.

WHY MEN GET OVERLOOKED

There's a good reason why the osteoporosis spotlight focuses directly on women. Virtually all women experience plummeting levels of bone-protective estrogen during menopause, leading to a significant decrease in bone density. In men, bone loss usually happens later in life and more slowly. But throw a risk factor or two into the mix, and the odds for osteoporosis in men increase substantially. Unfortunately, few doctors test for it in men (let alone offer treatment). That can be a deadly mistake.

The real danger: In the first six months after a hip fracture, the mortality rate in men is approximately double that of similar-aged women, according to the International Osteoporosis Foundation. Even after suffering a hip fracture, men are far less likely than women to be tested or treated for osteoporosis.

SHOULD YOU GET TESTED?

Doctors routinely test women's bone mineral density (BMD) starting at about age 65—or even younger if they have risk factors—but the same testing is rarely ordered for men...even if they have glaring risk factors. The best way to stay ahead of osteoporosis is to get tested before you break a bone.

Factors that increase your risk...

•**Long-term steroid use.** When used for two or more months, corticosteroids (such as prednisone), commonly prescribed for chronic conditions like chronic obstructive pulmonary disease (COPD) and rheumatoid arthritis, are the number-one cause of non–age-related osteoporosis.

•**Regular use of bone-depleting medications.** Several prescription and over-the-counter (OTC) drugs deplete bone density, including proton pump inhibitors (PPIs) used for heartburn ...selective serotonin reuptake inhibitor (SSRI) antidepressants...aluminum-based antacids...blood thinners...and diuretics. Exactly when the risk for bone loss kicks in depends upon the drug being used. For PPIs, for example, research has shown that risk for fracture occurs after two years and continues to increase over four years.

•**Celiac disease.** This condition blocks the absorption of nutrients, including calcium, making it a common "silent" cause of osteoporosis—even in people who get plenty of calcium.

•**Low testosterone.** Testosterone levels decline when a man ages, and that can be accompanied by lower levels of *estradiol* (a form of the female hormone estrogen). Low levels of bioavailable estradiol can increase fracture risk in men. In some studies, low testosterone alone has been shown to increase the risk for osteoporosis and fracture in men.

•**High cholesterol.** A direct link between high cholesterol (above 200 mg/dL) and low BMD in men was identified in a study published in *Molecular Medicine Reports* in 2019. High cholesterol damages bone microstructure and accelerates bone turnover, so more old bone is resorbed than new bone is created.

•**Gastrointestinal disease.** People with conditions such as ulcerative colitis, Crohn's disease and inflammatory bowel disease (IBD) face a higher risk for osteoporosis and fractures, according to research published in *Advances in Clinical and Experimental Medicine*. These diseases reduce absorption of essential vitamins and minerals that are needed for healthy bones.

•**Vitamin D deficiency.** A low vitamin D level, which research has shown affects 85% of older adults, leads to lower BMD and higher fracture risk.

•**Family history.** A family history of fractures—even if a relative was never diagnosed with osteoporosis—increases your risk for low bone density.

In addition to these risk factors, if you've lost height (about two or more inches)…suffered a low-trauma fracture (such as a fall from standing height or less)…or experienced sudden, severe back pain, you may have osteoporosis and should get tested immediately (see below).

GET TESTED

Doctors rarely test men (especially those under age 70) for osteoporosis, even if they've already broken bones. If you have one or more of the risk factors listed earlier, talk to your doctor about ordering the following tests…*

*Check with your insurer to see if these tests will be covered.

•**Central DEXA (dual-energy X-ray absorptiometry)** is the primary tool for diagnosing osteoporosis by measuring BMD in the hip and spine. Your bone density will be reported as a T-score and classified as normal…low (for osteopenia, a precursor to osteoporosis)…or osteoporosis.

Normal: T-score of –1.0 or higher

Low (osteopenia): T-score between –1.0 and –2.5

Osteoporosis: T-score of –2.5 or lower

•**Vitamin D (serum 25-hydroxy-vitamin D) level is a key indicator of fracture risk.** Many professional groups consider a vitamin D level of at least 30 ng/mL to be adequate, but osteoporosis experts recommend aiming for at least 40 ng/mL.

Other blood tests to consider…

•**Complete blood count**

•**Sex hormones,** particularly free testosterone and free estradiol

•**Calcium and phosphorous levels**

•**Kidney, liver and thyroid functions** (related disorders can increase risk for osteoporosis in men)

BONE-STRENGTHENING STEPS

To prevent fractures, you must keep your bones healthy and strong. *What helps…*

•**Take calcium and vitamin D supplements.** It's always best to get vital nutrients from food. However, it's often difficult to get adequate levels.

Recommended supplement dosages: For calcium, 500 mg to 600 mg taken twice daily with food…and 1,000 international units (IU) up to 5,000 IU of vitamin D daily. (Consult your doctor for the dosage that's right for you.)

Good brands: Vitamin D supplements from Douglas Laboratories and calcium supplements from Citracal or Caltrate. To boost absorption, take calcium supplements with a meal.

•**Get plenty of weight-bearing exercise.** That doesn't mean you have to hit the gym and lift weights (though resistance exercise can be helpful). Many everyday activities fit the bill, such as walking, hiking and climbing stairs. If you've been diagnosed with low bone density, avoid high-impact exercises (such as running) and twisting motions (like swinging a golf club). Aim for 30 minutes of weight-bearing exercise most days of the week to help keep your bones strong.

• **Consider appropriate osteoporosis medication.** While many drugs have been approved to treat osteoporosis, only a few have been approved for use in men. These include *alendronate* (Fosamax), *risedronate* (Actonel) and *IV zoledronic acid* (Reclast). A man may need one of these drugs if he has osteoporosis...is over age 50 and suffers a fracture from a low-trauma injury...or if a screening DEXA of the spine or hip shows osteopenia and there is a family history of low-trauma fracture. Side effects of these drugs may include upset stomach and back pain.

Caffeine/Blood Clot Danger

Paul R. Nagelkirk, PhD, director, Integrative Exercise Physiology Laboratory, Ball State University, Muncie, Indiana.

When men drank a caffeinated drink before a high-intensity cycling workout, caffeine increased the coagulation factor in their blood, leaving them at higher risk for blood clots, which can lead to stroke, heart attack and pulmonary embolism.

Bottom line: Caffeine is safe for most people, but consuming it before exercise may be detrimental, especially for those with a family or personal history of heart disease.

Next Breakthrough in Male Infertility

Elizabeth Williams, PhD, senior lecturer at The University of Sheffield Medical School, UK, and coauthor of the study published in *European Journal of Nutrition*.

Recent study: 56 men with no known fertility issues took either a placebo or a supplement with 14 mg of the antioxidant lycopene for 12 weeks. Men who took the supplement had significant improvements in the proportion of fast-swimming and normal-looking sperm, both indicators of sperm quality and important factors in conception. Lycopene can be found naturally in tomatoes and other red fruits.

Paternal Postpartum Depression

Study by researchers at University of Cambridge, UK, published in *JAMA Psychiatry*.

Paternal postpartum depression is underdiagnosed and undertreated, although it may affect 25% to 50% of new fathers. Now a study from University of Cambridge in the UK finds that postpartum depression in fathers increases the risk for daughters to have depression at age 18. (The same effect was not seen for boys.) The reason for the association was not clear, although the researchers suspect several factors may be involved. Earlier research by the same team found that fathers' postpartum depression is linked to behavioral problems in both genders at ages three and a half and seven. These results emphasize the need to address depression in both parents after a child is born.

CHAPTER 15

Natural Healers

Help Your Body Fight COVID-19—Naturally

Strengthening the immune system is one of the best ways to stay healthy, particularly in this time of the new coronavirus.

To add natural measures to that fight, here is integrative medicine specialist Dr. Joseph Feuerstein's approach—he himself is a COVID-19 survivor.

Important: You don't want to take all of these supplements. These are just options—good to have since certain supplements have been in short supply. And any of these supplements can interact with medications you are taking for other conditions, so never start taking one without consulting your doctor.

PREVENTION

Taking vitamin C (one gram daily) and vitamin D (2,000 to 5,000 IU) is a good way to keep your body strong and reduce the risk of getting sick. In fact, an early study by British researchers suggests that people who are deficient in vitamin D are at increased risk for COVID-19.

Additionally, 30 milligrams (mg) of zinc daily may kill the virus and can help stave off infection.

Astragalus (250 mg twice per day), quercetin (500 mg twice per day), elderberry (250 mg twice per day) and zinc help prevent the virus from entering your cells by blocking the receptors where it tries to dig in.

WHEN YOU'RE SHOWING SYMPTOMS

If you have a sore throat, headache and other potential symptoms but do not have a high fever or severe breathing problems, hospitals are instructing people to convalesce at home with rest and hydration. If you feel like you need it,

Joseph Feuerstein, MD, assistant professor of clinical medicine at Columbia University in New York City and director of integrative medicine at Stamford Health in Stamford, Connecticut, where he has been working directly with COVID-19 patients. Dr. Feuerstein is certified in clinical hypnosis, clinical acupuncture and homeopathy. He is author of *Dr. Joe's Man Diet*. DrFeuerstein.com

Power Up Your Immune System with Ginseng

When nursing home residents took a 200-mg capsule of an American ginseng extract product called COLD-FX twice daily, their risk for the flu was 89% lower than a placebo group, according to research published in *Journal of the American Geriatrics Society*.

My advice: Talk to your doctor about trying American ginseng. Be sure it's American ginseng—not Asian, Siberian or other ginseng varieties. *Important:* American ginseng may interact with medication, including blood thinners, diabetes drugs and monoamine oxidase inhibitor (MAOI) antidepressants, so be sure to consult your doctor. -Joseph Feuerstein

you can take Tylenol for fever above 100.4°F or headache.

In addition, zinc or elderberry (taken in the same doses stated earlier) may be effective at killing the virus inside your body.

If the virus does succeed at replicating, your body's natural defenses create an inflammatory response in an effort to rid the virus. But too strong a response—the so-called cytokine storm—is potentially deadly, and so at this point you don't want to boost your immune system.

ONCE YOU ARE RECOVERING

When you are starting to feel a bit better every day—no more fever and less fatigue, malaise and muscle and joint pain—then anti-inflammatory supplements may help speed healing. These include curcumin (500 mg twice daily)… Boswellia (100 mg daily)…quercetin (500 mg twice daily and also found naturally in brightly colored produce such as apple peel, berries and broccoli)…EGCG (found in in green tea)…and garlic.

Studies on elderberry extract (250 mg twice per day) and influenza suggest that it also may be helpful by reducing inflammation in the lungs.

Recovery from COVID-19 is individualized and takes weeks for many people.

Note that most of this advice is based on preclinical studies on animals or studies on humans with other similar viruses. There are no broad-scale, peer-reviewed COVID-19 studies yet due to the newness of the virus.

Try Turkey Tail to Boost Your Immunity

Laurie Steelsmith, ND, LAc, licensed naturopathic physician and acupuncturist in private practice in Honolulu. She writes Bottom Line's "Natural Healing Secrets for Women" blog and is coauthor of three books—*Natural Choices for Women's Health, Great Sex, Naturally* and *Growing Younger Every Day*. DrSteelsmith.com

Technically called Coriolus Versicolor, turkey tail is a medicinal mushroom whose healing uses date back to the Ming Dynasty. Then, it was used to bolster energy and reduce phlegm—precisely what you need when the mercury drops and germs are in the air. Since gaining recognition in Western medicine in the 1960s, the mushroom has been noted for its ability to improve immunity and stave off infections. Turkey tail is available in supplement form. It can also be consumed, such as in tea—add turmeric and lemon for an extra dose of immune power.

Best Nondrug Ways to Fight Autoimmune Disease

Mark Hyman, MD, director of the Cleveland Clinic Center for Functional Medicine in Ohio. Dr. Hyman is also board president of clinical affairs of The Institute for Functional Medicine and founder and director of The UltraWellness Center, based in Lenox, Massachusetts. He is author of several books, including *Food: What the Heck Should I Eat?* DrHyman.com

Americans are facing an autoimmune epidemic. More than 24 million of us are currently affected by autoimmune disorders, which encompass 80-plus conditions including psoriasis, rheumatoid arthritis, lupus, inflammatory bowel disease and multiple sclerosis.

Conventional medicine attempts to tackle these tricky conditions with treatments such as powerful immune suppressant medications, steroids and over-the-counter anti-inflammatory drugs like aspirin or ibuprofen to reduce inflammation and alleviate symptoms such as joint pain, skin rashes, abdominal pain and tingling limbs. But these drugs can be hit or miss and lead to side effects as extreme as bone and muscle loss, diabetes, depression, liver problems and kidney failure. And they don't address the root cause of the problem.

A MUCH BETTER WAY

Thanks to groundbreaking research in the last decade, functional medicine—which aims to treat medical problems at the root cause—now provides an effective plan to prevent and reverse autoimmune diseases.

The various autoimmune diseases are really just one disorder with countless variations based on a patient's genetic weak link and a common denominator of systemic inflammation that prompts the body to attack its own tissues.

Aside from genetics, most autoimmune diseases stem from environmental or lifestyle triggers, which include hidden infections…allergies or sensitivities to foods…toxins such as chemicals or heavy metals…and physical or psychological stress.

On top of that, the body may be missing factors it needs to regulate itself, such as certain vitamins, hormones, rest and relaxation, and/or exercise. One autoimmune patient's root cause could be chronic stress and a vitamin deficiency while another's might be high mercury levels in the body.

Try these strategies to treat or ward off autoimmune diseases…

•**Make changes to your diet.** Unearthing possible food allergies or sensitivities that contribute to autoimmune problems starts with eliminating grains…legumes…dairy…eggs…nightshades such as tomatoes, potatoes, eggplant and peppers…alcohol and coffee…flour…and processed sugar for six weeks.

Food groups can be added back into your diet one by one while monitoring how your body responds. If you experience symptoms such as fatigue, joint pain, digestive upset, headaches and/or sinus congestion when adding a particular food back into your diet, that food is likely a problem for you and should be eliminated from your diet.

Note: While some lab tests are very helpful in detecting food allergies and sensitivities, the elimination method described here is best.

Beneficial foods for autoimmune disease: Whole and unprocessed foods including vegetables…small amounts of meat and other proteins…and healthy fats such as extra-virgin coconut, olive, avocado, macadamia, walnut and almond oils, organic coconut milk, avocados, fatty fish like sardines, wild salmon, mackerel and herring, nuts (except peanuts) and seeds, olives and grass-fed or clarified butter or ghee.

These foods are nutrient dense with high levels of anti-inflammatory phytonutrients and omega-3 fatty acids.

•**Add these supplements.** Vitamin D, fish oil, vitamin C and probiotics connect with immune receptors to calm the immune response naturally. Also, consider taking a turmeric or curcumin supplement, which research credits with powerful antioxidant and anti-inflammatory properties.

Note: Check with your doctor before taking any new supplement and for the dosage that is best for you.

•**Get more exercise.** Regular physical activity is a proven disease-fighter, largely because it's extremely effective at reducing systemic inflammation. For those with autoimmune diseases, the best types depend on your possible limitations. Cardiovascular exercise such as jogging, biking, hiking or interval training for 30 minutes, six times a week is ideal…but even taking a brisk, 30-minute walk several days a week can make a real difference.

•**Try a variety of relaxation techniques.** We know that stress creates inflammation…so cutting stress is key to fighting autoimmune disorders. Try meditation, massage or even journaling for 20 minutes a day. Yoga can be relaxing as well.

•**Improve sleep.** It's worth a reminder that good immune function and stress reduction are both linked to getting high-quality, deep sleep. To promote optimal sleep, go to bed and wake up at the same time each day, use your bed only for sleep or sex, forgo caffeine after the morning hours, avoid vigorous exercise after dinner, and stop cell-phone and computer use within a couple hours of turning in.

ADDITIONAL STRATEGIES

From my experience, astoundingly, about 80% of autoimmune disease cases will improve solely by making dietary changes. But if you're not feeling dramatically better within six weeks of making changes to your diet, get tested for other underlying causes of inflammation. *Simple blood tests or other tests can check for...*

•**Infections such as Lyme disease, bacteria, viruses and yeast**

•**Celiac disease**

•**Heavy metal toxicity such as mercury exposure from fish consumption**

Also helpful: Talk to your doctor about multiple systemic infectious disease syndrome (MSIDS). MSIDS is a persistent illness caused by Lyme disease and/or related tick-borne coinfections, parasitic or fungal infections, allergies, environmental toxicity and compromised immune function. Symptoms can include joint and muscle pain, dizziness and sleep problems.

To access the questionnaire, go to Lyme ActionNetwork.org and click on MSIDS. If your score is moderate to high, you will be advised to consult your doctor.

New—and Natural—Ways to Power Up Your Energy Levels

Jacob Teitelbaum, MD, a Kona, Hawaii–based board-certified internist and nationally known expert in chronic fatigue syndrome, fibromyalgia, sleep and pain. He is author of numerous books, including *From Fatigued to Fantastic.* Learn more at EnergyAnalysisProgram.com

---

Are you in an "energy crisis"—with a bad diet, poor sleep habits, too many commitments and too much stress causing you to feel exhausted and depleted? You don't have to live that way! Here are seven natural, easy-to-do energy hacks that can dramatically restore your vim and vigor...

HACK #1: **Check your magnesium— you're likely deficient.** Low magnesium is linked to low energy and even to chronic fatigue syndrome (CFS). Magnesium is essential to many body functions (especially muscle function), regulates heartbeat and helps convert food into energy. Since the mineral is not produced in our bodies, we need to get it from dietary sources. The typical heavily processed American diet does not provide the daily Recommended Dietary Allowance of magnesium—420 mg for men and 320 mg for women.

Power up: Cut back or eliminate processed food. Stick to fresh foods or foods with less than five ingredients on their labels. Good dietary sources of magnesium include leafy greens, seeds, nuts and whole grains. Also consider taking a 150-mg to 200-mg magnesium supplement daily.

Bonus: Taking the supplement at night can help improve sleep quality.

Note: Magnesium supplements are generally considered safe but can cause diarrhea in some people. If that happens, cut back the daily dose to 75 mg. Magnesium glycinate and magnesium aspartate are good forms to take. Check with your doctor before starting magnesium if you take medication or have a chronic medical condition.

HACK #2: **Get more D-ribose.** D-ribose, a type of sugar produced by the body, plays a key role in production of adenosine triphosphate (ATP), the primary molecule that provides energy to every cell in the body. Our bodies manufacture some D-ribose naturally, but you may need more.

Power up: D-ribose supplements are available in a powder that can be stirred into coffee, tea or a smoothie. Look online or in health-food stores for brands with "Bioenergy Ribose" on the label, such as Doctor's Best Pure D-Ribose Powder, NOW D-Ribose Powder or my own brand, SHINE Ribose. Bioenergy Ribose is formulated to be more bioavailable—other kinds may not offer the same results.

Typical dose: 5 g every morning.

Note: D-ribose can lower blood sugar, which may affect dosing of diabetes drugs.

HACK #3: Cut out or minimize toxic relationships. Being around people we enjoy or engaging in activities that bring us pleasure gives us energy. Doing things we loathe, or being with angry, abusive, manipulative or pessimistic people, depletes our energy levels.

Power up: Keep healthy boundaries. If spending time with a particular friend, colleague or family member drains you, find ways to limit or cut out interactions with that person. Of course, it may be easier to cut off a strained friendship than a relative. Simply learn to say "no" to interactions that feel bad. This can often be done without disconnecting from the person.

Simple trick: For difficult people whom you would like to (or need to) keep around, focus only on aspects of them that make you feel good and ignore the rest. After about eight weeks, it's very likely that only those aspects will show up in your relationship—or the person will no longer be part of your life.

HACK #4: Hydrate with cold water. According to the Natural Hydration Council in the UK, symptoms such as fatigue and lack of energy account for one in five doctor visits…and for one out of 10 of such patients, dehydration is the primary culprit. Afternoon energy slumps are especially common—partly because we get busy and forget to drink…or a heavy lunch can put our parasympathetic nervous system into "rest and digest mode."

Power up: When you feel your energy dipping, drink 12 ounces of cold water. Or splash cold water on your face. The cold temperature stimulates adrenaline receptors in your skin, which signals your heart to pump harder and drives an energizing blood flow to your brain… while the water hydrates you.

HACK #5: Check your medications. Statins, such as *atorvastatin* (Lipitor), *rosuvastatin* (Crestor) and *simvastatin* (Zocor), lower cholesterol…but also lower levels of coenzyme Q10 (CoQ10), a vitamin-like substance that helps maintain energy levels. Proton pump inhibitors (PPIs) for heartburn, gastroesophageal reflux disease and ulcers, such as *omeprazole* (Prilosec) and *esomeprazole* (Nexium), cut stomach acid production. But long-term use impairs absorption of key energy-producing nutrients, including magnesium, vitamin B-12 and iron.

Power up: If you need a statin, ask your doctor about taking a CoQ10 supplement as well. A typical dose is 200 mg per day taken with a meal that contains fat to boost absorption. If you take a PPI, ask your doctor if you can switch to an H2-blocker, such as *ranitidine* (Zantac) or *cimetidine* (Tagamet). Research shows that they are far safer. These drugs reduce stomach acid but don't block it as completely as PPIs do, so nutrient deficiencies are less likely to occur.

HACK #6: Caffeinate…strategically. Caffeine is considered to be an adenosine blocker. (Adenosine triggers sleep and is not the same as energy-producing ATP.) Caffeine attaches to the same receptors in the brain that adenosine attaches to and prevents the drowsiness that occurs as adenosine levels rise during the day. But coffee also can cause a jittery, wired feeling and stomach upset.

Power up: Green tea is gentler than coffee, with about 25 mg of caffeine per cup versus 100 mg to 200 mg for coffee—enough to still kick your energy up a notch. According to a review of nearly 50 studies, just 40 mg of caffeine is enough to provide stimulating effects. Green tea is also rich in theanine, an amino acid that promotes calm alertness and improves deep sleep.

HACK #7: Wind down wisely. You've probably heard a lot of sleep-hygiene advice, such as powering down electronics an hour or two before bed and sleeping in a cool room. *Also try…*

Power up #1: Soak in a warm bath with two cups of Epsom salts added an hour before bedtime. The magnesium from the Epsom salts soothes tired muscles and eases stress, promoting a good night's sleep.

Note: Soaking in a warm bath can lower blood pressure and might make you feel light-headed. Be careful getting out of the bath, especially if you already have low blood pressure.

Power up #2: Eat a small protein-rich snack, such as a hard-boiled egg or a few tablespoons of cottage cheese, before bedtime to prevent blood sugar drops that often wake people up in the middle of the night.

Homemade Sore Throat Remedies

Carrie Runde, ND, naturopathic physician, Charm City Natural Health, Baltimore. She is an active member of the American Association of Naturopathic Physicians, where she served on the organization's board of directors for five years. CharmCityNaturalHealth.com

Your throat is so sore that it's agony just to swallow…yet you can't bear the thought of trekking to the drugstore for medicine to ease the pain…

Good news: There's no need to leave the comfort of home—just head for your kitchen. Chances are that your pantry or fridge contains what you need to soothe your poor sore throat…safely, naturally, effectively and economically.

Here is what Carrie Runde, ND, a naturopathic physician in Baltimore, often recommends for her own patients with sore throats…

FOUR FIXES FOR THROAT PAIN

You can use any or all of the following remedies (depending on the supplies you have at hand) in any order you like and as often as you like…

•**Licorice root tea.** Licorice root reduces inflammation, which gives some immediate relief from a sore throat. Consuming the herb in tea form also helps keep you hydrated and temporarily speeds up the movement of mucus, alleviating the nasal congestion that forces you to mouth-breathe and makes your throat dry and scratchy. In addition, licorice root stimulates the immune system and has antiviral properties that help your body combat the cold, flu or other ailment that's causing your throat pain.

Though licorice root is available in various forms, the easiest thing to do is to keep licorice root tea bags on hand (find them in health-food stores and many grocery stores). Steep the tea bag in eight ounces of very hot water for five to seven minutes, keeping it covered to preserve the active constituents that vaporize. Then sip.

Caution: Do not use licorice root if you have high blood pressure.

•**Carrot poultice.** You'll need one or two large carrots or the equivalent in smaller carrots…a dry cotton handkerchief, cheesecloth or similarly sized thin cloth…plastic wrap…and a scarf. (It's best to wear an old shirt in case it gets stained orange.) Finely grate the carrot using a food processor or hand grater. Place the grated carrot in the center of the handkerchief, then fold the sides of the cloth up and over to create a packet (like a Hot Pocket) about two to three inches wide and five to six inches long. Lie down and position the packet horizontally against the front of your neck so that the single thickness of cloth is against your skin. Secure the poultice in place by wrapping (not tying) a layer of plastic wrap around your neck—loosely enough that you're comfortable but snugly enough that the poultice doesn't fall off. Then wrap the scarf around your neck and leave everything in place for 20 to 40 minutes.

What does it do? When you're sick, white blood cells collect viruses and bacteria, then travel to your lymph glands to be filtered out. Carrots have a "cleaning" action on lymph glands. The carrot poultice increases circulation of blood and lymph fluid to the throat, bringing more healing oxygen, nutrients and white blood cells to the area and helping to clear away toxins.

•**Washcloth hydrotherapy.** All you need for this remedy is a washcloth and the kitchen sink. Wet the washcloth with cold tap water, and wring it out so it's not dripping. Place the wet cloth over your throat and rest, sitting or lying down, for 30 minutes. Initially this remedy helps ease the pain by cooling the entire area… then, as your body heat warms the cloth, there's an increase of healing circulation to the throat.

•**"Bone broth" chicken soup.** There are lots of reasons why this is a time-honored remedy. Chicken soup acts as an anti-inflammatory, inhibiting immune system cells that participate in the body's inflammatory response. It also alleviates nasal congestion and throat dryness. In addition, the zinc in the chicken improves your absorption of the nutrients in the soup's vegetables and gives your immune system a boost.

The most effective chicken soup has a "bone broth" base made with chicken bones, vinegar and vegetables such as carrots and celery—all simmered for six or more hours so that the nutrients in the bones and vegetables infuse the broth. (Chicken soup that you buy in a supermarket probably isn't as beneficial, because valuable compounds in the chicken bones may not make their way into store-bought broths and bouillon cubes.)

Best: Make a big batch of homemade chicken soup, and keep it in your freezer so you'll have it on hand when you need it. If your throat is too sore to handle soup with chunks of chicken and vegetables, you can sip on the broth and still get the healing benefits.

When professional medical help is warranted: Alert your doctor immediately if throat pain is severe or is accompanied by a fever of higher than 101°F, headache, stomachache, rash, joint pain and/or trouble swallowing or speaking—you may have an infection or some other condition that requires more treatment. Otherwise, contact your physician if a sore throat lasts for more than three days and is getting worse rather than better.

Reflexology for Better Health: Relieve Allergies, Gut Woes and More

Deborah Flanagan, clinical reflexologist and founder of Center for True Health in New York City. CenterTrue Health.com

Did you know that the answer to your sinus congestion problem might be found in your fingers? Or the cure for constipation found in your feet? Reflexology is based on the concept that our hands and feet contain nerve endings that form a map of the entire body. You can learn to do this safe therapy at home for relief from common health concerns such as back pain, allergy symptoms and even insomnia.

How it works: When you apply pressure to key points on your hands and feet, you activate nerve endings and help your nervous and circulatory systems get your body into better balance. Our nerve endings are connected to spinal nerves as well as to corresponding organs. Each can be reached by a point on the feet or hands. (For instance, the side of your thumb matches up with your spine.)

Reflexology has solid scientific research behind it. Back in 1993, the first US reflexology study published in a peer-reviewed medical journal, *Obstetrics & Gynecology*, studied the effects of reflexology on premenstrual syndrome (PMS). The study showed a 46% reduction in premenstrual symptoms.

More recently, the National Center for Complementary and Integrative Health awarded a second round of funding to Michigan State University researchers to continue studying the impact of reflexology on women undergoing chemotherapy for advanced breast cancer. So far, patients have shown improvement in shortness of breath, as well as in 10 areas of physical activity. Meanwhile, preliminary research out of The Ohio State University's Comprehensive Cancer Center is looking at the effect of reflexology and aromatherapy in women undergoing breast cancer radiation treatment—it suggests that the combo reduces pain by 60% and anxiety by 20%.

As a clinical reflexologist trained in this noninvasive, holistic therapy, I see the benefits in my clients every day. While reflexology generally is very safe, there are a few caveats. If you have unchecked diabetes, a blood clot or foot injuries or sores, you should check with your doctor first. And of course, remember that reflexology is a complementary therapy, not a substitute for medical care.

These are some of my favorite techniques that you can do at home for common health complaints. Relax, take off your socks and get hands-on for better health.

FIX GUT WOES

This move regulates and supports your GI system to help with constipation, gas and indigestion.

Equipment: Golf ball (or other similarly sized hard ball).

How to do it: Interlock your fingers.

1. Roll the ball around the lower area of your palms, or heels, of your hands. This corresponds to the digestive reflexes for the small and large intestines.

2. Continue rolling the ball for one minute.

Credit:Gettyimages/ sam74100

Rx: Do this once or twice a week for two weeks. Then, as needed.

ROLL AWAY A BLOATED BELLY

Rolling the soles of your feet is great for gastric distress and relieving bloating in particular. This is one of my personal favorite self-help techniques.

Equipment: Wooden foot roller.

How to do it: Roll underneath your arches on the soles of your feet with a wooden foot roller.

Rx: Do this after a big meal when you're feeling puffy. Do this for one to two minutes on each foot.

BEAT INSOMNIA

This technique is great if you're having trouble sleeping. You press a point on your thumb that is the reflex for the pituitary gland. The pituitary gland oversees the entire endocrine system (especially the adrenals, which are involved with cortisol levels and stress), so this is a really important point to help the body balance itself.

Equipment: None.

How to do it…

1. Find the middle of the whorl of your thumbprint. This is the reflex for the pituitary gland.

Credit:Gettyimages/alvarez

2. Using the side of one thumb, press that thumb's nail firmly into the center of the whorl of the other thumbprint and hold for 45 seconds. How do you know if you found the right spot?

Here are some clues: It might feel like a little metal ball under the skin. Or it might feel like you stuck a needle in your thumb. This area might feel more sensitive if you've had trouble sleeping lately.

3. Repeat with the other thumb.

Rx: Press this spot on both thumbs two to three times a day to sleep more soundly on a regular basis. And next time you wake up in the middle of the night, you'll know what to do.

RELIEVE ALLERGY AND SINUS CONGESTION

The fingers contain the reflexes for the head and sinuses. This move alleviates any kind of congestion—and the best part is that it often works right away.

Equipment: Just your hands!

How to do it…

1. Turn your hand palm-up. Press and rub from the base of each finger to the tip.

2. Switch hands, and repeat until you've done all 10 fingers.

Rx: Do this on each finger on both hands a few times, and repeat three or four times a day or as needed.

BANISH BACK PAIN

When you frequently have a sore back, it's hard to find DIY solutions that help ease the pain, so this move is a great one to know. Since this reflex area covers your whole spine, this trick helps alleviate upper- and lower-back pain.

Equipment: None.

How to do it…

1. The outside of the thumb down to the wrist contains the spine reflex. Starting with the left hand, press there with the

Credit: iStock.com/GCapture

right thumb, inching along from the top of the thumb down to the wrist.

2. Repeat on the right hand using the left thumb to press. Anywhere tender? That's normal if you're experiencing back pain. Spend more time on tender areas, but don't apply a lot of pressure if it hurts. "No pain no gain" doesn't apply with reflexology!

Rx: Do this on both hands, go down this area three or four times, and repeat three or four times a day.

TREAT PMS OR MENOPAUSE COMPLAINTS

This move, the Wrist Twist, helps women with symptoms such as cramping from PMS and hot flashes during perimenopause and menopause. The reflexes for the ovaries and uterus are on the sides of the wrist. Just don't expect instant relief—addressing hormonal imbalances and reproductive issues takes time, usually three months of weekly sessions. I also use the Wrist Twist on men who have issues with their testes or prostate.

Equipment: None.

How to do it…

1. Using your right thumb and forefinger, create a loose bracelet around your left wrist. Rotate your left wrist and forearm.

2. Do the same on the right wrist.

Rx: Rotate each wrist 20 times or so, two or three times a day.

For Better Health, Balance Your Hormones With Food

Neal D. Barnard, MD, FACC, adjunct associate professor of medicine at George Washington University School of Medicine, president of Physicians Committee for Responsible Medicine and founder of Barnard Medical Center, all in Washington, DC. Dr. Barnard's scientific research has been widely published in *JAMA, The Lancet* and other leading professional journals. He is also author of 20 books, including, most recently, *Your Body in Balance: The New Science of Food, Hormones and Health.* PCRM.org

Most people equate hormonal imbalances with hot flashes and mood swings in menopausal women. But scratch the surface, and you'll see that out-of-whack hormones also can set the stage for a wide range of conditions, including cancer, diabetes and depression.

Prevent GERD

To reduce your risk for heartburn, you may want to drink less during meals. Water—or any other liquids—can dilute the stomach acid and enzymes that are needed to aid food digestion.

Andrew Rubman, ND, founder and medical director, Southbury Clinic for Traditional Medicines, Southbury, Connecticut. SouthburyClinic.com

Now: A growing body of evidence shows that potentially dangerous hormonal imbalances respond quickly to changes in diet.

WHY HORMONES MATTER

Most people don't realize the crucial role that hormones play in overall health. You can think of it this way—it's your hormones that provide the "operating instructions" for every organ in your body to work effectively.

Secreted by one of many endocrine glands—from the pineal gland within the brain, to the testicles and ovaries of the reproductive system—hormones speed and slow your metabolism…determine how you store and burn fat…control reproduction and sexuality…affect your moods…and more.

Research shows that compounds in certain foods are the single biggest factor in balancing hormones to create clear instructions within the body.

HORMONE-BALANCING FOODS

The hormone-balancing diet I recommend is plant based, consisting of four primary food groups—vegetables, fruits, whole grains and legumes (beans, lentils, peas). As both research and clinical experience show, this vegan diet works in many ways to balance hormones.

While you might imagine that a vegan diet is challenging to follow, it turns out to be surprisingly easy. It is simple to have bean chili instead of meat chili or to enjoy a tasty tomato-based sauce on your pasta instead of a meat or cream sauce. For complete nutrition, get vegetables, fruits, whole grains and legumes…and add a B-12 supplement (at least 2.4 mcg daily).

Here's how to select the foods you need to help prevent, control and even reverse these hormone-related conditions...

BREAST CANCER

Breast cancer is a serious condition. A combination of treatments is often necessary, so you should see your doctor and follow his/her guidance. Even so, hormone-balancing foods can play a vital role.

Excess estrogen is a common driver of breast cancer. For example, women with higher levels of the estrogen estradiol in the bloodstream have twice the cancer risk as women with lower levels.

In breast cells, estrogen can damage DNA—turning a healthy cell into a cancer cell. Once a cancer cell arises, high levels of estrogen can stimulate it to multiply. *To balance estrogen...*

•**Cut the fat.** There is evidence to suggest that any type of fatty food increases estrogen. And fat cells themselves are hormone factories, producing even more estrogen. Avoid animal fats, as well as coconut and palm oils, which are also high in saturated fat. Skip margarine and butter, too. Go easy on vegetable oils, including olive oil.

Instead, use non-oil cooking methods, such as steaming, boiling, baking or sautéing in vegetable broth. For an alternative to oily salad dressings, try lemon juice, flavorful vinegars or nonfat dressings. Fruits, veggies, legumes and whole grains are naturally very low in fat. For packaged foods, check the label and favor those with 3 g of fat or less per serving.

•**Eliminate dairy.** Research on dairy's link to breast cancer has been mixed. However, recent evidence has increasingly found that it plays an important role in how women do after a breast cancer diagnosis. For example, women previously diagnosed with breast cancer who consumed one or more daily servings of high-fat dairy products had a 49% higher risk of dying of their cancer compared with breast cancer patients who ate fewer servings of full-fat dairy or low-fat dairy, according to a study published in *Journal of the National Cancer Institute*. If you really love milk or yogurt, choose nondairy varieties, such as almond milk or soy yogurt.

•**Boost fiber.** Fiber helps protect against breast cancer. Women with breast cancer who ate at least five servings a day of fiber-rich fruits and vegetables (and were also physically active) cut their risk of dying from the disease by 50%, according to a study published in *Journal of Clinical Oncology*. Aim for 40 g of fiber a day—daily servings of beans, vegetables, fruits and grains will get you there.

•**Add soy.** Soybeans contain isoflavones that reduce the risk of developing breast cancer and, for women who have breast cancer already, improve cancer survival. In numerous studies, women in Asian countries who consume the most soy (about two servings a day) have about a 30% lower risk of developing breast cancer than those who consume less soy. Good choices include tofu, miso soup and soy milk.

DIABETES

Blood sugar (glucose) is transported into your cells by insulin, a hormone made in the pancreas. If you have type 2 diabetes, your insulin isn't working right—a problem called insulin resistance. From a dietary perspective, the culprit is fat—beef fat, chicken fat, fryer grease, you name it.

Here's why: Dietary fat turns into microscopic fat particles that block insulin action in muscle and liver cells, interfering with its ability to work. *To balance insulin...*

•**Skip animal products such as meat, fish, poultry, eggs and dairy products.** Limit vegetable oils, too.

•**Avoid plant-based foods that are high in fat.** It turns out that any type of fat can interfere with insulin action—even "good" fats. This includes nuts, peanut butter, seeds and avocados.

•**Eat more raw foods, such as fresh fruits and salads.** They promote weight loss—and fat loss. Certain vegetables—such as broccoli and kale—are hard to digest raw. But others, such as carrots and salad greens, are easier.

•**Don't exclude healthy carbohydrate-rich foods, such as sweet potatoes, beans and fruit.** Remember, the cause of insulin resistance is fat buildup—carbohydrates from whole plant foods are not a problem. In my

Fast and Tasty Recipes for a Hormone-Balancing Diet

A plant-based diet focusing on vegetables, fruits, whole grains and legumes can significantly improve the body's hormonal balance, according to an increasing body of scientific evidence.

For a sampling of delicious, easy-to-prepare recipes that incorporate these foods, try the following for…

BREAKFAST

Green Smoothie Muffins

2 cups flour
½ cup brown or raw sugar
1 teaspoon baking soda
½ teaspoon ground cinnamon (optional)
Zest of 1 lemon
1½ cups (8 ounces) pineapple chunks (fresh or frozen)
2 cups fresh spinach
1-2 very ripe bananas
1 Tablespoon vanilla extract
¼ cup plain soy or almond milk

Preheat oven to 375°F and line a muffin pan with paper liners or silicone cups, or use a non-stick pan.

In a large bowl, whisk together flour, sugar, baking soda, cinnamon and lemon zest. Set aside. In a blender, combine pineapple, spinach, bananas, vanilla and milk. Blend until creamy. Pour wet mixture into dry ingredients and stir until just combined. If the batter is dry, add 2-4 tablespoons milk. Spoon batter evenly into muffin cups.

Bake 20-25 minutes or until an inserted toothpick comes out clean. Let cool completely before serving.

Makes 12 muffins.

Per muffin: 124 calories…3 g protein…27 g carbohydrates…10 g sugar…0.5 g total fat…2% calories from fat…1 g fiber…113 mg sodium.

SANDWICH OR WRAP

BBQ Bean Tortas

8 (6-inch) corn tortillas or 4 hamburger buns
1 (15-ounce) can low-sodium black beans, drained and rinsed
½ cup barbecue sauce
½ cup chopped pineapple
1 cup fresh salsa (or diced tomato)
Guacamole (optional)

If using tortillas, preheat oven to 375°F. Bake corn tortillas for 5-10 minutes or until crisp. If using hamburger buns, toast in oven.

Warm beans with barbecue sauce. Spoon onto tortillas or buns and top with pineapple, salsa and guacamole, if desired.

Makes 4 servings.

Per serving: 293 calories…9 g protein…61 g carbohydrate…18 g sugar…2 g total fat…6% calories from fat…11 g fiber…579 mg sodium.

MAIN DISH

Butternut Pasta

3-4 cups diced butternut squash (about 1 medium squash)
1 cup sliced mushrooms
1½ cups uncooked pasta
4 chopped dry-pack sun-dried tomatoes
1 cup canned low-sodium chickpeas (or navy beans), drained and rinsed
2 cups fresh arugula (or spinach)
¼ cup fat-free balsamic vinaigrette
Vegan parmesan (optional)

Preheat oven to 375°F and line a baking sheet with parchment paper. Place squash cubes in a single layer in the pan. Roast for 20-30 minutes or until fork tender and browning at the edges, turning halfway. Add mushrooms to the pan halfway through roasting the squash.

Cook pasta as directed on package, adding sun-dried tomatoes and chickpeas (or navy beans) to the water with the pasta. Drain and transfer to a bowl. Immediately add roasted squash and mushrooms and toss. Serve over (or mix in) arugula (or spinach) and drizzle with balsamic vinaigrette. Sprinkle with vegan parmesan, if desired.

Makes 2 servings.

Per serving: 642 calories…25 g protein…126 g carbohydrate…13 g sugar…6 g total fat…7% calories from fat…17 g fiber…351 mg sodium.

Excerpted from the book *Your Body in Balance: The New Science of Food, Hormones, and Health* by Neal D. Barnard, MD, FACC, with Menus and Recipes by Lindsay S. Nixon. Copyright © 2020 by Neal D. Barnard, MD. Recipe text copyright © 2020 by Lindsay S. Nixon. Reprinted with permission of Grand Central Publishing. All rights reserved.

approach to balancing hormones in diabetes, there are no limits on healthful carbohydrates, but I recommend avoiding high glycemic-index foods that cause blood sugar to spike.

Examples: Instead of wheat bread, opt for rye and pumpernickel, which have less effect on blood sugar. Instead of cold cereals, choose old-fashioned oatmeal.

PROSTATE CANCER

Being overweight and consuming certain foods have both been linked to prostate cancer. A hormone-taming, plant-based diet can help. *To balance hormones that affect the prostate…*

•**Go dairy-free.** A large body of evidence links dairy products to prostate cancer. Look for dairy and cheese substitutes.

Examples: Use nutritional yeast in salads, casseroles and pizza instead of cheese. Wherever you use milk, try soy, almond, rice or oat milk instead.

•**Eat more tomatoes.** They're rich in prostate-protecting lycopene. Research published in *Journal of the National Cancer Institute* shows that men who have 10 or more servings of tomato products each week have 35% less risk of developing prostate cancer, compared with men who have tomatoes less often. Even ketchup and pizza sauce were protective. In fact, cooking helps release lycopene from the tomatoes, making it easier to absorb.

•**Get more soy.** As in breast cancer, soybeans have protective hormonal effects, balancing estrogen and testosterone. Research published in *Nutrients* shows that men who consume the most soy have 29% less risk of developing prostate cancer, compared with their soy-avoiding counterparts.

DEPRESSION AND NOREPINEPHRINE

The scientific link between hormones and depression is intriguing, but not definitive. However, research shows that the hormones that control blood pressure—such as norepinephrine (noradrenaline, from the adrenal gland)—also control your emotional state. And low levels of norepinephrine can cause depression. *To balance norepinephrine…*

•**Eat more vegetables.** A study in *Public Health Nutrition* found that people who eat the most vegetables are 62% less likely to develop depression than people who eat the least.

•**Get more soy.** Consuming two to four soy servings per day may have a significant anti-depressant effect, according to research published in *Menopause*. This perhaps explains the low prevalence of depression among Japanese people on traditional soy-rich diets. Have two servings per day. A serving would be a cup of soy milk or two to three-and-a-half ounces of tofu.

Digestive Supplements— Here Are the Ones That Really Work…

Tamara Duker Freuman, RD, CDN, an expert in digestive health in private practice and a clinical preceptor for the Dietetic Internship Program at Teachers College, Columbia University, both in New York City. She is author of *The Bloated Belly Whisperer: See Results Within a Week and Tame Digestive Distress Once & for All.* TheBloated BellyWhisperer.com

Supermarkets, pharmacies, health-food stores and the Internet offer a confusing array of digestive-support products that promise relief from bloating, gas, abdominal discomfort…and more.

The fact is, many of these don't work as claimed—and might contribute to other health problems. In spite of rave reviews, scientific evidence does not back the claims of many digestive supplements. Dietary supplements do not need Food and Drug Administration (FDA) approval that they are safe, nor do supplement makers need to test their products to prove marketing claims.

To help ensure that you get the digestive support you need, here's a quick primer on products that really can help…

•**Magnesium—for constipation.** This essential mineral plays a critical role in maintaining nerve and muscle function…regulating blood pressure and blood sugar levels…and may help prevent migraines and stroke. Doses of 350 mg or more stimulate bowel movements by drawing water into the gastrointestinal tract.

Use any form of magnesium (citrate, sulfate, oxide, hydroxide). Typically, 400 mg taken at night with a full glass of water (with or without food) produces an easy, cramp-free bowel movement the next morning. If it doesn't, increase the dose by 200 mg/night up to 1,000 mg. If 1,000 mg isn't helpful, talk to your doctor about other options.

Good product to try: Phillips' Milk of Magnesia (500 mg magnesium per liquid or caplet dose).

•**Lactose-digesting enzyme (lactase)—for lactose intolerance.** Digestion of the milk sugar lactose requires lactase, an enzyme that is deficient in about 65% of adults worldwide. Lactase supplements allow people who are deficient in lactase to still enjoy dairy foods.

Key: Consume enough lactase with the first bite of dairy-containing food to handle the full amount of lactose in the dairy meal/snack. Lactase products on the market typically recommend 9,000 acid lactase units (ALU) per dose, which should be sufficient for most dairy-containing meals.

Good product to try: One that does not contain the gas-producing sugar alcohols sorbitol or mannitol, such as Puritan's Pride–brand lactase.

•**Alpha-galactosidase—for gas, bloating and abdominal discomfort from eating certain foods.** In order to digest the highly fermentable fibers in certain healthy foods, including legumes (chickpeas, beans), cabbage, broccoli and brussels sprouts, you need to have enough of the enzyme *alpha-galactosidase*. If these foods cause you excess gas, bloating and abdominal distress, you may be able to comfortably eat them if you also consume alpha-galactosidase, the active ingredient in Bean-zyme and Beano.

Note: This enzyme may reduce the effectiveness of the diabetes medication *acarbose* (Precose).

Research finding: In a small study from University of Pavia in Italy, participants who consumed alpha-galactosidase while eating a meal that contained about two cups of beans produced significantly less gas afterward, compared with those who received a placebo with their beans.

A serving size of Beano (two capsules) or Bean-zyme (one capsule) contains 300 alpha-galactosidase units (GalU). Participants in the study who got the most intestinal relief consumed 1,200 GalU—but they also ate a lot more beans than you're likely to eat in one meal. How much to take varies by individual. Try 300 GalU with your first bite of a problem food. I often recommend two Bean-zyme pills per half cup of beans, adjusting as needed.

Note: Look for alpha-galactosidase supplements that do not contain sugar alcohols, such as mannitol (or other ingredients that end in ol). As noted earlier, these can cause gas.

10 Natural Ways to Take Care of Your Eyes

Marc Grossman, OD, LAc, doctor of optometry and licensed acupuncturist in New Paltz and Somers, New York. He is coauthor of *Natural Eye Care: Your Guide to Healthy Vision.* A holistic eye doctor, his multidisciplinary approach uses nutrition, lifestyle changes and Traditional Chinese Medicine to tackle eye problems. NaturalEyeCare.com

You think you take good care of your eyes. You wear sunglasses outdoors and get regular eye exams. But did you know that exercise, stress and even mindfulness practices can impact eye health? Holistic optometrist Dr. Marc Grossman suggests 10 natural ways to show your eyes some love—and see your way to healthy vision for years to come.

•**Pay attention to your posture.** The eyes are extensions of the brain and part of our central nervous system. Signals and messages are sent from the eyes to the visual cortex in the brain, which processes and sends the information down the spinal cord to the rest of the body. Poor posture can disrupt these connections and lead to blurred vision, and conversely, visual strain can result in poor posture. To avoid this, when sitting, keep your chest up, shoulders back and weight over your seat so that both eyes are at task level and an equal distance from what is being seen. Always sit upright while reading or watching television instead of lying on your back, side or stomach.

•**Seek out sunlight.** Walking is one of the best things we can do for exercise, and depending where you walk, it has another benefit—natural sunlight. The eyes are light-sensing organs. It's important to get enough sunlight so that your eyes operate optimally. In fact, a recent study published in *JAMA Ophthalmology* found that increased exposure to sunlight reduces your risk for myopia (nearsightedness). Aim for at least 20 minutes of natural sunlight a day—just be sure to wear sunglasses that provide 100% UV protection and filter out both UVA and UVB rays.

•**Go Mediterranean.** The health-promoting effects of the Mediterranean diet—which emphasizes eating mostly vegetables, fruits, legumes, whole grains, nuts and seeds…and limiting animal products and sweets—are well-known. Yet few people realize that adhering to this eating plan also can greatly reduce their risk for age-related macular degeneration (AMD), the leading cause of irreversible vision loss and blindness after age 50. Most recently, a large-scale European study published in *Ophthalmology* investigated the connection between genes and lifestyle on the development of AMD and found that those who ate a primarily Mediterranean diet were 41% less likely to develop AMD than those who did not. Interestingly, it wasn't any of the specific components that lowered AMD risk. Rather, it was the overall pattern of consistently consuming a nutrient-rich diet that mattered.

•**Cut back on sugar.** Sugar is lurking in so much of what we consume—from beverages to processed foods to desserts—and it's not just bad for your teeth and your weight. Higher sugar intake also is associated with an increased risk of developing—as well as worsening—most eye conditions, such as cataracts, glaucoma and AMD. In the case of cataracts, high blood sugar levels limit the ability of the eye to keep the lens clear. High blood sugar also can cause the blood vessels in the eye to narrow, creating a buildup of fluid that can lead to glaucoma. And people with type 2 diabetes are at risk for a condition known as diabetic retinopathy. Their blood sugar levels have to be carefully regulated with the right amount of insulin or the blood vessels in the eye can leak, which may cause spots in their vision that can lead to severe impairment or blindness.

•**Get moving.** Aerobic exercise not only benefits your heart, it also has been linked to improved retinal health and prevention of eye disease. Exercise raises oxygen levels in the cells and increases lymph and blood circulation. This increased circulation is a prerequisite for good vision. In addition, research published in *The Journal of Neuroscience* has found that moderate aerobic exercise may be able to delay the progression of AMD by preserving the structure and function of the nerve cells in the retina. Get 20 minutes of aerobic exercise daily by walking, swimming or doing any other activity that you enjoy.

•**Don't forget about vision fitness.** Simple eye exercises will ease discomfort and support healthy vision. *Try figure eights to increase the flexibility of your eye muscles in a relaxed way…*

•Stand or sit with your feet shoulder-width apart, hands at your sides.

•Imagine a horizontal figure eight (as wide as is comfortable) about 10 feet away.

•Without moving your head, trace the figure eight with your eyes in one direction, then in the opposite direction. Remember to breathe normally and blink your eyes regularly as they move along the figure eight. Repeat several times. Do this for two minutes twice a day.

•**Change focus.** Don't keep your eyes locked on a computer or television or any other screen for a sustained period of time. Doing so causes tension on the visual system. We don't blink as much when we're staring at something, which dries out the cornea and exhausts the eye muscles. To change your focus when you're doing close-up work, look up and away often—such as out a window—to give your eyes a break.

Try the 20-20-20 rule: Every 20 minutes, look at something 20 feet away for 20 seconds.

•**Relax your eyes.** Relax the muscles around your eyes, and bring healing energy to your eyes through increased circulation and energy flow with a technique called palming. This is especially useful after long periods of computer use. *How to do it…*

• Remove your glasses or contact lenses, and sit leaning forward with your elbows resting on a table and your eyes closed.

• Place the palm of your left hand over your left eye, with your fingers on your forehead, the hollow of your palm directly over your eye (but not touching it), and the heel of your hand resting on your left cheekbone.

• Do the same thing with your right palm over the right eye and the right fingers crossing over the fingers of your left hand and the heel of your hand resting on your right cheekbone.

• Remain this way for three minutes, remembering to breathe normally.

• **Go the distance.** The eye muscles are most relaxed when using our distance vision because that's what they were designed for. Nowadays, to keep your eyes in top shape, make an effort to perform outdoor activities that require seeing at a distance, such as playing golf or tennis, riding a bike or just walking. When walking, keep your head up and scan the horizon. Indoors, do reading, writing or close-up work with an eye-to-activity distance of roughly 14 to 16 inches for adults. Watch TV from a distance of about eight to 10 feet for most large-screen TVs.

• **Be mindful.** It's no secret that mental stress affects the immune and respiratory systems and causes inflammation throughout the body. But did you know that stress-reduction techniques can have a specific impact on glaucoma? Your body can't deliver essential nutrients to your eyes if stress is impairing circulation and digestion. Destress by practicing proven mindfulness techniques such as meditation, deep breathing and yoga. Inversion poses in yoga, such as downward dog, also benefit vision because they increase blood flow to the head (consult your doctor first if you have glaucoma or high blood pressure).

An intriguing new study published in *Journal of Glaucoma* found that meditation in particular may be especially helpful for glaucoma patients. Hour-long, daily mindful-meditation sessions for just three weeks resulted in a significant reduction in eye pressure and in levels of the stress hormone cortisol, helping to minimize optic damage. Even five to 20 minutes a day can be very helpful.

Use Your Sense of Smell to Improve Your Health

Alan R. Hirsch, MD, board-certified neurologist and psychiatrist specializing in the treatment of smell and taste loss, and neurological director of Smell & Taste Treatment and Research Foundation, Ltd., in Chicago. He has published hundreds of studies on smell in journals such as *Neurology, Headache* and *International Journal of Aromatherapy.* SmellAndTaste.org

We've all heard that smell is our "most powerful" sense—touching our hearts with the fond memory of the aroma of Grandma's famous lasagna or Mom's perfume or bringing us the heady whiff of new-car leather. Beyond triggering memories, scents and aromas actually can affect our energy levels, improve memory and even enrich relationships.

It's not surprising that people tend to be happier and more optimistic in environments that smell pleasing to them. Most everyone can smell, and with a little guidance, you can tap into scents' true potentials. *Here's how to use scent to your advantage…*

TO IMPROVE YOUR LOVE LIFE

Did you know that purposefully inhaling certain scents may help fuel your libido? Perhaps not surprisingly, sweet scents are associated with arousal in both men and women.

As odd as it sounds, however, it is a combination of donuts and black licorice that increased male sexual arousal, boosting penile blood flow by more than 30%, per research from the Smell & Taste Treatment and Research Foundation. For another sexy combo, try pumpkin pie and donuts. These scents combined increased penile blood flow by 20%.

Women also are affected by black licorice. A blend of the scents of Good & Plenty licorice candy and banana-nut bread enhanced female sexual arousal by 18%. Oddly, a lone vegetable makes it onto the sexiest scents list—a combination of cucumber and Good & Plenty stimulated women.

Scientists theorize that these odors work by reducing anxiety, which in turn reduces inhibitions. That can lead to enhanced sexual desire.

TO RESIST CRAVINGS

Go ahead and breathe in those freshly baked smells at the grocery store. A 2019 University of South Florida study found that smelling indulgent foods such as pizza or cookies for an extended period of time actually can help ward off cravings. Subjects who were exposed to these ambient scents for longer than two minutes while in a supermarket were less likely to purchase "unhealthy foods," compared with those who shopped with no ambient scent or in the presence of a "nonindulgent food–related ambient scent" such as strawberry or roast turkey.

Scientists hypothesize that the brain may derive sufficient sensory pleasure from the aroma of the food alone, without even tasting it. In essence, you can fool the brain into thinking that you have eaten the goodie already.

Helpful idea: If you're trying to avoid sugary indulgences at an office meeting or party, just wait a few minutes before you lift anything to your lips. The first 30 seconds will be hard—the study showed that a very brief whiff of the cookie scent left subjects more likely to want to eat a cookie. But after that, it became easy to ignore the cookies.

Don't want to stick your nose in a cookie platter or get that close to tempting treats? Study authors theorize that using a cookie-scented extract or cookie-scented candle (or any other indulgent scent) might be just as effective at beating those cravings.

TO EASE STRESS

Many people know that lavender is a major de-stressor, hence it often is used to scent candles, body lotions, fabric softeners and more. The mere smell of lavender increases alpha-wave activity in the brain, indicative of a more relaxed state. A 2018 Japanese study suggests that the calming effect may be due to linalool, a fragrant alcohol compound that gives lavender its distinct aroma. The calming qualities also improve sleep—a study published in *Journal*

of Alternative and Complementary Medicine found that study participants who slept with a chest patch imbued with lavender essential oil for five consecutive nights (Noctilessence, 10 patches for $24.99) experienced better overall sleep quality, compared with people wearing unscented patches. Even more impressive, the sleep benefits remained after two weeks of sleeping patch-free.

But a much more surprising de-stressor can be found right in your laundry basket or on your closet floor. Try breathing in a piece of clothing recently worn by your romantic partner to help calm your nerves. Recent research from University of British Columbia, published in *Journal of Personality and Social Psychology,* showed that women who were asked to smell a shirt recently worn by their partner (without being told that it had been worn by their partner) felt less stressed both before and after a challenging math test or mock interview.

TO WAKE UP

You know that a cup of coffee can help you wake up in the morning. But did you know that you may be able to derive just as much of an energizing effect from sniffing it as you do from sipping it? Simply smelling coffee can make you feel more awake.

Helpful idea: Program your coffee maker to start percolating 10 minutes before your alarm is set to go off if you want to wake up feeling energized before you've even had your first cup of Joe.

Whether or not you're a coffee drinker, the next time you need to perform at your best—while taking an exam, for instance, or before a job interview—inhale a deep whiff of coffee beans to feel instantly more alert.

TO IMPROVE YOUR MEMORY

Rosemary oil contains several compounds shown in test tube studies to facilitate activity of the chemical messengers in the brain that are involved in memory.

In a British study, people over the age of 65 were divided among three rooms. One room was scented by placing four drops of rosemary essential oil on an aroma diffuser that ran for five minutes before participants entered...one was lavender-scented…and one was unscented. The participants were presented with a series of challenges designed to assess prospective memory—the type of memory that helps us plan for the future, such as mailing a letter after seeing a mailbox. Rosemary's woody aroma improved prospective memory by 15% across the tasks.

Note: When purchasing essential oils, don't be fooled into thinking that more expensive means more effective. In my experience, more costly brands typically perform on par with less expensive ones. Surprisingly, artificially created oils also perform similarly to ones labeled "natural."

How to Improve Your Sense of Smell

Sense of smell declines with age, but it may be possible to retain it—or even regain it—by purposefully inhaling potent odors several times a day for three months. A 2009 study found that when 40 anosmic volunteers sniffed "Sniffin' Sticks" of rose, eucalyptus, citronella and clove twice a day for 12 weeks, nearly one-third of them ended up with improved olfactory functioning overall. Subsequent studies have replicated the effects. It may work with age-related smell loss, as well as with individuals who have lost their sense of smell from head trauma, a virus or another condition.

What to do: Choose three odors that you currently have difficulty detecting—cologne, cinnamon, roast chicken, for example—and sniff them (one at a time) three times per nostril, four times a day, for three months.

Note: Many medications used for hypertension, high cholesterol, cancer and depression can cause smell loss because they affect your taste receptors…or cause dry mouth, which in turn can diminish your sense of smell. If you are experiencing a loss of smell, talk to your doctor about whether it is a possible side effect of your current medications. You may be able to take a lower dose or a different drug. Smell typically resumes within a few months.

How Healthy Is Your Mouth? Natural Ways to Build Up Good Bacteria

Gerald P. Curatola, DDS, founder of Rejuvenation Dentistry, a biologic restorative dental practice and adjunct clinical associate professor at New York University College of Dentistry, both in New York City. He is also executive director of Bioregulatory Dentistry at the Providence, Rhode Island–based American Center of Bioregulatory Medicine and Dentistry, which provides holistic dental services that address the oral microbiome. He is author of *The Mouth-Body Connection*.

For years, doctors and dentists have recognized that gum disease and heart disease often go hand-in-hand. Statistically speaking, gum disease is linked to a 25% to 90% higher risk for heart disease.

Latest development: Emerging research is now linking oral health with a host of other systemic conditions, including diabetes, pneumonia, erectile dysfunction, Alzheimer's disease and more. On top of that, a study published in *The Lancet Oncology* found that men with gum disease, also known as periodontitis, have a 50% higher risk of developing kidney cancer and are about 30% more likely to be diagnosed with lung or blood cancers.

Inflammation is the likely culprit. Scientists theorize that the body interprets inflammation as a sign that something is injuring its cells. In the case of a flu virus or a scraped knee, that's helpful—it mobilizes the immune system to fight the virus or heal the wound. But chronic low-grade inflammation, like that caused by gum disease, puts the body into a constant state of high alert for perceived threats, wearing down organ systems in the process.

Something else is at play, too. When bacteria in the mouth express themselves in a harmful way, they also can "hijack" our immune system, hampering our ability to fight diseases and predisposing people to chronic systemic illness or complicating existing chronic conditions.

There's plenty we can do to prevent these health-sabotaging bacteria from running wild. The key lies in nourishing and protecting your oral microbiome.

WHAT IS THE ORAL MICROBIOME?

Most people associate the term "microbiome" with the gut. But the mouth ranks second behind the gut as the most diverse community of microbes in the body. More than 800 bacterial species reside in the average mouth…and that's a good thing!

Ideally, when this grand community of bacteria is in balance, the good bacteria outnumber the bad, optimizing an environment that not only fosters oral health but also limits the likelihood of inflammation and bad-for-you bacteria spreading from the mouth to other parts of the body.

That balance is elusive, though. The most popular conventional oral hygiene products have adopted a scorched-earth policy of killing all bacteria. In the process of eradicating the bugs that cause bad breath and cavities, they disturb the entire terrain, including the beneficial microbes needed to rein them in.

For example, in a healthy mouth, *fusobacterium nucleatum* is a common oral bacteria, but more or less well behaved. But when the community is disturbed, this microbe can cause trouble—it's the main bacteria identified in colorectal tumors and a host of other serious diseases. *Fusobacterium nucleatum* can act like a "key that opens a door" in human blood vessels and can cause other bacteria to enter the blood and travel to almost any destination in the human body, like a bus loaded with passengers.

We also need good bacteria to "remineralize" (or strengthen) teeth (bacteria transport minerals from the saliva to the surfaces of teeth) and oxygenate gums—both important for fighting tooth decay and gum disease.

Because the importance of the oral microbiome is still under-recognized, many people make mistakes that are putting their overall health at risk. *Among the most common missteps—and the healthy habits to follow instead…*

MISTAKE #1: **Using a detergent-based toothpaste and harsh mouthwash.** Detergent-based toothpastes contain many ingredients, including the foaming agent *sodium lauryl sulfate* (SLS), that have a laundry list of harmful effects on the body. Mouthwashes containing alcohol or antimicrobial agents essentially sterilize your mouth. Listerine, for example, was originally invented as a surgical disinfectant… and to clean floors! But while you might temporarily enjoy minty fresh breath, you've also killed off helpful microbes, clearing the way for opportunistic pathogens to multiply.

A note about fluoride: This mineral is supposed to bind to tooth enamel so that the tooth becomes resistant to damaging acids from bacteria. However, there is conflicting evidence on the ability of fluoride to prevent tooth decay…and fluoride is considered a poisonous ingredient, which explains why labels for widely used over-the-counter (OTC) toothpastes warn against swallowing toothpaste after brushing.

Meanwhile, fluoridated water combined with other sources of fluoride have led to an increase in *fluorosis*, a discoloring of the teeth, and in some cases, rough, pitted enamel. My belief is that a far superior approach to preventing tooth decay focuses on a healthy balance of the oral microbiome—along with good nutrition.

My advice: Opt for a gentler detergent-free toothpaste and alcohol-free mouthwash. If you're concerned about bad breath, harsh antiseptic mouthwashes aren't the right option. Bad breath and cavities are caused by an imbalance in the oral microbiome—not from an individual bacterium, as was once thought. It's all about promoting balance—or what is known as *microbial homeostasis.*

Toothpastes I recommend: Auromere Ayurvedic Licorice Toothpaste…Weleda Calendula Toothpaste…and Revitin Prebiotic Toothpaste.* You can make your own mouthwash (look online for recipes)…or look for a gentle OTC product. For example, Hello Mouthwash and Aesop Mouthwash do not have harsh ingredients or alcohol. All of these products are available online.

MISTAKE #2: **Eating the wrong foods.** The Standard American Diet, aptly known as "SAD," is filled with foods (such as sweets and refined carbs, fried foods and alcohol) that shift the pH balance of the mouth to a more acidic level. An acid-leaning oral pH level helps promote the overgrowth of harmful bacteria.

*Dr. Curatola is the creator of Revitin Prebiotic Toothpaste.

My advice: Increase your intake of alkalizing foods. Whole, natural foods such as fresh produce, lean protein and beans and seeds are considered alkalizing, and they keep the oral pH balance in check. One surprising microbiome-friendly pick is celery. Besides its alkalizing effect, celery is a rising "superfood" with a host of medical benefits, such as improving cholesterol levels. It's highly anti-inflammatory, contains more than a dozen antioxidants and is known to help the gut microbiome by restoring levels of hydrochloric acid in the stomach, which are often depleted by acid-suppressing medications.

Helpful: To distinguish acidic foods from alkalizing, remember this hint—alkalizing items can spoil, as opposed to acidic, packaged products, which have unnaturally long shelf lives.

Exception: Fermented foods, such as kefir, kimchi and sauerkraut, are alkalizing while also having long shelf lives.

MISTAKE #3: **Taking medication that dries out your mouth.** Saliva is the "life blood" of the mouth and essential for oral health. Yet more than 400 drugs, including antidepressants, antihistamines, narcotic painkillers and blood pressure drugs, can cause dry mouth, depriving teeth and gums of nourishing saliva and promoting periodontitis.

My advice: If you have dry mouth and take one of the medications that causes this, ask your doctor if another drug can be used. For a list of medications and their side effects, including dry mouth, go to MedlinePlus.gov/druginformation.html.

Also, sip water throughout the day and promote saliva production with sugar-free candy or gum. Avoid caffeine and alcohol (both contribute to dry mouth)…and consider sleeping with a humidifier.

MISTAKE #4: **Not moving enough.** Regular exercise is irrefutably good for us. But what does it have to do with the microbes in our bodies? Emerging evidence suggests that exercise can have a positive effect on the microbiome. High-intensity resistance training is especially helpful. Besides enhancing circulation, contracting muscles cause the body to release *myokines*, anti-inflammatory proteins that help dampen chronic inflammation throughout the body.

My advice: Get 15 minutes of high-intensity resistance training, twice a week. When combined with proper nutrition and rest, this regimen will help turn off the inflammatory cascade that can lead to periodontitis.

You need super-slow, high-intensity movement to fatigue each muscle group in order to get the biggest anti-inflammatory payoff.

In general, you'll want moves that work all muscle groups—such exercises as squats, seated rows and chest presses—while using a high-quality resistance band.

Each rep (usually 15 to 20 reps per exercise are done each session) should take 20 seconds…10 seconds up and 10 seconds down, continuing until your muscles burn and shake. You can work with a trainer to develop a routine.

Also, build movement into your daily routine.

What helps: Get up every other hour to grab a glass of water. Hide your TV's remote control. Stand or pace when talking on the phone. Stand for part of the time when commuting via bus or train.

And don't forget: Regular dental visits are the backbone of oral health. Adults should get cleanings at least twice a year.

Saffron for ADHD

Study by researchers at Tehran University of Medical Sciences, Iran, published in *Journal of Child and Adolescent Psychopharmacology.*

Saffron may be an alternative to Ritalin for children and teens who do not respond to medication commonly used to treat attention-deficit/hyperactivity disorder (ADHD). In a preliminary short-term study of patients ages six to 17, the herb, which was given in a 20-mg to 30-mg capsule, was as effective at controlling symptoms as *methylphenidate*—the generic term for Ritalin. Saffron also has antidepressant and memory-enhancing properties, which may be beneficial to those not diagnosed with ADHD.

Conquer Your Pain with These Ancient Healing Secrets

Catherine Browne, DAOM, LAc, DipLAc, RH, a holistic practitioner in Harmony, North Carolina, who specializes in the treatment of pain, emotional imbalances and opioid dependency. She is author of *Natural Therapies for Overcoming Opioid Dependency: Control Pain and Recover from Addiction.* InHarmonyWellnessClinic.com

Whether it's due to arthritis, headache, an injury or some other agonizing condition, chronic pain is endemic in the US. A whopping 116 million Americans live with this dark cloud—more people than heart disease, cancer and diabetes combined.

Treatment for chronic pain runs the gamut from physical therapy and chiropractic care to powerful—often dangerous—painkillers and even surgery. But one approach that can be highly effective isn't even on the radar of most Americans: Traditional Chinese Medicine (TCM).

HOW TCM WORKS

TCM treatments focus on underlying imbalances and blockages that lead to pain. According to TCM principles, pain is caused by stagnation in yin (substance, or blood) and yang (movement, or qi, the body's vital energy).

The natural therapies of TCM treat pain by unblocking qi stagnation, restoring blood flow and enhancing qi. A TCM diagnosis is determined in many ways, including the location of the pain…pulse diagnosis…and tongue diagnosis. The location indicates what acupuncture channel(s) the pain is affecting. The pulse and tongue diagnoses help to reveal the body's internal state of qi. These clues help the practitioner form a treatment plan.

TOP TCM THERAPIES

TCM offers a variety of therapies. Among the most effective…

•**Acupuncture.** TCM describes qi as flowing through 20 channels or meridians in the body, most of which are matched with organ systems, such as the kidneys, liver, lungs, spleen and stomach. The meridians are covered by about 400 acupoints, the energy points that are targeted by acupuncture. To resolve stagnation and move qi, an acupuncturist inserts hair-thin, disposable needles at the appropriate acupoints chosen as part of the patient evaluation and diagnosis.

Don't expect immediate results from acupuncture—it is a healing therapy that takes consistent treatment to resolve chronic pain conditions in most instances. An average course of treatment ranges from 12 to 22 sessions, depending on the severity of the chronic condition.

Also, let your acupuncturist know if there's been a change in the intensity and/or frequency of your pain. These valuable clues can indicate that the treatment is working, even if the pain is not yet entirely eliminated.

Compelling research: When scientists reviewed the evidence on acupuncture for chronic pain, this treatment was found to be an "effective, safe and cost-effective" solution for relieving many types of chronic pain, including low back, neck, shoulder, knee and headache, according to a research review published in *Current Opinion in Anaesthesiology.*

Look for a licensed acupuncturist (LAc) who is board-certified through the National Certification Commission for Acupuncture and Oriental Medicine, NCCAOM.org—a process that requires an average of approximately 2,000 hours of training specifically in Oriental medicine.

•**Emotional therapy.** In TCM theory, emotions such as chronic anger—which is very common in our society—create stagnation in the liver, which controls the flow of blood and qi throughout the body.

Liver qi stagnation can cause chronic joint pain, headaches, muscle spasms, and generalized aches and pains. Many other chronic negative emotions—such as chronic worry or depression—also can play a role in chronic pain.

Self-care option: In addition to acupuncture, you can use herbs such as yellow dock root, bupleurum root or milk thistle seed—all of which soothe the liver and are available individually online. Bupleurum, however, is more widely found in a combination formula such as Xiao Yao Wan, also called "Free and Easy Wanderer," which is available online as well. Follow the dosage recommendation on the label.

Important: Be sure to consult your doctor before taking any herbal formula—especially if you have a chronic medical condition or take medication.

Yoga Breathing: The Surprising Secrets to Its Benefits

Sundar Balasubramanian, PhD, C-IAYT, a cell biologist and assistant professor of research in the department of radiation oncology at Medical University of South Carolina in Charleston. He is also founding director of Prana-Science Institute, PranaScience.com, a website dedicated to research and education on yoga breathing.

Most health-savvy people know that deep breathing has a wide range of mind-body benefits backed by loads of scientific evidence.

But cell biologist and certified yoga therapist Sundar Balasubramanian, PhD, was inspired to investigate further after a realization that he produced an abundance of saliva while practicing controlled yoga breathing exercises collectively known as *pranayama*. He has since conducted pioneering research into the role that spittle (aka "spit") plays in the healing effects of deep breathing.

HIDDEN POWERS OF SALIVA

Hundreds of studies have demonstrated the benefits of yoga breathing—ranging from lower blood pressure and less depression to better concentration and improved lung function—but it's not known why saliva is produced so abundantly during pranayama.

Recognized mainly for its role in promoting healthy digestion, saliva is comprised of about 98% water and various other substances, such as enzymes that help break down food. When people go about their daily activities, they produce about 25 to 50 ounces of saliva daily. However, if you're stressed, your mouth becomes dry. So it makes sense that when your body is extremely relaxed—as occurs during yoga breathing—you produce more saliva than you ordinarily would.

But how does that boost in saliva production contribute to pranayama's benefits? It's been established that saliva contains more than 1,000 proteins along with other crucial molecules, such as neurohormones. And it's been shown that the specific makeup of each person's saliva is unique, and it can change from day to day—even moment to moment based on one's emotional and physiological responses. *Saliva is believed to contribute to the healing effects of yoga breathing by…*

• **Increasing brain-boosting proteins.** Through our research published in *International Psychogeriatrics,* we discovered that a protein called *nerve growth factor* (NGF) increased 10 times more in the saliva of people practicing pranayama for a single 20-minute session compared with study participants who quietly read an article for the same length of time. This is significant because NGF goes straight to the brain, where it encourages brain cell growth. NGF levels are substantially lower in Alzheimer's patients.

• **Elevating cancer-suppressing proteins.** With a study published in *Evidence-Based Complementary and Alternative Medicine,* we confirmed that pranayama not only stimulates saliva production but also elevates levels of proteins with immunity-building and cancer-suppressing properties.

• **Reducing inflammatory markers.** Pranayama also reduces production of inflammatory biomarkers in saliva that are linked to such conditions as pain, depression and diseases, such as scleroderma and post-traumatic stress disorder (PTSD), according to research we published in *BMC Complementary and Alternative Medicine.*

TWO EXERCISES TO GET STARTED

With such varied health benefits—and a new understanding of saliva's crucial role in delivering them—you may be eager to try pranayama.

If you're just starting out with yoga breathing, it's common to worry that you'll "do it wrong." But the truth is, all you have to do is breathe, count and pay attention to how you're feeling. If you don't force an uncomfortable breathing practice or hold your breath for too long, there's nothing about pranayama that you can do wrong.

Natural Ways to Get Some Shut Eye

Rock to Sleep. A gentle rocking motion helps people—even those who are already good sleepers—fall asleep more quickly and have longer periods of deep sleep, during which the mind consolidates memory. A bed that gently rocks all night also preserves sleep continuity—people get up less often.

Editor's note: Rocking bed frames can be found online at RockingBed.com.

Studies by researchers at University of Geneva and University of Lausanne, both in Switzerland, both reported in *Current Biology*.

Simple Sleep Mask. How can something as simple as a sleep mask help insomnia? Even when we turn out the lights, our blinking and backlit gizmos—cell phones, cable-TV boxes, clock radios, smoke alarms, etc.—often allow light to enter our bedrooms. This is a problem because melatonin, a hormone that regulates both sleepiness and the quality of sleep, is highly sensitive to light. A study reported in *The Journal of Clinical Endocrinology & Metabolism* found that light exposure during normal sleeping hours reduced melatonin production by more than 50%.

A sleep mask blocks ambient light—even if it's just a sliver of light from a streetlamp that slips through your bedroom curtains. Try a sleep mask before pills. It may be the best $10 you could have spent.

Rebecca Shannonhouse, editor-in-chief, health conteny, Bottom Line Inc.

Important: If you have a respiratory disorder, such as emphysema or chronic obstructive pulmonary disease (COPD), consult your physician and/or a yoga therapist on the right exercises for your condition.

Even though there are numerous approaches to yoga breathing, here are two simple exercises to get you started—for best results, sit up straight, close your eyes and do one or both of the following throughout the day...

•**Beginner humming breath.** Also called "bee breath" because of the buzzing sound you make, this exercise is a good introduction to yoga breathing. It's quick, easy and doesn't require you to hold your breath.

What to do: Breathe deeply and inhale as much as you can comfortably. Then hum as you slowly exhale at a rate that is comfortable for you. Repeat this exercise for a minute or two when you wake up...and before eating breakfast and your other meals or snacks throughout the day to stimulate your saliva flow.

•**Cooling breath.** This exercise promotes copious saliva production by stimulating the glands in your oral cavity.

What to do: Roll your tongue in a U-shape. Inhale slowly through your tongue, then exhale through your nostrils. Repeat for five to 10 minutes. If you can't roll your tongue, inhale through your mouth while smiling and exhale through your nostrils.

To learn more about yoga breathing, go to PranaScience.com.

Peppermint Eases Painful Swallowing

Mohamed Khalaf, MD, esophageal disorders research fellow, Medical University of South Carolina Health Digestive Disease Center, Charleston.

When participants with swallowing difficulties and noncardiac chest pain took two peppermint oil tablets before meals, 73% reported improvement. Of those with just chest pain or swallowing problems, 63% and 53%, respectively, reported feeling better. Participants with swallowing issues took peppermint before every meal and those with chest pain took it during an attack. Peppermint oil, available in health-food stores, relaxes the smooth muscles of the lower esophagus.

Important: Consult your doctor first to rule out obstruction of the esophagus or heart disease.

Natural Ways to Relieve Shingles Pain

Andrew Rubman, ND, medical director of Southbury Clinic for Traditional Medicines in Southbury, Connecticut. He is author of Bottom Line's "Nature Doc's Patient Diary" blog. SouthburyClinic.com

If you had chicken pox as a child, you still have the *varicella zoster* virus in your nerve tissue, which can lead to shingles years later. People whose immunity is weakened by cancer or a chronic health problem, such as diabetes, are more likely to get shingles. The itchy, painful rash and fluid-filled blisters can last for up to six weeks.

Medical doctors (MDs) often prescribe an antiviral, such as a*cyclovir* (Zovirax) or *valacyclovir* (Valtrex), as soon as symptoms begin, to shorten the course of the illness and lessen associated nerve pain. Other commonly prescribed medications include over-the-counter (OTC) painkillers, such as *ibuprofen* (Motrin)… numbing topical agents, including lidocaine… powerful prescription antidepressants, such as *nortriptyline* (Pamelor)…nerve pain medication, including the antiseizure drug *gabapentin* (Neurontin)…and opioid pain medications.

However: Prescription antivirals do not affect the frequency of shingles recurrence, and drugs used to treat shingles-related pain can have side effects, ranging from liver and kidney damage to opioid-related addiction.

Simple self-care steps I recommend…

•**Wear loose, comfortable clothing until the pain eases.** If the pain is too intense to leave the house, wear a lightweight cotton robe until you get relief.

•**Soak in a lukewarm bath for 15 minutes.** Add to bathwater a cup or two of colloidal oatmeal or baking soda, which can ease pain and itchy blisters.

Important: Avoid bathing or showering in hot water during an outbreak of shingles—heat increases blood flow to the skin, which can worsen pain.

•**Try a cool washcloth.** Soak a washcloth in cool water, wring it out and hold it on the rash for several minutes to ease pain.

•**Use a soothing topical.** Mix two tablespoons of baking soda or cornstarch and one tablespoon of water. Gently apply it to the rash, and rinse off with cool water after 15 minutes.

Also helpful: Freshly squeezed aloe gel, as needed, or *capsicum*, also known as capsaicin, a popular topical nerve-pain blocker derived from hot peppers.

Beyond self-care: As a naturopathic doctor (ND), I often prescribe natural therapies instead of prescription medications to help ease symptoms and restore the body's self-healing capacities following shingles.

Important: These therapies should not be self-administered. An ND* or other health-care practitioner who is knowledgeable in the use of botanical medicines should be consulted for proper dosing and monitoring.

What I often prescribe for shingles…

•**Chinese liniment (Zheng Gu Shui)** or efficascent oil, a Filipino remedy, can be helpful for pain. (I advise my patients to avoid using either product near the eyes, nose or mouth.) Most NDs can boost the effectiveness of efficascent oil by using an ultrasonic device to help the active components penetrate affected areas more deeply.

•**Lomatium** is a potent herbal anti-viral that reduces the risk for recurrence of shingles. An oral supplement of an isolate of lomatium can be taken…or a few drops of lomatium tincture can be added to an eight-ounce glass of water.

Caution: Lomatium can cause a rash in some people, so a small dose usually is prescribed initially and stopped if there are any signs of a new rash.

Best practice: An MD and ND should collaborate on the most effective therapies for you, based on your age, medical history, chronic conditions and use of any medications. To reduce risk for lingering shingles pain (postherpetic neuralgia), prescription antiviral medication is advisable (within 48 to 72 hours of the onset of shingles symptoms).

*To find a naturopathic doctor (ND) near you, consult the American Association of Naturopathic Physicians at Naturopathic.org.

Restless Legs Syndrome: 8 Best Ways to Get Relief

Brian B. Koo, MD, associate professor of neurology at Yale School of Medicine and director of the Yale Center for Restless Legs Syndrome (certified as a Quality Care Center by the Restless Legs Syndrome Foundation), both in New Haven, Connecticut. He is also director of the Sleep Medicine Laboratory at Connecticut Veterans Affairs Health System.

If you have ever suffered from an irresistible urge to move your legs when, say, relaxing in front of the TV at night—or, even worse, when you're in bed trying to sleep—you know that restless legs syndrome (RLS) can drive you batty.

The condition, which affects up to 10% of people in the US, is so frustrating that some sufferers pace the floor, toss and turn in bed or even consider suicide, according to research recently published in *Sleep Medicine.*

To get relief, many people who would prefer to forgo pharmaceuticals think they have no choice but to turn to drugs that are commonly prescribed for RLS, including medications for seizures or so-called dopamine-agonist drugs mainly used to treat Parkinson's disease. But these drugs can lead to side effects such as nausea and dizziness…and sometimes cause RLS symptoms to worsen (see Step #6).

Good news: You may not have to take medication to relieve RLS. There are lesser-known strategies that can restore your precious sleep…and your sanity. *Eight of the most effective steps…*

STEP #1: Ask to have your ferritin level tested. If it's low or even borderline (still within normal, but on the low end), iron supplements could be all you need to reduce RLS symptoms. Though this has been known for some time among RLS specialists, many primary care physicians aren't aware of it.

Note: Checking ferritin, a protein that stores iron in your body's cells, is not the same as checking your iron level. An iron blood test can still come back normal even after ferritin stores have started to decline.

Some people with an iron deficiency respond best to an iron infusion (through an IV) every few months or even two or three times over a few weeks.

Note: RLS may accompany end-stage kidney disease and peripheral neuropathy, too. Your physician should also check to see if either condition is contributing to your RLS.

STEP #2: Get a "medication checkup." A number of medications can make RLS worse. These range from over-the-counter (OTC) antihistamines and sleep aids, such as melatonin, to prescription antidepressants, antipsychotics and antinausea drugs. If you take one of these, you may sleep better without it, but consult your doctor before stopping a medication. If the drug was prescribed by a psychiatrist, he/she should confer with your RLS doctor to look for alternatives.

STEP #3: Review your sleep quality and quantity. You know that getting a good night's sleep can improve RLS, and you may already be practicing good sleep hygiene by keeping your bedroom cool and turning off all electronic gadgets at least an hour before bedtime. Just be sure to get enough sleep—seven to eight hours nightly.

Important: If you snore (ask your bed partner if you aren't sure or set your smartphone to record yourself while sleeping), talk to your doctor about scheduling a sleep study to check for sleep apnea. Correcting apnea often improves RLS symptoms.

STEP #4: Exercise the right way. Physical activity can help if it's performed during the day or early evening at the latest. Vigorous exercise, such as running many miles at any time of day, may worsen RLS symptoms. If that's true for you, opt for walking, slower and less intense jogging, slow cycling and/or swimming. Research has also found yoga to be a good option for RLS.

STEP #5: Reduce stress. If, like many people with RLS, stress worsens your symptoms, try relaxation techniques, such as a warm bath…massage…acupressure or acupuncture…and/or meditation. These therapies may calm down the brain arousal systems that appear to be overactive in RLS.

STEP #6: Get help for augmentation. The same drugs that can help RLS at first, such as the dopamine-agonist medications mentioned earlier, can worsen symptoms over time. The initial dose may become less effective, and RLS symptoms can grow more intense. Called augmentation, this medication-related phenomenon usually happens after six months. When the drug is discontinued, symptoms typically improve. However, you'll need to work with your doctor to identify augmentation and then treat it, often with a gradual switchover to a different drug, such as *gabapentin* (Neurontin).

STEP #7: Ask your doctor about RLS devices. Two devices that require a doctor's prescription can be used whenever you're lying down. Both were relatively recently cleared by the FDA and are eligible for FSA/HSA reimbursement. Restiffic is a vibrating foot wrap that exerts gentle pressure on strategic muscles in the foot. The device costs $199 online at Restiffic.com. Relaxis is a vibrating pad that you place beneath your legs for better sleep. It costs about $600 online at MyRelaxis.com.

STEP #8: Go to an RLS center. As frustrated as you might feel, RLS is very treatable. If you suffer from this condition on most nights or your symptoms have worsened after using an RLS drug, contact one of the nine Quality Care Centers in the US that are certified by the Restless Legs Syndrome Foundation.*

At these centers, specialists take a comprehensive look at your sensory, motor, psychological and sleep symptoms...do a detailed analysis of factors that could be affecting your symptoms (including sleep, diet and medication)...and then personalize treatment to your unique situation.

Also helpful: Consider joining the Restless Legs Syndrome Foundation to share ideas with other patients in its forums and be in the loop on new developments.

*To find a center, go to RLS.org and click on "Treatment."

Kick Gout Out the Natural Way

Jacob Teitelbaum, MD, holistic physician and nationally recognized expert in the fields of pain, sleep, chronic fatigue syndrome and fibromyalgia. He is author of numerous books, including *Real Cause, Real Cure...From Fatigued to Fantastic!...*and *Beat Sugar Addiction Now!...*and the free app Cures A-Z (available for iPhone and Android). He is founder of the Practitioners Alliance Network (PAN). Vitality101.com

The pain of a gout attack can feel like tiny shards of glass piercing your big toe. Even the slightest brush of a bedsheet on your skin can be excruciating. Sufferers limp with agony and are simultaneously plagued by fever and chills.

Once called the "disease of kings" because only the wealthy had the means to overindulge in the rich foods that are commonly associated with gout, the disease has since reached mass proportions. Incidence has more than doubled in the last 20 years to more than eight million people according to a study published in *The Journal of Rheumatology*. Gout is caused by a buildup of uric acid, which congeals into sharp crystals causing pain and destroying joints.

Doctors commonly suggest that you lower levels of uric acid and prevent future attacks with medications such as *allopurinol* (Zyloprim, Aloprim). Beware—newer anti-gout drugs such as *lesinurad* (Zurampic) and *pegloticase* (Krystexxa) do not have proven safety records and do not provide more therapeutic benefit than allopurinol.

You can avoid dependence on medication and prevent gout flare-ups with successful natural treatments that can get to the root of the problem—excess uric acid and the inflammation that it causes. Since flare-ups are mainly diet-related, treatment also centers around changes in your diet.

Here's what works best for preventing and treating this disease...

•**Eat plain yogurt.** You may already love yogurt because it is high in protein, calcium and vitamins, but now it has also been associated with lowering gout attack risk. In new research published in *Modern Rheumatology,* Japanese scientists studied 25 people with high uric acid (hyperuricemia) and/or gout. Half the patients consumed daily yogurt drinks rich in the probiotic *lactobacillus gasseri*, and half did not.

After eight weeks, patients who ate yogurt had lower levels of uric acid. Even though it was a small study, the results were significant. If you don't like yogurt, a probiotic supplement may help.

•**Avoid high-fructose corn syrup.** It may not surprise you to learn that uric acid levels have risen along with the skyrocketing consumption of high-fructose corn syrup (HFCS). In a landmark study published in *Diabetes,* scientists from University of Colorado specifically blame rising uric acid levels on the HFCS found in sodas, juice drinks, candy, ice cream, baked goods (including breads), commercial salad dressings and many other processed foods. Although HFCS consumption seems to have peaked and is starting to fall, Americans still consume unhealthy amounts. Beware of other sugars as well. Fructose-rich fruit is OK to eat, but commercial fruit juices deliver too much fructose—even if they don't contain HFCS.

•**For sweetness, consider using stevia.** You're probably already familiar with the sweetener stevia—made from the leaves of the stevia plant and typically available as a powder or liquid extract. It is a safe, healthy and calorie-free natural sweetener. But now there's a new benefit to using stevia—recent scientific research shows stevia lowers uric acid. There are hundreds of stevia-sweetened products on the market, including sodas, chocolate bars, candies, puddings, jams, etc.

Latest research finding: In an animal study conducted by Chinese scientists and published in *Journal of Food Biochemistry*, a stevia extract lowered fructose-caused high uric acid levels and inflammation. And it worked even better when combined with the prescription drug *allopurinol.*

•**Add more fatty fish to your diet.** The omega-3 fatty acids in fatty fish such as salmon, trout, mackerel, sardines and anchovies are powerfully anti-inflammatory and can help prevent gout attacks.

Important new finding: Researchers at Harvard Medical School looked at more than 700 people with gout. Those who ate omega-3–rich servings of fish were 26% less likely to have a gout attack.

Note: Many doctors and organizations such as the Mayo Clinic and the Arthritis Foundation routinely recommend that patients with gout avoid purine-rich foods, including seafood, organ meats and wild game. But this recommendation is becoming outdated. The most recent scientific research shows that avoiding purines is unlikely to help you avoid gout attacks and only serves to remove potentially healthful foods from your diet.

Try this: It's better to add anti-gout foods to your diet rather than eliminate healthy foods for a questionable benefit.

•**Take the powerful anti-inflammatory curcumin**—the active ingredient in the spice turmeric.

New research finding: In a study published in *Arthritis Research and Therapy*, Chinese scientists successfully used curcumin to stop inflammation caused by uric acid crystals. Researchers concluded that curcumin is so effective, it could be considered a new "drug" for the treatment of gout. Gout attacks often can be stopped with the curcumin-containing supplement Curamin* from Terry Naturally, which contains a highly absorbable form of the same compound.

Directions: Take two or three capsules two to three times daily until you feel better. For a maintenance dose that can help prevent future attacks, take three capsules daily.

•**Take a tart cherry supplement.** You also can treat gout attacks with the supplement End Pain* from Enzymatic Therapy, which contains an extract of tart cherry (as well as boswellia and willow bark, two anti-inflammatory herbs). During a gout attack, take two tablets of End Pain three times daily. For maintenance to prevent gout attacks, take one tablet three times daily.

New research finding: In a study published in *Current Developments in Nutrition,* researchers had 26 overweight people drink either tart cherry juice or a placebo beverage

---

*Dr. Teitelbaum works on the scientific advisory board of the company that makes Curamin, and he designed and sells End Pain. He donates all financial compensation for both products to charity.

over a four-week period and then switch—so that each group tried both tart cherry juice and the placebo. Tart cherry juice lowered both uric acid and C-reactive protein (an inflammatory biomarker) by 19%.

Caution: Regular intake of tart cherry juice to prevent or control gout is not recommended because it delivers too much fructose, so it is better to use a supplement such as End Pain instead.

Note: Drinking a lot of water every day can dilute uric acid levels by helping you stay hydrated but will not stop an acute gout attack. You also can take supplements of omega-3s and antioxidants—these essential fatty acids are crucial for your body's health, but they won't do as much for gout as actual changes in your diet and lifestyle.

Green Space Linked to Lower Healthcare Costs

Analysis of county-level health and environmental data from 3,086 of the 3,103 counties in the continental US by researchers at University of Illinois at Urbana-Champaign, published in *Urban Forestry and Urban Greening*.

Medicare costs tend to be lower in counties with more trees and shrubs than in counties with other types of land cover. Counties with the lowest socioeconomic status seem to benefit the most from increases in forests and shrubs. The study does not show a cause-and-effect relationship, but it is one of several recent ones linking green space to better health in people living nearby.

Music as Medicine

Barbara Else, MT-BC, board-certified music therapist and managing editor of Journal of Music Therapy. She is a consultant who serves as senior adviser, research and policy, to the American Music Therapy Association (AMTA), based in Silver Spring, Maryland. MusicTherapy.org

It's no secret that listening to a mellow song can calm us or that listening to an upbeat song can make us feel energized. But music's power over our minds and bodies runs deeper than people tend to realize. Music can trigger the release of mood-altering neurochemicals in the brain and activate brain regions associated with memory, emotion and creativity. Researchers have discovered that music can reduce pain...pull people out of depressed moods... spur recall of long-ago events...and more.

But you might not reap the potential benefits of music simply by flipping on the radio. The songs you select matter, as does the way you interact with those songs—participating in the creation of music tends to be more effective than just listening. Don't worry if you can't play an instrument or carry a tune—even humming, singing privately in the shower and/or drumming a couple of pencils on a table can convey the benefits of music creation.

Here are four ways to use music therapy to improve your life...

USE MUSIC TO REDUCE PAIN

In 2016, researchers conducted a meta-analysis of 97 earlier studies that examined the effect music has on pain.

Their conclusion: Preferred music can reduce the pain patients report on the one-to-10 pain scale by an average of more than one point, which is enough to lower someone's pain level from "distressing" to "tolerable." This reduction in pain tends to reduce people's use of addictive opioids and other painkillers.

What to do: If you're experiencing a low-to-moderate level of pain—something closer to discomfort than agony—listen to (or better yet hum or sing) music that you find relaxing. The calming effect that this music has on your brain is likely to lessen your sensation of pain. Which songs and genres to choose varies from person to person—the music someone else finds relaxing, you might find irritating. Still, if you're not sure where to start, you could enter words such as "mellow" or "relaxing" into a music-streaming website or app such as Spotify (Spotify.com, free for the ad-supported version to $9.99 per month for the ad-free premium version) or Amazon Prime Music (Amazon.com, included with Amazon Prime, which costs about $13 a month or $119 a year). Listen to the songs that these searches turn up, and create a playlist of only those that are calming for you.

If you experience substantial pain, instead listen to songs that you consider extremely engaging. These are songs that you cannot help but sing or hum along with every time you hear them—whether it's a show tune such as "Seventy-six Trombones" or classic rock such as The Isley Brothers' "Shout." They're songs that pull your attention away from other thoughts when they come on the radio. These songs are so powerful that they actually can distract your mind from your pain, to a degree. (Relaxing songs tend not to capture the attention sufficiently to overcome substantial pain.)

You probably already know what songs you find especially engaging—they're likely the songs that you've been listening to over and over again for years. There's a good chance that many of them date back to when you were in your teens, 20s or early 30s—the music people listen to during this stage of life can become so deeply ingrained that it has special power over the mind. Create a playlist of these engaging songs to listen to during painful medical or dental procedures…while waiting for treatment in hospital emergency rooms…while waiting for painkillers to take effect…and during other times of significant pain.

USE MUSIC
TO REMEMBER THE PAST

Researchers have determined that among the regions of the brain activated when we listen to or create music are regions associated with autobiographical memories. That's why when we hear a song we heard frequently many years earlier, the song isn't all we remember—we often recall events from our own lives that happened around the time when the song was new to us.

What to do: Couples who have been together for many decades often feel closer to each other when they listen to (or sing or play) songs they originally listened to together long ago. The songs revive memories of experiences and adventures they enjoyed together. This can be especially beneficial when one partner is suffering from dementia—remarkably, music has the power to recover autobiographical memories even for these people who are slowly losing their past. The songs people listened to in their teens, 20s and early 30s are especially likely to be tied to personal memories.

Try this: If you're caring for someone who has late-stage dementia and you need to get a message through, such as "it's time for dinner," see if you can capture his/her attention using the melodies or lyrics you know he loved. They are most likely to be effective.

This music also can be useful for reminiscing about the old days with friends…or when trying to reconstruct family history and life reviews for descendants.

USE MUSIC
TO REMEMBER THINGS LATER

Music doesn't just help us recall the distant past. It also can help us remember day-to-day details. A study published in *Memory & Cognition* determined that people are more likely to recall a phrase if it is sung as a song lyric than if it is simply spoken. That finding hints at a useful trick for remembering any detail.

What to do: Rather than tell yourself to remember, *The car is parked on 12th Street*, as you walk away from it, sing that line to yourself a few times—any melody will do. And if there's something you chronically misplace or forget to do, create a habit of singing about it.

Example: If you frequently misplace your car keys, you might sing, "I'm hanging my keys on the hook by the door," each time you enter your house.

USE MUSIC
TO IMPROVE YOUR MOOD

A 2011 study published in *Nature Neuroscience* found that listening to music can stimulate the release of dopamine in the brain—the same mood-lifting neurochemical that gets released when people have sex, use drugs or enjoy a favorite food. In fact, music doesn't just pick us up when we're feeling a little down—it actually can help overcome clinical depression.

Findings: A 2017 analysis of nine earlier studies concluded that music therapy accompanied by other depression treatments was more effective than those other treatments on their own.

What to do: When you hear a song that makes you want to sing…makes you want to get up and move…and/or simply makes you feel good, make note of it—these are the songs that are especially likely to trigger the release of mood-improving neurochemicals for you. Create a playlist of these songs, and listen to it when you feel low. Sing, hum, drum or dance along to these songs—an article in *British Journal of Psychiatry* speculated that the potential physicality of music might contribute to its ability to lift depression.

A board-certified music therapist can provide guidance about how to take full advantage of the benefits of music. To find a music therapist in your area, visit MusicTherapy.org/about/find.

Try These Medicines Made by Bees!

Jamison Starbuck, ND, is a naturopathic physician in family practice in Missoula, Montana, and producer of *Dr. Starbuck's Health Tips for Kids,* a weekly program on Montana Public Radio, MTPR.org. DrJamisonStarbuck. com

I have a fondness for bees. Beekeeping itself is good medicine—and not that hard to do. I find being around bees and watching their activity to be relaxing and interesting. But there are easier ways to get health benefits from bees. *Bee products with natural medicinal value…**

•**Honey.** I like to use honey instead of sugar as a sweetener because it metabolizes slowly, reducing the "sugar rush" and subsequent crash people often experience when consuming "regular" sugar. Also, honey has some nutritional value that sugar lacks—it contains potassium and magnesium, B vitamins, amino acids and enzymes. Both honey and sugar are composed of fructose and glucose, but honey contains the enzymes needed to break down these compounds, making it easier for the body to di-

**Caution:* While allergic reactions to honey, pollen or propolis are rare, consuming these products may not be advisable for those with severe plant allergies. All of these products contain some pollen, which comes from plants. Honey should never be given to children younger than one-year-old due to the risk for botulism poisoning.

gest and less irritating to the stomach. Honey soothes respiratory inflammation from a sore throat, cough or bronchitis. Add one teaspoon of honey to a cup of tea (I like slippery elm and mullein for respiratory ailments).

Because of its antibacterial and anti-inflammatory properties, honey also can be used topically for healing wounds, burns and eczema. Simply smooth some honey over a wound, burn or patch of dry, scaly skin, then cover it with dry, sterile gauze. Change the gauze, and reapply honey daily until the area is healed. See your doctor for a deep wound or if you have signs of infection such as redness and/or swelling.

Best types of honey: To get the full benefits of honey, your best bet is to use raw, unpasteurized honey (check the label). For topical use, consider Manuka honey, a type of honey made by bees using the nectar from the wild manuka bush found in New Zealand. Manuka honey is available in most natural-food stores.

•**Pollen is primarily used to treat mild seasonal allergies.** The theory is that ingesting very small amounts of pollen, made from plants to which one is mildly allergic, will improve tolerance to those plants—similar to the way allergy shots or homeopathic allergy remedies work.

To use as an allergy medicine, pollen must be obtained from plants grown in your environment, which you can obtain from a local natural-food store or from a beekeeper directly. I typically recommend taking one-quarter teaspoon of bee pollen granules daily for a month or more before allergy season begins. You can sprinkle it on cereal or toast or add to yogurt or smoothies.

•**Propolis is a resinlike material that bees produce to protect their hives.** It's made from saliva, beeswax and material gathered from trees, including aspen, birch and poplar. I combine tinctures of propolis and slippery elm in a 50:50 ratio to make a soothing sore throat medicine. Spray this mix on the back of your throat every two hours as needed. You can also buy this premade in natural-food stores.

Case Study: Weak Voice Restored Naturally

Andrew Rubman, ND, naturopathic physician and founder and medical director of Southbury Clinic for Traditional Medicines, Southbury, Connecticut. A consultant or adviser to numerous organizations, including the National Center for Complementary and Integrative Health, Dr. Rubman is a member of the National Center for Homeopathy and the Science National Honor Society, among other groups. He is author of the blog, *Nature Doc's Patient Diary*, at BottomLineInc.com

The patient: "Buster" is a pilot of a Sikorsky UH-60 "Black Hawk" who was not "disposed to discuss his employer or missions."

Why he came to see me: He had been suffering from sinus congestion and mild gastric reflux that had made his voice occasionally "scratchy and high-pitched." As a pilot presumably involved with some serious duty and operators, this problem was "unacceptable."

How I evaluated him: We reviewed his past treatments and attempted interventions as well as his upper GI studies and ENT exam, which were entirely normal except for "boggy slightly irritated" vocal cords. I prescribed some dietary suggestions that seemed appropriate as the cause appeared to be a combination of a slight persistent post-nasal drip related to dairy protein allergies and airborne particulates and a production of stomach acid between meals (there isn't supposed to be much of any) that was not enough to cause pathological changes observed in the endoscopy, but enough to create acid vapor rising up and bothering his vocal cords, causing the voice distortion.

How we addressed his problem: I provided a digestive enzyme formula to be taken at the start of meals to increase his mid-meal acid concentration to help improve digestion and thereby decrease microbes residing in his stomach (the probable source of his between-meal acid vapors), a botanical mixture containing small amounts of ephedrine and atropine alkaloids from natural sources, among other components, to help reduce his nasal congestion and post-nasal drip. I also gave Buster another botanical mixture featuring slippery elm, horehound and gentian that I instructed him to inhale—a drop or two from the tip of the dropper—a few times per day to coat his vocal cords with a soothing solution. This unusual procedure sounded intimidating to him, so I demonstrated how to perform it, which helped gain his trust in my prescription.

The patient's progress: I'm happy to report that Buster called a few days after and was delighted with the results.

CHAPTER 16

Pain Relief

How to Explain Your Pain—the Secret to Finally Getting Relief

When you're in pain, it's often difficult to find just the right words to describe it. But it's worth the effort. Accurately describing the "quality" of your pain is one of the most important—yet underappreciated—steps in getting the best treatment.

Now: Pain specialists are giving pain sufferers new methods to help them communicate exactly how they are feeling.

What you need to know...

BEYOND THE 0-TO-10 SCALE

It's no surprise that there's huge variability in how pain is experienced. One person's low-back pain, for example, might be "dull and bearable," while another's might be "sharp and unbearable."

That's why telling your doctor that you have "low-back pain" is not descriptive. Rather, you must be specific when describing your pain.

While the location of pain is a useful starting point, indicating whether it radiates, what makes it start and stop and describing the quality of the pain are often important clues in determining the source—and planning a way to treat the underlying cause. *Seven key elements to describe...*

•**The intensity of your pain.** The most common way to describe pain intensity is with the classic 0-to-10 pain intensity scale—with 0 being no pain...1 to 3, mild...4 to 6, moderate...and 7 to 10, severe (10 being the worst pain possible). Unfortunately, far too many people rely solely on this pain scale. This is where your pain description should start, not end.

Seth A. Waldman, MD, director of the Pain Management Division at Hospital for Special Surgery and clinical assistant professor of anesthesiology at Weill Cornell Medical College, both in New York City. He is also the former director-at-large for the New York Society of Interventional Pain Physicians. His scientific articles have appeared in *Anesthesia & Analgesia* and other leading journals in the field of pain and pain management.

Both patients and doctors tend to overuse this tool, overlooking more effective ways to verbally describe pain with stories and words (see below). The 0-to-10 scale has only "modest accuracy," according to a study published in *Journal of General Internal Medicine.*

Also, using the 0-to-10 scale leads patients and doctors to both underestimate and overestimate pain. A person with high pain tolerance may say that his/her pain is a "3"—but that pain should be treated. On the other hand, a person who says, My pain is 30 out of 10, isn't accurately communicating the level of his pain—he is communicating that he urgently wants the pain treated. What's more, that exaggeration poses a real danger—a well-intentioned clinician might try to help with a pain medication that's stronger than needed.

Interesting recent finding: Researchers from McGill University and University of Toronto conducted experiments that showed that men—not women, as previously believed—are more stressed by pain and more hypersensitive to repeated pain. This study was published in *Current Biology.*

•**What your pain feels like.** Words and stories about pain give your doctor important clues as to the pain's real cause and optimal treatment. In fact, your doctor should ask you to tell your story about your pain—because you most likely have something you want to say...and you want to get better. Telling your story meets both needs.

Example: *I've had an aching back for more than a decade that started after a car accident. Last week, I had a sudden sharp pain in my back—and then the back pain went away! But right after that, I started to have stabbing leg pain.* This story tells the doctor that it's likely you have a herniated disk in your spine.

Some of the most descriptive pain words to use in your story include: Burning...sharp...dull...throbbing...sore...stabbing...shooting...aching...cramping...tingling...stinging...gnawing...dragging...unbearable...intermittent...brief...steady...and constant.

Also, tell your doctor if you have nonpain symptoms that accompany your pain, such as nausea, numbness or weakness. Such symptoms often help clarify the cause of your pain.

•**The location of your pain.** Tell your doctor exactly where the pain occurs...or if it travels from its site of origin to other parts of your body.

Example: Say, *I have a pain in my back that moves into my right buttock, right knee and right foot.* Or *I have a pain on the left side of my neck that goes down into the top of my left arm.*

Helpful: Ask your doctor for a "Body Chart" that shows front, back and side views of the body—and make marks on the chart that show exactly where you experience pain.

What not to do: In describing the location of your pain, don't diagnose yourself by saying, for example, *I have sciatic pain* or *I think I have a hernia.* It's actually dangerous to use words such as "sciatica" that you may have read on the Internet or heard from a health professional—they may be wrong and may lead the doctor to a misdiagnosis.

•**The duration of your pain.** Tell the doctor whether your pain has been occurring for days, weeks or months at a time. If it's chronic, does it come and go throughout the day or is it constant? Is it more severe during the week than on the weekend? Has it worsened over time?

•**What makes your pain better and what makes it worse.** This information is very useful to your doctor in creating a personalized protocol to control and relieve your pain.

Examples: I have pain every time I walk on a hard surface. I have pain when I stand up. I always feel better while sitting. My pain is worse (or better) when I—drink alcohol...eat...have a cup of coffee...go out in cold weather...get a massage...feel tense...go to work...exercise...am fatigued...or don't sleep well.

Also tell the doctor the environments where your pain occurs—for example, while at work or at home.

•**The psychological impact of your pain.** This tells your doctor what pain means to you—that is, how much it makes you suffer, which can vary significantly in people who have the same type and degree of pain. With this information, your doctor can determine what additional treatments might be beneficial for you, such as psychological or medical support for depression and anxiety (both of which are common in people with chronic pain).

•The medications you're taking. Tell the doctor each medication you're taking for pain—the dose, how long you've been taking it and the extent to which each medication helps with the pain. You should also talk about any pain medication you've tried and discontinued…and why you stopped it—either because it didn't help or because of side effects.

Also: Be sure to mention any other medication you're taking, which could interact with pain medication.

KEEPING A PAIN DIARY

Keeping a pain diary (see page 282) for at least a week before your doctor appointment is another important way to clearly communicate the details of your pain to your doctor. *You should note the following factors…*

When the pain occurs…where it hurts…what it felt like…what you were doing when the pain hit…how severe the pain was on a 0-to-10 scale…what you did to try to reduce the pain… and the result of what you did.

A common mistake: Logging too many entries. It's important to keep your diary focused. If you describe every incident of pain, hour by hour, day after day, your doctor will have a hard time making sense of your diary.

Better: Set a specific interval for making diary entries about your pain—a few times a day (*Example*: morning, afternoon and evening) or once a day.

Important: If you have pain, it's always best to start with your primary care doctor. If necessary, he will refer you to a pain specialist.

Facial Pain a Symptom of Headaches

Arne May, MD, PhD, professor of neurology and head, headache outpatient clinic, University of Hamburg, Germany.

When nearly 3,000 people with headaches, including migraines and cluster head-aches, completed questionnaires about their symptoms, 10% reported facial pain—a previously under-recognized headache symptom.

Takeaway: If you experience facial pain—with or without predominant head pain—be sure to tell your doctor so that you can get properly diagnosed and treated.

Coffee Triggers Migraine

Elizabeth Mostofsky, ScD, instructor, department of epidemiology, Harvard T.H. Chan School of Public Health, Boston.

While caffeine is known to help relieve headaches and is found in some migraine medications, too much of a good thing can backfire.

New finding: Drinking three or more servings of a caffeinated beverage (one serving is six to eight ounces of coffee or tea or 12 ounces of caffeinated soda) increases the risk for headache that day or the next, according to a study of nearly 100 adults who suffer from episodic migraine.

Gender Gap in Pain Evaluation

Study in which 264 adults were asked to rate the pain of a child during a doctor's finger-prick test, by researchers at Yale University, New Haven, Connecticut, published in *Journal of Pediatric Psychology.*

Boys' pain is taken more seriously than the same pain felt by girls. Women, in particular, rated boys' pain higher—while men rated boys' and girls' pain more similarly. The reason is unknown, but researchers hope that the findings will add insight into the role of gender bias in pain management and health care.

WEEKLY PAIN DIARY

	MONDAY	TUESDAY	WEDNESDAY	THURSDAY	FRIDAY	SATURDAY	SUNDAY
Duration of Your Pain	Start: ____ Stop: ____ Intermittent: ____	Start: ____ Stop: ____ Intermittent: ____	Start: ____ Stop: ____ Intermittent: ____	Start: ____ Stop: ____ Intermittent: ____	Start: ____ Stop: ____ Intermittent: ____	Start: ____ Stop: ____ Intermittent: ____	Start: ____ Stop: ____ Intermittent: ____
Location of Your Pain (e.g., back, hip, knee)							
Description of Your Pain (e.g., stabbing, dull, throbbing, burning, etc.)*							
Possible Triggers (e.g., missed medication, sleep problems, etc.)							
Intensity of Your Pain (0 to 10)							
What You Did to Relieve Your Pain…and How It Worked (e.g., yoga, massage, ice pack, pain reliever, etc.)	Exercise: ____ Complementary Therapy: ____ Self-Care: ____ Medication: ____	Exercise: ____ Complementary Therapy: ____ Self-Care: ____ Medication: ____	Exercise: ____ Complementary Therapy: ____ Self-Care: ____ Medication: ____	Exercise: ____ Complementary Therapy: ____ Self-Care: ____ Medication: ____	Exercise: ____ Complementary Therapy: ____ Self-Care: ____ Medication: ____	Exercise: ____ Complementary Therapy: ____ Self-Care: ____ Medication: ____	Exercise: ____ Complementary Therapy: ____ Self-Care: ____ Medication: ____

***Examples of words to describe your pain:** Sharp…pounding…pulsing…searing…heavy…radiating… tingling…
piercing…squeezing…excrutiating…mild…quivering…crushing…pulling.

High-Tech Help for Migraine Pain

Brian M. Grosberg, MD, director of Hartford Health-Care Headache Center, Ayer Neuroscience Institute, and professor of neurology at University of Connecticut School of Medicine, Farmington. He is principal investigator of a study on the Nerivio published in *Headache: The Journal of Head and Face Pain.*

Medications have helped many people impacted by migraines, but now there's a new FDA-approved non-drug treatment that offers relief. It's a wearable electric-stimulation device for people who prefer nondrug relief...don't get relief (or enough relief) from treatments such as triptans or non-specific migraine medications...or experience unwanted side effects from those drugs. Called Nerivio, it also can be used in tandem with medications for greater pain relief.

Unlike earlier stimulation devices that are placed on the head, Nerivio goes on the upper arm and can be discreetly covered by clothing. It works by delivering electrical stimulation to the peripheral nerves in the arm. This relays pain-sensitive information to the brain, triggering the release of chemicals to reduce the pain signals that occur during a migraine.

Important: Start treatment as early as possible, but always within 60 minutes of migraine headache or aura onset.

Participants who wore the armbands in a recent clinical trial experienced relief lasting up to 48 hours after the treatment.

Through an app on your smartphone, you set the intensity level yourself. It should feel strong but comfortable and not painful. Available by prescription, each armband delivers 12 45-minute treatments and costs $99. (There are no rechargeable versions yet.)

Note that Nervio is not for people with chronic migraine.* Also, the device is not recommended for anyone with a severe heart condition, uncontrolled epilepsy or any implanted medical device.

*Defined as having a migraine at least eight days a month and a total of at least 15 headaches a month for more than three months.

Got Painful Hand Arthritis? Get Relief Without Drugs

Carole Dodge, OTR, CHT, who supervises the occupational hand therapy program at University of Michigan Health System in Ann Arbor. She specializes in osteoarthritis, rheumatoid arthritis, joint replacements and traumatic hand injuries. She is also director of the Michigan Medicine Hand Fellowship program.

If turning a doorknob or a key, opening a jar or gripping buttons, zippers or other clothes fasteners is painful—even unbearable—you're probably coping with osteoarthritis (OA) in your hands.

The hands often bear the brunt of this "wear and tear" arthritis. The good news is, there are plenty of under-the-radar nondrug strategies that can ease the pain of hand arthritis.

BEYOND THE PILL BOTTLE

Many people don't know about the approaches that follow because they're not heavily advertised and few doctors talk about them. While the benefits may be temporary, these tactics can be used as often as desired—with no downsides. *Among the best nondrug therapies to relieve hand OA...*

•**Arthritis gloves.** Gentle compression from arthritis gloves, which are not the same as those used for burns or lymphedema, eases pain and lessens OA swelling. The gloves can be worn all day and night, if needed, for pain relief—even in the summer, since they are lightweight. *Good products...*

•Norco Compression Gloves. A soft, nylon-and-spandex blend, these gloves are sold individually for left and right hands and come in two fingertip styles (full-finger and tipless for easy smartphone use) and wrist lengths. A built-in wrist slit makes them easy to slide on, and they're sold in three sizes. The soft compression gets raves from patients who've tried them for symptom relief. *Cost:* $9.95 each.

•IMAK Compression Arthritis Gloves. Endorsed by the Arthritis Foundation, these mostly cotton, part spandex gloves are breathable, flexible and have open fingertips. Sold in three sizes. *Cost:* About $20 a pair.

•**Splints and braces.** These devices, known as orthotics, provide more structure than arthritis gloves and can stabilize the entire hand or just individual knuckles…and are particularly useful for arthritis affecting the base of the thumb. *Good product…*

•Comfort Cool Thumb CMC Restriction Splint. This splint supports the arthritic thumb while offering flexibility and freedom for the fingers. It's made of spongy, thin neoprene and lined with terry cloth for softness against the hand and wrist. Since it's pliable, it can be trimmed if desired. It should be worn during the day when performing activities that increase pain. *Cost:* About $26.

•**Paraffin baths.** Paraffin baths are an easy way to get moist heat deeply into the soft tissues of the hand and joints. Paraffin should be heated to 120°F to 130°F. After dipping your hand(s) in warm paraffin, wrap the hand in a plastic bag and place in an oven mitt or towel, keeping it still for 15 to 20 minutes. The paraffin then peels off easily. Paraffin gives immediate relief that lasts about two hours. *Good products…*

•GiGi Digital Paraffin Bath. A somewhat pricey but highly effective option, the GiGi has a quick-melt feature with an easily adjustable digital temperature control. The oversized steel tank also has a see-through and spill-resistant lid. *Cost:* About $150 (including six pounds of paraffin).

•HoMedics ParaSpa Paraffin Bath. This lower-priced product has a light to let you know when the wax is ready for use, along with a locking safety lid. You can monitor the temperature with a meat or candy thermometer. *Cost:* $39.99 (including three pounds of paraffin).

•**Topical pain relievers.** To avoid the potential side effects, such as upset stomach and stomach ulcers, of oral nonsteroidal anti-inflammatory drugs (NSAIDs), many doctors recommend topical treatments for hand OA—especially capsaicin cream, which uses the key ingredient in chili peppers to help block pain messages to nerves. Over-the-counter arnica and Biofreeze are other good topical products. Ask your doctor for advice.

•**Hand therapy.** Hand therapists are specially trained to teach strategies that will enable you to use your hands with less achiness and stiffness. The therapy usually involves four visits, including evaluation of self-care, management of assistive devices, orthotic fabrication and management, and instruction in a home exercise program. Many health insurers cover hand therapy. To find a qualified hand therapist near you, consult the Hand Therapy Certification Commission website at HTCC.org.

4 Simple Exercises That Ease Hand Arthritis

If you're struggling with arthritis pain in your hands, you may not want to move them much, but resist that temptation! You need to do exactly the opposite.

Daily exercises that specifically target affected joints can improve pain, range of motion and hand strength by promoting blood flow to damaged cartilage and increasing the natural joint lubrication that occurs with movement.

Try these hand exercises…

•**Make an "O" by touching the tip of your thumb to the tip of your index finger and hold for three seconds. This will increase thumb stabilization.**

•**Handle coins and other small objects to improve pinch and finger manipulation.**

•**Flip and shuffle cards to increase the flexibility of your fingers.**

•**Squeeze putty to strengthen all the muscles of your hand. This will increase both your grip and pinch strength for opening jars and containers, opening doors and for lifting and carrying items.**

My advice: Do these exercises for 10 to 15 minutes, twice daily.

—Carole Dodge, OTR, CHT

Osteoarthritis Raises Risk for Social Isolation

Analysis of data on 1,967 people, all around age 73, from six European countries by researchers from the American Geriatrics Society and published in *Journal of the American Geriatrics Society.*

About 30% of adults over age 65 have the painful joint disease. Because they have difficulty moving around, it is harder for them to stay in social contact with others or make new friends. The pain of osteoarthritis also is associated with anxiety, depression and physical inactivity—all factors contributing to social isolation.

When Dental Cleanings Hurt

Louis Siegelman, DDS, a dentist in New York City who treats patients who fear dental procedures, and clinical assistant professor, NYU College of Dentistry, also in New York City. DentalPhobia.com

There are a variety of strategies that can significantly ease the discomfort from painful dental cleanings.

If your teeth are sensitive, be sure to ask your dental professional to be very gentle. You also can ask for a topical numbing agent (such as *benzocaine*), a numbing oral rinse or an injection of a more powerful anesthetic. Some people find that listening to relaxing music can help, too.

Your teeth become more sensitive when tooth enamel erodes, so it helps to avoid acidic beverages, like sodas, seltzers, fruit juices and tomato juice, which weaken enamel, especially several days before your visit. Using certain over-the-counter (OTC) remineralizing toothpastes, rinses, gels and creams also can help ease sensitivity. Ask your dentist which products he/she advises for you. Taking an OTC pain reliever—*ibuprofen* (Motrin) or *acetaminophen* (Tylenol)—about an hour before the appointment helps to ease discomfort as well.

If these steps don't give adequate relief, you may want sedation, such as laughing gas (*nitrous oxide*). It can cause nausea and vomiting, so don't eat immediately prior to the appointment, and I don't advise driving immediately afterward. Check with your insurance carrier to see if the cost will be covered.

Also, some dentists now offer a pain-management method called *transcutaneous electrical nerve stimulation* (TENS) in which pads are placed on the face where the numbing is needed, and the patient uses a remote to control the level of electrical stimulation.

Beware of Steroid Shots

In a study of nearly 500 patients who received a corticosteroid injection for hip or knee osteoarthritis, the complication rate was 8%—much higher than expected. Serious complications included accelerated joint damage, insufficiency fractures beneath the joint cartilage, bone death and rapid joint destruction that may hasten the need for total hip or knee replacement. Before getting a steroid injection, discuss the risks and benefits with your doctor. Also, ask about getting an X-ray before the injection to determine whether you are at increased risk for complications.

Ali Guermazi, MD, PhD, chief of radiology, VA Boston Healthcare System.

The Fascia Fix

Warren I. Hammer, DC, MS, a chiropractor who has been in private practice in Norwalk, Connecticut, for 60 years. Dr. Hammer lectures internationally on the treatment of soft-tissue problems and is editor of three editions of the textbook *Functional Soft-Tissue Examination and Treatment by Manual Methods.* He is the English editor of *Functional Atlas of the Human Fascial System* by Carla Stecco, MD. WarrenHammer.com

This soft-tissue problem goes undetected by most doctors. You wake up feeling stiff and achy. When you walk, your joints might crackle or pop, and you may even feel a bit uncoordinated. Odds are you are suffering from chronic hip, knee, leg, shoulder or spinal pain.

Most people would be quick to blame an injury or osteoarthritis. But for many of those with chronic pain and immobility, the culprit is myofascial pain syndrome (MPS), a soft-tissue problem that most people—including the majority of those suffering from it—have never even heard of.

With MPS, pain originates within the fascia, the thin, white or nearly transparent connective tissue that covers every muscle fiber, blood vessel, nerve and organ in our bodies. Often, the fascia can stiffen, thicken or lose flexibility due to past injuries, inactivity or mismanaged pain.

Unfortunately, most doctors are unable to diagnose MPS because there is no standard diagnostic criteria or lab test to indicate that you have this condition. It can only be diagnosed with a physical exam that reveals a loss of motion in joints and/or diminished muscle strength related to painful nodules, especially in areas from which pain is referred.

That's why you've probably treated only the symptoms of your pain rather than the root cause. Or perhaps you have simply lived with it. Either way, you need to know that long-lasting relief is possible for people with MPS.

4 WAYS TO KEEP YOUR FASCIA HEALTHY

If you have MPS, you need to…

•**Do one-minute stretches.** Your brain communicates with an army of receptors in the fascia every time you move your body. Whenever you use your muscles, the fascia receptors must stretch. If pain or injury inhibits that stretch, muscle fibers don't work at full capacity, leading to more stress on the joint.

Stretching is critical to ensure that your muscle fibers continue firing properly. The good news is, just one minute of static stretching (holding the stretch in place) can effectively activate the fascia in an affected area, such as the neck, shoulders, legs and arms.

My advice: To wake up your muscle fibers, start your day with a hot shower. Throughout the day, remember to do one-minute stretches, targeting areas that are particularly painful. For best results, consult a fascial stretch therapist. Some physical therapists, massage therapists and personal trainers are certified in fascial stretch therapy. Check with your doctor or search "fascial stretch therapy" online for a practitioner near you.

•**Move your body.** Immobility leads to stiffness, pain and more immobility. That's why you have to move your body. The specific type of exercise is not that important—just remember to back off when you feel pain. When you move, your body is talking to you. If you listen, you'll be more likely to avoid injury.

My advice: Walking is often the easiest and most convenient form of physical activity. If you've been sedentary, start by doing just five to 10 minutes daily and gradually increase your distance by a quarter mile at a time until you are walking a mile or more daily. Other good exercise options include swimming and tai chi.

•**Try this supplement.** A good way to support your fascia is to get more hyaluronic acid (HA). Our bodies naturally produce this gooey substance to retain water and lubricate our joints, muscles and connective tissues, including fascia. But HA production declines with age.

Up to 80% of my patients experience significant relief after using an oral HA supplement called Baxyl, which should provide relief within the first month.

Typical dose: For the first week, take one teaspoon in the morning and another at night. After the first week, take just one-half teaspoon twice a day.*

Note: For people with bone-on-bone damage and severe cartilage degeneration, HA injections, which are administered by some rheumatologists and orthopedic surgeons, can be given. An injection can provide three to six months of pain relief.

•**Get Fascial Manipulation.** The goal of this therapy is to release restrictions, mobilize areas that are stuck and restore function to your

*Consult your doctor before taking this—or any other—supplement.

fascia. It is based on myofascial pathways, which are similar to the meridians (energy pathways or channels) of traditional Chinese medicine.

Before treatment, the practitioner (usually a chiropractor, physical therapist or massage therapist) will examine you to find the affected pathways. The practitioner then uses his/her knuckles, elbows and/or hands to manipulate the fascia and muscle using vertical pressure. In some cases, there may be increased pain for a day or two due to the inflammatory process that's needed to heal local fascial points.

Most of my patients show increased mobility after just one or two treatments. Others require three to five treatments before they experience noticeable pain reduction. Check with your health insurer to see whether Fascial Manipulation is covered. For about an hour-long session, the cost will be approximately $125 and up, depending on your location.

TO FIND A CERTIFIED FASCIAL

Manipulation practitioner: Go to Fascial ManipulationWorkshops.com or FascialManipulation.com/en (for practitioners worldwide). Certified practitioners have passed a test after taking the 96-hour Fascial Manipulation course, which originated in Italy and has been taught in 47 countries.

Rebuilding Powerhouse Muscles Helps Conquer Pain

Eric Goodman, DC, founder and creator of Foundation Training. Based in Carpinteria, California, he is author of *True to Form: How to Use Foundation Training for Sustained Pain Relief and Everyday Fitness* and coauthor of *Foundation: Redefine Your Core, Conquer Back Pain, and Move with Confidence.* FoundationTraining.com

Not surprisingly, all the hunching, slumping and slouching of modern-day life are taking a toll on our bodies. Reading and working on our computers and smartphones…spending large amounts of time in the car…watching TV on the couch. Life in the 21st century is filled with many pleasurable conveniences and one giant modern-day nuisance—chronic pain.

Specifically, the sitting and slumping compress the spine and overtax the joints. Over time, poor posture weakens the muscles along the back of the body known as the *posterior chain*. These powerhouse muscles—the back, glutes and hamstrings—are intended to do the heavy lifting, working to protect the joints and skeleton.

Excess sitting and inactivity cause the posterior chain to weaken, while the chest and quadriceps overdevelop to compensate. This causes joint degeneration and all of its debilitating symptoms, such as headache, neck, back and hip pain, carpal tunnel syndrome, plantar fasciitis and more. Compression squeezes the internal organs, too, impacting your breathing, your digestion and your immune function.

I created Foundation Training, a series of corrective body-weight exercises that allows you to use gravity to counterbalance the physical changes caused by inactivity. It healed my own chronic back pain, and I've watched as thousands of patients—from former professional basketball players in their 40s to decorated Air Force veterans in their 70s—have experienced great success and eventual pain relief with this system.

When you reactivate and strengthen the chain, your body rediscovers how to move properly, the pain dissipates and, eventually, stops.

CORE MOVEMENTS

Here are four good starter exercises that will help engage your posterior chain and reactivate neglected muscles—without going to the gym or investing in any special equipment.

•**Decompression breathing.** The first of these exercises, called decompression breathing, is present in every future Foundation Training pose. It is the standard way to enter and exit the positions for all of the exercises.

A curled or hunched stance hinders the lungs' ability to expand and contract, leading to shallow breathing, which in turn shortchanges every other organ and process in the body. Decompression breathing works to actively lift and widen the rib cage while simultaneously strengthening all of the muscles that are required to keep the rib cage there.

Stand tall, toes touching, an inch or so between the heels. Place your thumbs on the bottoms of your rib cage, pinkie fingers on the tops of your pelvic bones. Inhale deeply, broadening and elevating the rib cage as much as possible, and trying to increase the distance between your thumbs and pinkies. As your chest lifts up and expands, you begin to experience a widening of the rib cage in all directions. Remember to keep the back of your neck long and shoulders down.

As you exhale, imagine your rib cage remaining in its expanded state. The goal is to maintain that upper-torso expansion when you exhale. Inhale again, filling out even further, using slow and controlled breaths. Breathe in for three to five seconds, and breathe out for five to seven seconds with every decompression breath. Do this for 10 breaths, and you should instantly feel taller and more energized.

•**Supine decompression.** As with the previous move, this is about strengthening and expanding your lungs and lifting your chest so that your internal organs are no longer squished. Begin by lying down on a yoga mat, face up, with your hands resting on your chest and your legs and feet touching each other. Your neck should be long—imagine lots of space between the bottom of your head and the base of your neck. Move your

hands to the ground, slightly away from your sides with your palms up.

Start to squeeze your knees together, engaging the leg muscles. At the same time, flex your feet so that your toes point toward the ceiling (heels remain on the floor), and press your hands into the ground (try to get every fingernail touching the floor).

Keeping your knees squeezed and feet together and flexed, lift both knees a few inches off the ground—your knees will bend, and your

heels will naturally move a few inches closer to your rear end as you do this. Extend your arms above your chest with your fingertips touching, forming a ball. Continue to lift your extended arms overhead with your fingertips still in the ball position, lifting your chest higher with each breath. You should feel tension in your pelvis, shins, arms and neck. Repeat the move 10 times, with the same breath count as you used for the standing decompression breathing.

REAWAKEN YOUR POSTERIOR CHAIN

Even active people can have weak posterior chains—back muscles, glutes and hamstrings—if they spend the majority of their time sitting or have chronic poor posture. Every time they exercise or go for a stroll, they're exercising the wrong muscles. The muscles in the front of the body end up doing the heavy lifting, so to speak, fighting gravity every step of the way. At the same time, the powerful muscles along the back of the legs and hips learn to live in a short, tight, underutilized position.

To shift the burden of supporting your body back to the strong posterior chain, you need to challenge those long-neglected glutes, hams and back muscles with these two very effective exercises…

•**The Founder.** Stand with your feet wide, about three feet apart. Your weight should be in your heels, arms down at your sides, chest up, shoulders down. Your chest should be fully expanded and held high (higher than what might feel natural or comfortable). Face forward and take a deep decompression breath, expanding the rib cage.

Next, begin to hinge at the hips, knees very slightly bent, extending your hips back behind

you, as if you were starting to sit down in a chair. At the same time, reach your arms in front of you, as if you were pretending to touch the top of an imaginary doorway. (You'll be in a pose similar to a chair pose in yoga.) Look straight ahead, keeping your head in line with your spine. Hold for 10 seconds, breathing deeply while keeping your chest elevated. Let your back muscles burn—they're getting stronger! Lift your arms up a few more inches, pointing toward the seam where the wall meets the ceiling. Your gaze remains straight ahead. Hold for 10 more seconds. A few Founders a day will strengthen your muscles. When done well, it's a powerful pose.

•**The 8-point plank.** Begin by lying on a yoga mat, stomach down, head and upper body propped up as if you are in a sphinx pose. You'll be propped up on your forearms, hands flat on the floor, elbows a few inches in front of your shoulders. Your forearms will point straight ahead, and your palms should be flat on the floor. Flex your feet so that your toes press into the ground. Your knees should continue touching the ground.

Note: You now have eight points of contact with the floor—two hands, two elbows, two knees, two feet.

Start decompression breathing. With each inhale, feel your ribs expand—you'll feel a lifting sensation in your upper body, almost as if your back is floating up toward the ceiling. Continue pressing your palms, forearms, knees and toes into the ground as your upper back lifts. Eventually, your pelvis will follow, lifting a few inches off the ground.

Note: The eight points all stay on the ground. Allow your head to sag—keep your neck long and your chin back, and gaze at your hands. Continue decompression breathing for five to 10 breaths, then gently lower yourself back down.

Perform several of these planks a day for three to six months to elicit a major shift in your posture, pain and overall health. The exercises will activate muscle connections. Each time you practice, you are improving upon a neurological pattern. You won't just get stronger, you'll get better.

You can find free tutorials for each of the exercises shown in this article by searching "Foundation Training" at YouTube.com.

Exercise images courtesy of Eric Goodman.

Roll Away Tight Muscles

Joel Harper, a New York City–based personal trainer whose clients include several Olympic medalists. The creator of the PBS DVD *Joel Harper's Firming After 50*, he designed all of the personal workout chapters for Dr. Mehmet C. Oz and Dr. Michael F. Roizen's YOU series of books and accompanying workout DVDs. He is author of *Mind Your Body: 4 Weeks to a Leaner, Healthier Life* and the Bottom Line blog "Your Personal Mind-Body Coach." JoelHarperFitness.com

Foam rollers are great for easing muscle tightness and relieving soreness by releasing knots in fascia, which surround the muscles, and increasing blood flow to enhance recovery. *Roll away muscle stiffness and pain in three common tight spots…*

TIGHT-MUSCLE MOVES

Roll back and forth from the top to the bottom of each target muscle 25 times. Do one set per muscle. Repeat all exercises on both sides of your body. Never roll over joints.

•**IT Band Roll**—for the iliotibial band that runs along the outside of your thighs and helps keep your hips and knees stable. Lie on your right side with the roller under the middle of your thigh. Support your upper body with your right forearm on the ground and your left hand on the floor in front of your stomach. Keep your chin up and right elbow pressed back so that you stay on your side and avoid tilting forward with your upper body. Legs are together, ankles crossed. If this is too difficult, cross the top leg over the bottom one and anchor your left foot on the floor for balance. Use your hands and your core to shift your weight and help you roll along the full length of your quad.

•**Lat Roll**—releases tension in the muscles on the upper sides of your back. Lie on your right side, legs together and bent at right angles. Place the roller just below your armpit, perpendicular to your body. Your right elbow is bent in the air, and your right hand is holding your head. Using your left hand as a prop, use your hips and legs to roll two inches up and down along the muscles wherever you feel it is most needed. You also can tilt your body forward and back to get a cross-muscle massage as well.

● **Calf Roll.** Sit on the floor with legs straight, and place the roller under your calves (or under only your right calf with your left leg to the side if that is easier), just above the ankle. Lean your upper body back slightly, and place your hands flat on the floor for support, arms slightly bent. Use your hands and hips to help you roll up and down the length of your calves, tilting your legs slightly from side to side as you roll to find the area that needs it most. To add pressure, cross one leg over the other, bending the upper leg so that your foot is on the top of your calf...or for even more pressure, slide your foot down your calf to rest on your ankle. Switch legs and repeat.

The Best Workouts If You Have Hip Pain

Robert Klapper, MD, director, joint replacement program orthopaedic surgery at Cedars-Sinai in Los Angeles. He hosts a weekly radio show "Weekend Warrior" on ESPN. Dr. Klapper is co-author with Lynda Huey of *Heal Your Hips: How to Prevent Hip Surgery and What to Do If You Need It.*

I f you want a workout that won't hurt your hips, head for the pool instead of the machines! Simply walking in water that is navel-high is all you need to do to get an effective, pain-free workout that's good for your heart and your hips.

The best way to do this is to walk forward and then backward in the shallow end of the pool for 30 minutes three times a week. The buoyancy of the water eases stress on hip and knee joints (both of which are weight-bearing) while adding resistance that helps build key muscles that can function as "shock absorbers" to curb hip pain.

If you want to vary the routine, you can alternate walking with marching. Bend your arms and lift your right arm while your left knee bends, and vice versa. If your hip starts to hurt while you're marching, just lower your knees a bit.

If you don't have access to a pool...prefer to exercise in the gym...or just want to mix up your exercise regimen, choose a stationary bike. Pedaling gently rotates the hip joints, which helps improve range of motion and relieves pain by increasing blood flow to hips. An elliptical trainer also is a good choice for a person with hip pain since it is low-impact. Thirty minutes on either of these machines will help build bone density and prevent osteoporosis. You can gradually increase the resistance/elevation on these machines, just be careful to not overdo it. If your hips are hurting, skip the treadmill or stair climber—both can be hard on your joints, including your hips.

A mat Pilates or yoga class is also beneficial for sore hips since it will strengthen your core and build flexibility. Pilates moves, such as leg lifts while lying on each side, will help strengthen your hips. Yoga poses such as the one-legged pigeon, which involves extending one leg straight behind you and bending the other leg so that the outside thigh is on the mat and your foot points the other direction, releases tightness around your hips but should be avoided if you have knee problems. If any Pilates move or yoga pose seems too difficult, your teacher can help you modify the exercises to help you avoid injury. I advise my patients to skip full forward bends, squats and lunges since these exercises can sometimes place too much stress on hips. But if any move causes pain, stop!

A go-easy regimen: Many people age 50 and older love to hike and play tennis on weekends, even though their hips and knees ache afterward. I advise them to exercise gently during the week so that their higher-impact weekend activities will be more comfortable. This might include, for example, a combination of pool walking three days a week, followed by one weekend day of a higher-impact activity such as tennis or skiing.

Is a "Slipping Rib" Causing Your Pain?

Cassidy Foley Davelaar, DO, FAAP, CAQSM, division of orthopedics and sports medicine, Nemours Children's Hospital, and assistant professor, University of Central Florida College of Medicine, both in Orlando. She is also clinical care provider for the United States Tennis Association.

The cause of abdominal pain can be hard to figure out, with so many key organs, muscles and skeletal parts located between the shoulders and hips. But if your belly, back or chest hurts when you move certain ways—and other conditions have been ruled out—you might have slipping rib syndrome. Here's what happens…and what to do about it.

You probably think that your ribs expand enough to allow breathing, but they basically stay in place. And that's mostly true. However, your eighth, ninth and 10th ribs are not attached directly to your sternum (the flat bone at the center front of the chest, aka the breastbone). Instead, they are attached to cartilage that attaches to the sternum.

The cartilage itself can weaken because of trauma from activities that involve major movement of the rib cage. Or the cartilage attachments can weaken from unknown causes. The weakening allows one of the ribs to slip from its proper position during normal movements of the abdominal muscles.

Most often, the slipping rib is the 10th one… and 90% of the time it occurs on just one side of the body. The slippage compresses and irritates the intercostal nerve that runs through the tissue between the ribs. This causes pain that comes and goes, often worsening with exercise or certain movements. (More on that below.)

WHO'S AT RISK?

Slipping rib syndrome first came to medical attention about 60 years ago. While the condition is not considered common, it is so often missed or mistaken for other conditions—such as an ulcer, gallbladder disease, kidney stones or appendicitis—that it's hard to know exactly how common it really is. For instance, 54 cases were found at one sports medicine clinic between 1999 and 2014. And a recent study published in *Clinical Journal of Sports Medicine* found that the average person with this condition sees more than two specialists and takes more than 15 months to get a correct diagnosis.

Slipping rib can happen at any age and afflicts more women than men, particularly during reproductive years. (In the sports medicine clinic study mentioned above, 70% of cases were in women.) Certain sports, such as running, rowing, swimming and weight lifting… and conditions that cause chronic coughing, such as asthma or bronchitis, can make slipping rib syndrome more likely. Being hypermobile (the medical term for "double-jointed") also increases risk. About 20% of patients with slipping rib syndrome are hypermobile.

SYMPTOMS AND DIAGNOSIS

Upper-abdominal pain unrelated to an obvious injury is the most common symptom of slipping rib. The pain usually starts gradually and is described as sharp, severe or cramping…although over time it may fade to a dull ache. The pain usually is triggered by activities that involve upper-arm movement. However, coughing, getting up from a chair or just rolling over in bed also may cause pain.

Once other conditions have been ruled out and slipping rib is suspected, it's actually not hard to diagnose. This is often done with a simple test performed in the doctor's office called a "hooking maneuver." The doctor hooks his/her fingers under the edge of the lower rib cage and pulls upward and outward to see if that triggers pain. Ultrasound also can confirm the diagnosis.

TREATMENT OPTIONS

Depending on the patient's age, activity level and disability from the condition, treatment usually starts with less invasive treatments—nonsteroidal anti-inflammatory drugs (NSAIDs), Lidoderm patches, chiropractic treatment and acupuncture. Generally, noninvasive treatments are about 30% effective at relieving pain, although some work better than others. Diclofenac gel was found to be 60% effective, and osteopathic manipulative treatment (OMT) was 71% effective at relieving pain.

If these methods aren't effective or don't help enough, physical therapy and special home exercises can be beneficial for roughly half the patients who try these therapies.

For patients who still aren't getting adequate pain relief, an ultrasound-guided nerve block can be tried. Injections of numbing medication and/or steroids can provide full relief for several months…and may resolve the pain permanently.

For severe cases of slipping rib, surgery to remove the affected cartilage attached to the problematic rib can relieve the pain. Once healed, pain usually goes away permanently—and the patient can return to normal activities, including sports.

Ankle Weakness Can Remain After an Injury

Luke Donovan, PhD, ATC, assistant professor of kinesiology, University of North Carolina at Charlotte.

Years or even decades after an ankle sprain, some of the symptoms of the original injury can linger, and a person may feel like his/her ankle will give out at times and have cyclic swelling and pain. In fact, about 40% of people who suffer an ankle sprain develop this *chronic ankle instability* (CAI), which can affect a person of any age.

But aging also can be a primary cause of ankle instability. As we age, there's a natural decline in muscle and tendon function as well as neuromuscular control.

If you're experiencing ankle weakness, simple exercises help. The exercises below are best done barefoot and on both sides of the body. Perform them daily, doing strength exercises and balance exercises on alternating days.

To strengthen ankle-supporting muscles, stand on one foot and roll from heel to toes, then reverse and roll from your toes to heel. Repeat three sets of 10 to 15 reps three to four times a week. Next, walk a few feet just on your heels…then the insides of your feet…the outsides of your feet…and finally on your toes. When muscles start to tire, try to take a few

more steps and then work a new muscle group. Balance exercises, such as standing on each leg for 30 to 60 seconds up to three times a day, have been shown to improve neuromuscular control. To make this more challenging, close your eyes.

Note: If you have a balance disorder, check with a doctor before doing these exercises. Also, if any exercise starts to become painful, stop and try another time. And always be sure to stand next to something sturdy that you can grab onto in case you lose your balance.

Helpful: A lace-up ankle brace for support. And if your ankle is painful or swollen, *ibuprofen* (Motrin) or *naproxen* (Aleve) and/or icing the ankle for 15 minutes can relieve pain.

If your ankle worsens, see a foot and ankle surgeon, who may advise physical therapy or surgery to repair ligaments.

Aching Feet? It Could Be Arthritis

Kristen Lee, MD, a rheumatologist with the Joint Preservation and Arthritis Center at the NYU Langone Orthopedic Center and assistant professor in the department of medicine at NYU Langone Health, both in New York City. Her research has been published in *Clinical Rheumatology, Arthritis & Rheumatology* and other leading medical journals.

Standing on your feet all day and wearing tight shoes aren't the only causes of foot pain. You might be surprised to learn that the culprit could be arthritis—even if no other joint in your body is achy. There are 100 different types of arthritis (surprising in itself), and many of them can affect the feet, from the toes to the heel and ankle.

Among the most common forms that can trouble your tootsies…

•**Osteoarthritis (OA).** The same degenerative—or "wear and tear"—arthritis that, over time, leads to the deterioration of cartilage in frequently targeted joints, such as hips and knees, also can occur in the feet and ankles. OA might affect just one foot and even just one part of the foot, such as the big toe or the area from the arch to the front of the ankle. This form of degenerative arthritis can develop at the site of a past injury, like a fracture, so if you've ever broken a bone in your foot, arthritis can strike in that area some years later. OA typically causes pain and stiffness during weight-bearing activities, such as walking or jogging.

•**Gout.** The telltale sign of this inflammatory type of arthritis is sudden and excruciating pain in one big toe, the result of an accumulation of uric acid in the joint. Though gout affects more than eight million Americans, its association with overindulging in food and drink (such as organ meats and beer) leaves many people too embarrassed to seek medical help. But besides having to live with the pain unnecessarily, repeated attacks of unchecked gout can lead to secondary osteoarthritis in the big toe, and the resulting permanent loss of cartilage can cause its own pain, even if the gout is eventually controlled.

•**Rheumatoid arthritis (RA).** This is one of many autoimmune diseases that can affect the joints in the feet, causing them to feel hot and painful, swollen and stiff. An overwhelming 90% of people with RA experience foot pain. In fact, for some, this is the first sign of the disease.

Because RA affects the body symmetrically, you'll feel it in both feet, though the symptoms can alternate, and because RA can attack numerous joints, you may feel symptoms in many of your smaller toes and fingers. RA can lead to joint deformities and cartilage loss within months if severe, and this damage may be visible on an X-ray or MRI.

•**Psoriatic arthritis.** Even though this autoimmune disease is thought to have genetic links to the skin condition psoriasis, psoriatic arthritis can occur on its own in a very small percentage of those who develop arthritis before the psoriasis. Most often, the inflammatory arthritis manifests in people with current psoriasis, past psoriasis or a strong family history of psoriasis.

You may develop plantar fasciitis, which causes pain along the sole or Achilles tendinitis at the back of the heel. But because both of these foot conditions can occur for other reasons, people don't always connect the dots to psoriatic arthritis and attribute their pain to a sports injury or other mishap.

One telltale sign of psoriatic arthritis is a type of inflammation known as *dactylitis*, the intense swelling of an entire digit, including the joints in one or more toes (or fingers) that creates a sausagelike appearance. Foot pain can be excruciating, and joint damage can set in within a few months.

•**Ankylosing spondylitis.** This is a type of inflammatory arthritis that primarily affects the spine, leading to back pain, but symptoms also can occur in your feet and the heel area, in particular. It can look very similar to psoriatic arthritis. Inflammation can lead to Achilles tendinitis at the back of the heel and/or plantar fasciitis at the base of the heel, with severe pain and tenderness that can limit movement. Ankylosing spondylitis also can lead to sausagelike swelling of the toes.

HOW TO GET RELIEF

If you're experiencing foot pain, see your primary care physician, a podiatrist or a rheumatologist (if autoimmune conditions are suspected) for an evaluation. You need a proper diagnosis so you can start treatment early enough to help preserve your mobility.

However, getting a correct diagnosis can sometimes be challenging. Testing should include a careful physical exam, along with blood tests and imaging tests, such as X-rays, an MRI and/or an ultrasound. Seeing a rheumatologist sooner rather than later often helps ensure a proper diagnosis.

The types of arthritis described earlier are generally treated with a combination of medication (primarily anti-inflammatory drugs) and physical therapy to ease pain. Specialized drugs, such as *disease-modifying antirheumatic drugs* (DMARDs), designed to stop or slow the progression of the specific condition, also may be used depending on the diagnosis.

Whatever your treatment plan, make sure that specific foot care is part of it—despite how often feet are affected by these conditions, they're sometimes overlooked in a "big picture" approach.

Here are steps that can help…

• **Make ice your go-to for swelling.** Ice is great for reducing inflammation —alternate 10 minutes on with 10 minutes off until you feel relief. Mold a bag of frozen veggies over the affected part of your foot or simply put your foot in a bucket of icy water.

• **Go shoe shopping.** Arthritic feet will feel much better in shoes with a roomy toe box, a wider width and a lower heel. If you have plantar fasciitis or other soft-tissue involvement, you may benefit from a heel cup or an insert for arch support. See a podiatrist to get a formal biomechanics evaluation of the foot and recommendations for orthotics.

• **See an occupational therapist.** I suggest this to all my patients—there are techniques you can incorporate into your lifestyle to make everyday activities easier to do. Ask your doctor to refer you to an occupational therapist. Insurance typically covers a predetermined number of sessions.

• **Get a handle on stress.** There's a definite link between stress and pain. Diffusing that relationship is helpful whether you do it by practicing deep breathing…working one-on-one with a mental health professional…and/or joining a support group. To find an arthritis support group near you, consult the website CreakyJoints.org.

HEALTHY HABITS THAT HELP

Regardless of which type of arthritis *you have, the same good habits will help. What's most important…*

• **Eat a more nutritious diet.** Obesity, high blood pressure and diabetes often go hand-in-hand with gout and psoriatic arthritis. Rheumatoid arthritis increases risk for heart problems. People with ankylosing spondylitis may also suffer from Crohn's disease or ulcerative colitis, which are inflammatory diseases of the gut. Osteoarthritis is linked to depression. In every case, you'll benefit by avoiding foods that are high in saturated fat and added sugars…and adopting a diet that's rich in fiber with plenty of fruits, vegetables and whole grains.

With gout, you'll also want to avoid foods high in purine, a naturally occurring compound that forms uric acid. These foods include fatty red meats, organ meats and shellfish, as well as beer. Many people with psoriatic arthritis have fatty liver disease and should limit alcohol.

• **Stay active.** Exercise lubricates joints, and keeping ligaments limber and muscles strong reduces the physical load that joints have to bear. Arthritis pain can flare with strenuous activity, so find your personal "sweet spot" when it comes to intensity and duration—do enough to benefit joints without overtaxing them. Many people say strength training that targets the "core" muscles of the abdomen, chest and back makes them feel better.

With osteoarthritis, you might think that your exercise choices are limited because the more you move, the more stress and pain you feel. But listen to your body for ways to adapt, such as switching to low-impact walking if running is difficult.

• **Lose weight if necessary.** For every type of arthritis, carrying around extra pounds means you're putting additional stress on your joints. Losing just 10% of your body weight can make a big difference.

Botox May Treat Heel Pain

Plantar fasciitis is one of the most common causes of heel pain. It happens when the supportive ligament connected to the heel and its surrounding nerves become inflamed. Pain eventually becomes chronic if the condition is not treated. Standard treatments use orthotics, daily stretching and cortisone injections. But some doctors say Botox injections also can relieve the pain and pressure on the inflamed ligament, taking just three to seven days to have an effect.

Caution: Botox is not FDA-approved for this use, not all doctors agree with using it, and insurance may not cover the cost, which could be $500 per treatment.

Roundup of neurologists and podiatrists reported at Prevention.com.

Starting Physical Therapy? How to Get the Best Results

Mitchell Yass, DPT, a specialist in diagnosing and resolving pain and creator of the Yass Method for treating chronic pain. He is author of *Overpower Pain, The Pain Cure Rx* and *The Yass Method for Pain-Free Movement.* MitchellYass.com

If you're suffering from neck, back or knee pain, physical therapy is one of the most commonly recommended treatments. But often, it just doesn't work. There's a good reason for that, though very few people understand what goes wrong.

Typically, when pain is severe and/or chronic, doctors order an MRI, which often identifies a structural abnormality (such as a herniated disk, pinched nerve, arthritis or torn cartilage)—and that structural deviation is usually assumed to be causing the pain.

Here's where things get tricky: Most people—in pain or not—have these sorts of structural variations within their bodies. In fact, research shows that the overwhelming majority of people age 65 and older who are not in pain have some disk degeneration.

Based on my 25 years of treating thousands of patients with neck, back or knee pain, I have found that in more than 95% of the cases, the cause of pain was muscular—and not due to a disk, nerve or some other structural abnormality. Muscular problems often go undetected because they are not visible on an MRI or other diagnostic scans, and there are no medical specialists trained to diagnose and treat them.

Once you're in a physical therapist's (PT) office, he/she is not required to confirm or refute your doctor's diagnosis. If you're diagnosed with a pinched nerve or arthritis when you enter physical therapy, you'll be treated for that condition—even if that's not the real cause of your symptoms.

A complete physical evaluation can identify whether the cause of the pain is structural or muscular. When muscular, the simple tests below will reveal telltale clues to the underlying problem, which often can be corrected with the exercises that follow (typically performed in three sets of 10 reps each, three times a week, resting one minute between sets…until you are pain free).* *Give this information to your PT, who can use it to identify the true cause of your pain and help you perform the exercises…*

NECK AND UPPER-BACK PAIN

The likely culprit: Muscle weakness and/or imbalance of the neck and upper-torso muscles will lead to poor posture. Most neck and upper-back pain is felt a few inches away from one or both sides of the spine. However, a structural variation (such as a bulging disk or pinched nerve) would typically lead to a major loss of range of motion (ROM) and cause pain along the spine.

One common offender: The levator scapulae muscle, which attaches from the inside upper corner of each shoulder blade to the upper neck, supporting the head and stabilizing the shoulders. Because of rampant computer and smartphone use, hunched, rounded posture shortens and pulls the chest muscles forward, weakening and overstretching the levator scapulae muscle, causing neck and/or upper-back pain.

Ask your practitioner to…

• **Press on the spot where you typically experience pain.** For many patients, this will be at the top inner corner of one or both shoulder blades, where the levator scapulae originates. If pressing here triggers or intensifies your pain, this strongly suggests a muscular problem.

• **Evaluate your posture.** If your head and shoulders lean in front of your hips when standing, that's another indicator of weak muscles.

• **Check your ROM.** Tight, weak muscles can restrict motion and/or cause pain as you move your head side to side, touch your chin to your chest or lean your head back.

Try this test: Lie on your back on the exam table with your head hanging off the end but supported by the PT. As you completely relax your neck, ask the PT to gently move your head side to side…and up and down.

If your head can be easily and painlessly moved back and forth and up and down, the

*Ask your PT for guidance on any exercise regimen you take.

tight muscle theory is confirmed. If the PT has difficulty moving your head, and it feels like a bone is hitting another bone, this is a sign that a structural variation is limiting ROM and contributing to neck pain.

Exercises to perform to correct the muscular imbalance causing neck pain and poor posture: Lat pulldowns with a neutral grip and a lower trap exercise to strengthen the lower trapezius muscle, which extends from your neck and across your shoulder blade to the middle of your back. (Ask your PT to demonstrate.)

LOW-BACK PAIN

The likely culprit: Tight quads and hip flexors. Hip flexors are workhorse muscles that originate on either side of the lower spine and travel down the front of the pelvis, attaching at the hip joints. Sitting for hours at a time, day after day—at a desk, in a car or in front of a TV, for instance—weakens the hamstrings and shortens and strains the hip flexors. Tight hip flexors, along with weak hamstrings, cause the pelvis to tip forward, creating an excessive arch and back pain…none of which show up on an MRI.

Hint: If you typically need to push on your thighs with your hands to stand fully upright after sitting, you likely have tight hip flexors—your hands are helping to manually lengthen your hip flexors.

Ask your practitioner to…

• **Press on your hip flexors.** Tender? That's one sign they may be causing your low-back pain.

• **Evaluate your posture.** You want just a very mild curve in your lower spine, with the front and back of the pelvis at equal height.

• **Check for dominant quad muscles.** Again, lie on your back on the exam table, this time with your butt at the edge of the table and your legs hanging off. Pull one knee toward your chest as the other leg dangles. If the foot of the dangling leg is not perpendicular to the knee (less than a 90-degree angle with the foot pointing away from the table), the quad is dominant and overly tight, contributing to low-back pain.

Exercises to resolve the muscle imbalance leading to low-back pain: Hamstring curls, hip extensions and hip abductions. (Ask your PT to demonstrate.)

Note: Perform the exercises only on the painful side—or on both sides if pain affects both sides.

KNEE PAIN

The likely culprit: People with pain around the kneecap are frequently told they have meniscal tears or "bone-on-bone arthritis," which indicates a complete loss of cartilage in the joint between the base of the thighbone and the top of the shinbone. Both of these conditions limit ROM and can be treated only with surgery. Furthermore, neither of these conditions causes pain around the kneecap. If the real cause of your pain is muscle imbalance (with your quads being far stronger than your hamstrings)—and it likely is—surgery isn't necessary and won't even help.

Ask your practitioner to…

• **Check your ROM when you bend your knee if you've been told you have bone-on-bone arthritis or a meniscal tear.** If either condition is causing your pain, you will have a significant loss of ROM, and the end point of movement will feel like a bone is hitting another bone, preventing further motion. If pain occurs around the kneecap and you have full ROM, this rules out either bone-on-bone arthritis or a meniscal tear as the cause of pain.

• **Watch you negotiate stairs.** A muscular problem causes pain as the knee joint struggles to maintain alignment as you walk up or down stairs—as well as with standing and sometimes with sitting.

• **Check for dominant quad muscles.** (See earlier description.)

Exercises to resolve muscular imbalance and pain around the kneecap: Hamstring curls, hip extensions, knee extensions and quad stretches. (Ask your PT to demonstrate.) Do these exercises only on the side where the knee is painful. If you have pain in both knees, do the exercises on both sides.

Try Pain-Fighting Acupressure for Easy TCM Self-Care

Catherine Browne, DAOM, LAc, DipLAc, RH, a holistic practitioner in Harmony, North Carolina, who specializes in the treatment of pain, emotional imbalances and opioid dependency. She is author of *Natural Therapies for Overcoming Opioid Dependency: Control Pain and Recover from Addiction.* InHarmonyWellness-Clinic.com

When it comes to fighting pain, Traditional Chinese Medicine (TCM) offers a variety of therapies—some of which can be used as self-care.

For example, acupressure—in which pressure is applied with the fingers to acupoints (or "energy points")—is a simple, effective alternative to acupuncture, a TCM therapy commonly used to treat pain.

Two acupoints on the wrist—LU7 and LU9 (see below)—can help ease many types of chronic pain.

What to do: Starting with the left wrist, apply pressure with your thumb or fingers to each point, for one to three minutes. The pressure should be firm but not painful. Repeat on the right wrist. Do this several times daily.

LUNGS (LU)

Important: It takes regular, long-term acupressure treatments to affect chronic pain—often for several months. Even though acupuncture is generally considered more "potent" than acupressure, the latter can be an effective and convenient self-treatment option.

QUELL HARMFUL EMOTIONS TO EASE PAIN

Harmful emotions, such as chronic anger, create stagnation of the liver, which controls the flow of blood and qi (vital energy) throughout the body.

For liver qi stagnation—one of the most common imbalances in Western societies contributing to chronic pain syndromes—use the acupressure points LV2, LV3 and LI4 (using the steps described above).

LIVER (LV)

LARGE INTESTINE (LI)

To help energize or activate these points, you also can put a drop of diluted essential oil (use one to two drops of essential oil in one teaspoon of carrier oil, such as olive oil or grapeseed oil) on the areas that correspond with the liver prior to each acupressure session. Fennel, marjoram and mandarin orange/tangerine essential oil all correspond to the liver acupuncture channel, and you can combine them or choose one that appeals to you. *Note*: If you have allergies, test a small amount of diluted essential oil on your wrist before using to make sure there is no reaction.

Credit: Excerpted from *Natural Therapies for Overcoming Opioid Dependency* © by Dr. Catherine Browne, illustrations by Ilona Sherratt, used with permission from Storey Publishing.

What to Do About a Mysterious Bruise

Eric H. Kraut, MD, professor of internal medicine and director of benign hematology, The Ohio State University Wexner Medical Center, Columbus.

Small bruises on your hands or palms without any known cause are mysterious, especially if the finger above the bruise feels a bit numb. Should you be concerned?

Numbness in the hand (or any other part of an extremity) that lasts for more than a week, warrants a visit to a primary care physician. Hand numbness can signal an underlying condition not related to an injury, such as carpal tunnel syndrome, a pinched nerve or even diabetes, which can damage nerves—especially those leading to the extremities.

To investigate the cause of the numbness, your doctor should evaluate muscle strength and numbness in all your extremities and, depending on his/her findings, perhaps recommend further tests and/or refer you to a neurologist.

If you have only a bruise, you would probably not require medical attention. A bruise is a small bleed into the skin that typically occurs after some kind of physical trauma. Many people bruise easily and don't necessarily recall the injury that caused it.

Older adults tend to bruise more easily—their skin is thinner and blood vessels are more fragile. But people of all ages are often more likely to bruise if they take medications that thin the blood, such as aspirin or anticoagulants, or some supplements like fish oil or ginkgo biloba. Even a vigorous workout, such as weight lifting, could lead to bruising—overtaxed muscles can cause small tears in blood vessels.

It may be helpful to apply ice (a bag of frozen peas works fine) to a bruise for 15 to 20 minutes when it's first noticed. This can help to minimize it. For most people, a bruise takes about two weeks to heal, gradually lightening in color as the leaked blood is absorbed back into the body.

What to Do About a Fast-Growing Bunion

Harris H. McIlwain, MD, a board-certified rheumatologist, founder, McIlwain Medical Group, Tampa, and coauthor of *Pain-Free Arthritis*.

A bunion ordinarily takes years to develop, but sometimes in special situations one can develop in a matter of weeks. A bunion (the medical term is *hallux valgus*) is a deformity of the big toe joint. One forms when the first bone in the foot shifts outward and causes the big toe to turn inward and rotate toward the smaller toes. People with flat feet and low arches and those who stand a lot or engage in a high-impact physical activity, such as tennis or ballet, also are more likely to develop bunions. Even though wearing too-tight shoes and/or high heels can contribute to a bunion, this is not considered an underlying cause. Not surprisingly, women are at greater risk than men.

The fast-growing nature of some bunions suggests that something else may be going on.

It could be linked to rheumatoid arthritis (RA). RA is an inflammatory autoimmune condition that occurs when the immune system mistakenly attacks its own joints, causing pain and swelling. People with RA often develop deformities in their hands and feet.

A rheumatologist can diagnose RA with an imaging test, such as an X-ray or MRI, and a blood test. The condition is typically treated with an over-the-counter (OTC) nonsteroidal anti-inflammatory drug (NSAID), such as *naproxen* (Aleve) or *ibuprofen* (Motrin), a corticosteroid or *disease-modifying antirheumatic drugs* (DMARDs), such as *methotrexate* (Rheumatrex), and/or newer targeted medications, including *tofacitinib* (Xeljanz).

Lifestyle changes, such as maintaining a healthy body weight and eating lots of anti-inflammatory foods, including purple grapes, blueberries and dark cherries, also can help reduce pain and sometimes allow RA sufferers to limit or even avoid medication. If your bunion is linked to RA, it's possible that the RA treatments described above may slow down the bunion's progression.

For the bunion itself, there are various treatment options. If it's not continually painful, simply wearing wider, low-heeled shoes with orthotic inserts will improve foot alignment and provide support. OTC bunion pads may prevent irritation. Using an ice pack for 20 minutes at a time, when needed, and/or taking an NSAID will ease bunion pain after walking or other exercise.

However, if your bunion is large and/or very painful, surgery may be necessary. There are many different types of bunion surgery, which involve shaving the bony bump and/or moving the foot bone into its correct position. Your surgeon will recommend the procedure that is best for you. Surgery is the only way to correct a bunion deformity. To find a foot surgeon near you, consult the website of the American Orthopaedic Foot & Ankle Society. AOFAS.org

---

CHAPTER 17

Respiratory Health and Allergies

Is Your Medication Harming Your Lungs?

Maybe you've taken antibiotics to treat a urinary tract infection...or you regularly take medication to combat a chronic condition such as psoriasis or atrial fibrillation. If breathing problems (such as a hacking cough or shortness of breath) occur during that time, would you ever think that the culprit may be a drug you take for something entirely unrelated to your lungs or respiratory tract?

What most people don't realize: Everyday medications—including those prescribed for pain, common infections, heart conditions and cancer—can endanger your respiratory system.

Here's how to protect yourself...

A BIGGER PROBLEM THAN THOUGHT

Certain medications have been known to cause lung problems, including allergic reac-tions, abnormal buildup of fluid in the lungs and inflammation of the lung air sacs, but a recent systematic review of 156 research papers found that such complications are more com-mon than previously understood.

New finding: While more than 350 medica-tions have been associated with some type of drug-induced lung problems, a study published in October 2018 in *Journal of Clinical Medicine* implicated 27 drugs that are most often linked to *interstitial lung disease* (ILD).

What exactly is ILD? It's a fancy term for a group of disorders that cause scarring of the lungs. The culprit might be an irritant (such as asbestos or silica dust)...an autoimmune disease (such as rheumatoid arthritis or scleroderma) ...or a medication. While we may think that our lungs are safe when we take medication for, say,

Jack Fincham, PhD, RPh, professor of pharmaceuti-cal and administrative sciences at Presbyterian College School of Pharmacy in Clinton, South Carolina. He serves as a special appointee to the FDA's Peripheral and Cen-tral Nervous System Drugs Advisory Committee and an appointee to the Canadian Institutes of Health Research College of Reviewers.

arthritis pain or an irregular heartbeat, there's a catch—every organ in the body, including the lungs, has the ability to metabolize drugs.

This means that the lungs can be vulnerable to any toxic effects—even if the drug isn't inhaled. The result can be ILD or another illness such as pneumonia, pneumonitis (inflammation of lung tissue) or pulmonary fibrosis (lung scarring). Shockingly, up to 5% of ILD cases are drug-induced, according to this research, and death rates of 50% or higher for a handful of medications, including the colorectal cancer drug *panitumumab* (Vectibix), were reported in some of the multiple studies reviewed.

A TRICKY TIMELINE

While you might assume that a drug-induced lung problem would show up right after starting to take a medication, that's not always the case. Symptoms of ILD, which can include labored breathing and even general malaise, might develop shortly after starting a new medication (as might occur with an antibiotic, for example)…within days or weeks…or months or even years later—in some cases, even after the drug has been discontinued. This tricky timeline can make it far more difficult for you or your doctor to connect the dots.

Getting a correct diagnosis of drug-induced ILD generally involves a thorough clinical exam, listing all medications taken over the last several years…as well as X-rays or other imaging tests, which might show changes in the lungs. Pulmonary function tests might also be ordered. *In addition to blood tests to measure oxygen and carbon dioxide levels, other tests may include…*

•**Spirometry,** in which you breathe multiple times into a tube that is connected to a computer, to measure your rate of air flow.

•**Pulse oximetry,** in which a probe is placed on your fingertip or a skin surface such as your ear, to estimate oxygen levels in your blood.

Once ILD has taken hold, there's no way to rid the lungs of the telltale lesions that accompany this disease, but you can potentially stop it from progressing. A corticosteroid can reduce inflammation and ease symptoms, but this medication comes with its own potential side effects (such as weight gain, high blood pressure and bone damage) that need to be weighed against potential benefits. Lung transplants are a last-resort option for those who are most severely affected.

TOP THREATS

If a drug leads to ILD and an alternative medication exists, your doctor may recommend switching. Which medications are the worst offenders? *Watch out for these in particular…*

•**Chemotherapy drugs,** including *bleomycin* (Blenoxane)…*busulfan* (Myleran)…*cyclophosphamide* (Cytoxan)…and *panitumumab* (Vectibix), among others. Biologics used as cancer immunotherapies also appear on the list, including *bevacizumab* (Avastin) and *trastuzumab* (Herceptin).

•**Antiarrhythmic medications,** especially *amiodarone* (Cordarone), which treats atrial fibrillation and is the most common cardiovascular drug linked to lung problems. As many as 6% of people taking this drug develop ILD, and an estimated 10% to 20% of them die from its lung-related complications.

•**Antibiotics,** such as *nitrofurantoin* (Macrobid), which treats urinary tract infections… or *sulfamethoxazole/trimethoprim* (Bactrim), which fights ear infections, bronchitis and other bacterial infections.

•**Vasodilator drugs,** especially *hydralazine* (Apresoline), used for high blood pressure and heart failure.

•**Disease-modifying antirheumatic drugs (DMARDs),** especially *methotrexate* (Rheumatrex, Trexall, Rasuvo), which treat autoimmune conditions, such as rheumatoid arthritis and psoriasis, as well as cancer.

•**Seizure medications,** such as *phenytoin* (Dilantin) or *carbamazepine* (Tegretol).

•**Nonsteroidal anti-inflammatory drugs (NSAIDs),** such as aspirin, *ibuprofen* (Motrin) and *naproxen* (Aleve), used for pain.

Note: An NSAID user's vulnerability to ILD is highly individualized.

- **Beta-blockers,** such as *atenolol* (Tenormin) and *propranolol* (Inderal), for high blood pressure.

- **Statins,** such as *simvastatin* (Zocor) and *atorvastatin* (Lipitor), to lower cholesterol.

TAKE THESE PRECAUTIONS

It's unfortunate that drugs we need might wreak such havoc on our lungs. But there are smart precautions to take…

- **Know your baseline.** Be aware of your body's normal "feel" and function, and monitor all symptoms after you begin taking any new drug. Be alert for new or persistent trouble breathing, and consider getting a baseline spirometry test (described earlier) when starting a drug that may lead to ILD.

- **Get vaccinated.** Both the pneumococcal vaccine, which helps prevent pneumonia, and the flu vaccine, which is ideally received each year in early fall, before flu season begins, are important protections against ILD. Why? If you take a pill predisposing you to ILD and are then exposed to bacteria or viruses, it can spell double trouble for vulnerable lungs. By preventing pneumonia or the flu, the vaccines can mitigate any ripple effects from compromised lungs that may contribute to ILD.

Note: The CDC recommends the annual flu vaccine for all adults…and the pneumococcal vaccine for all adults age 65 and older and anyone ages two to 64 with certain medical conditions, such as heart disease, asthma or weakened immunity. Smokers also are advised to get the pneumococcal vaccine.

- **See your doctor promptly if you develop any breathing problems** (such as a cough, labored breathing, shallow breathing or wheezing) that seem acute or last longer than a few days. Bring a list of medications you take, and ask the doctor if your symptoms could be due to one of these drugs.

- **Get monitored.** If you take one of the drugs linked to ILD, ask your doctor to monitor your lungs with one or more of the tests described earlier.

Getting Over a Cold or the Flu?

Joseph Feuerstein, MD, assistant professor of clinical medicine at Columbia University in New York City and director of Integrative Medicine at Stamford Health in Stamford, Connecticut. He specializes in family medicine, focusing on nutrition and disease prevention. Dr. Feuerstein is also certified in clinical hypnosis, clinical acupuncture and homeopathy. He is author of *Dr. Joe's Man Diet.*

When you're sidelined by the fever and head-to-toe body aches of the flu or even the endless sneezing and coughing of a cold, it's tempting to want to get back to normal life at the first sign of feeling better. Wait! These illnesses take a toll on your body, and the flu, in particular, can set you up for serious complications.

When flu turns deadly: While the flu itself can quickly lead to lethal respiratory failure if the lungs are overtaken by inflammation, complications of the flu, such as pneumonia or sepsis, are often the actual cause of death. In some cases, being run down from a bad cold can even set the stage for pneumonia.

Whether you're battling the flu, a cold or even the recent coronavirus, here's a natural six-step recovery plan that will also help fortify you against serious complications…*

- **Get tested.** If you're sure you've got a cold, you might be able to tough it out on your own. But symptoms of the cold and flu can be similar. The distinguishing characteristics are typically the flu's rapid onset and extreme fatigue, but both illnesses can cause headache, coughing and a runny nose. A fever is more common with the flu, but not everyone with the flu will run a fever. COVID-19 symptoms are very similar to the flu.

That's why if you're not sure what's causing your illness—especially if you're over age 65…have had a heart attack or stroke…or have a chronic condition such as lung disease, diabetes or cancer—talk to your doctor about getting tested for the flu. Some nasal or throat swab tests can provide an answer in 30 minutes or less. If

*Check with your doctor before taking any supplement—especially if you have a chronic medical condition or take medications.

you do have the flu, your doctor may want to closely supervise your recovery—in some cases, with monitoring in a hospital if you're frail and/or have a chronic health problem.

Important: Don't assume that a cold is harmless. If it improves but then worsens…lingers for more than 10 days without getting better…and/or causes fever that lasts for more than three days, consult your physician. This could signal a complication such as bronchitis or pneumonia.

If you have a cold or the flu and experience shortness of breath, chest pain or a fever over 103°F, call your doctor or 911.

Caution: Respiratory infections (particularly the flu) are linked to increased risk for heart attack—especially in the week following a flu diagnosis.

•**Stay "horizontal."** There's a reason you're tired and feverish and have no appetite. Your body is forcing you to stop all activity so that it can wage an all-out effort to fight the virus. In most cases, fever is an integral part of the process—it actually stimulates your immune system to work harder than normal. What you need is lots of sleep, fluids (see next column) and bed rest!

Don't let a hectic schedule or guilt over missing obligations keep you from listening to your body. It usually takes about a week to get over a cold, but the flu can set you back for up to two weeks. It may take even longer if you were run down before getting sick or if you're managing a chronic condition, such as lung disease or diabetes, that was already stressing your system.

Important: When you must get up (to, say, go to the bathroom), do so in stages—sit up…swing your feet over the side of the bed…then stand for a few seconds before you start to walk. Prolonged bed rest can lower your blood pressure, which can cause dizziness and even fainting if you stand up too quickly.

•**Consider taking elderberry and echinacea.** Even though some people prefer to take a pharmaceutical such as *oseltamivir* (Tamiflu) for the flu, elderberry and echinacea are worth considering.

While some modern research on these botanicals has been mixed, both have been used for centuries to ease cold and flu symptoms, and a comprehensive 2017 study published in *Journal of Evidence-Based Complementary &* *Alternative Medicine* found that elderberry and echinacea were effective against cold and flu viruses.

The phytonutrients that give elderberry its deep black-purple color have been found to help stop virus cells from multiplying. Black elderberry extract is available in liquid, tablets and lozenges. Sambucol, Black Elderberry is particularly effective.

Echinacea purpurea (one of various species of echinacea) has been shown to have immune-stimulating properties. It's available in capsule, extract and liquid form.

Note: If you have allergies or asthma, be sure to check with your doctor before trying echinacea.

Some cold and flu products, such as Gaia Herbs' Quick Defense with Echinacea & Elderberry…and Solaray's Echinacea & Elderberry, contain both herbs. A combination tea, Echinacea Plus Elderberry, is available from Traditional Medicinals.

Also: To treat your fever, consider alternating the lowest possible dose of *acetaminophen* (Tylenol) and a nonsteroidal anti-inflammatory drug, such as *ibuprofen* (Motrin). This helps minimize the side effects of each medication.

Zinc supplements have been shown to significantly reduce the length and severity of cold symptoms. For a cold, try zinc lozenges within 24 hours of the start of your symptoms and for the duration of the illness.

•**Drink more fluids than you think you need.** You don't have to force yourself to eat solid foods, but liquids are essential—and you may not realize how much water you're losing when you're sweating from a fever. This can lead to dehydration, another reason for dizziness when you go from lying to standing.

My rule of thumb: Drink enough to make your urine clear. Listen to your body and stick with broth and other soups at first to avoid straining your digestive system.

•**Spice up your chicken soup.** To amp up the healing power of chicken soup, add immune-boosting, anti-inflammatory spices such as turmeric and ginger, along with garlic. Use as much as you can tolerate of each to taste. When you are ready for solid food, start with healthy starches such as oatmeal and whole-wheat toast. It takes more effort for your body to digest raw fruits and vegetables, so try to avoid them until you've recovered.

•**Pace your reentry.** The common rule of thumb is to wait at least 24 hours after your fever is gone before returning to your usual activities, but that can be too soon. Whether it's work, household chores or hobbies, the more physical activity that's involved—even standing for long periods of time—the more gradual your return should be.

As for resuming your exercise regimen, wait until you have gone back to your normal diet… and start with slow-to-moderate walking for 10 minutes. It could take a week or more to get back to your full workout schedule.

For more on natural help with COVID-19 recovery, see pages 83-84.

Surprising Ways That Winter Affects Your Health

Drew Koch, DO, FACOEP-D, MBA, a board-certified physician in emergency medicine at Guthrie Robert Packer Hospital in Sayre, Pennsylvania, and clinical assistant professor of emergency medicine in the department of clinical sciences at Geisinger Commonwealth School of Medicine in Scranton, Pennsylvania. He is a Distinguished Fellow of the American College of Osteopathic Emergency Physicians.

Cold weather is rough on health. Colds and cases of life-threatening flu are rampant. Ice and snow increase the risk for dangerous falls.

Those problems are bad enough. But there also are hidden health dangers of winter that few people know about—problems that can turn you into a seasonal statistic.

Death rates are 25% higher in winter than in summer—with winter triggering more circulatory, breathing, hormonal and digestive problems, according to recent research published in *The Journal of Steroid Biochemistry and Molecular Biology.*

Cold-weather risks to guard against…

•**Dehydration.** It sounds like a summer issue, but dehydration is a big cold weather risk, too, since the problem is less obvious this time of year.

For one thing, sweat evaporates more rapidly in cold, dry air, tricking you into thinking you're not losing a lot of water from your body. But you are.

The body's thirst response is reduced as well when temperatures are cooler, so you may not drink enough water.

Medications play a role, too. People who take fluid-draining drugs, such as diuretics, as well as other medications for high blood pressure, heart disease and kidney disorders are at increased risk for dehydration. *What to do…*

•Drink more water. If you have mild-to-moderate dehydration, marked by such symptoms as a dry, sticky mouth, sleepiness, dry skin, headache and/or dizziness, drink more water!

Chronic diseases—particularly diabetes, kidney disease and heart failure—put you at higher risk for dehydration year-round. If you have a chronic medical condition, ask your doctor for advice on how much fluid you should drink.

•Call 911. If you have symptoms of severe dehydration, such as extreme thirst…irritability and confusion…feeling faint…little or no urination…sunken eyes…shriveled and dry skin (it lacks elasticity and doesn't "bounce back" when pinched into a fold), this is a medical emergency, and you need to be rehydrated with intravenous fluids immediately.

•**High blood pressure.** When temperatures fall, your body conserves heat by constricting blood vessels—and those tightened vessels can lead to high blood pressure, which increases risk for heart attack and stroke.

Scientific evidence: The average systolic (top number) blood pressure reading was 5 mmHg higher in winter than in summer, according to a study of adults age 65 or older and published in *Archives of Internal Medicine.*

Even though everyone is at risk for cold weather increases in blood pressure, you're especially vulnerable if you've already been diagnosed with high blood pressure. *What to do…*

•Talk to your doctor if you take blood pressure medication. The dose of antihypertensive medication you take in the summer may not be high enough for winter control.

•Dress warmly. To avoid blood pressure spikes when you're outside in the winter, dress in layers and wear a hat, scarf and gloves. (Cold hands alone can spike blood pressure for hours.)

•Keep it toasty indoors. Cooler indoor temperatures have been linked to higher blood pressure, according to a study published in *Journal of Hypertension. Researchers* advise people with high blood pressure to keep indoor temperatures at around 70°F.

•Don't overexert yourself. People with high blood pressure can have a heart attack if they're unfit and try to shovel snow. *Smart step:* Ask your doctor to assess your overall health and give his/her OK for such activity before winter starts or initiating any exercise program. And if you do shovel snow, take breaks every 10 minutes or so and make sure you're dressed warmly and are well-hydrated.

•Get your vitamin D-3 level checked. Blood levels of this sunshine- produced vitamin can plummet during the winter—with research published in *Circulation* linking low levels to high blood pressure…and to nearly twice the risk for heart attack, stroke and heart failure. Ask your doctor to test your vitamin D-3 level. If it's lower than 30 ng/mL, take 2,000 international units (IU) of vitamin D daily throughout the winter.

•**Neuropathy.** Cold slows the flow of blood to your hands and feet. With this decreased circulation, there's an increase in symptoms of peripheral neuropathy—prickling, burning nerve pain in the hands and feet, along with numbness. The most common causes of peripheral neuropathy are diabetes and chemotherapy. *What to do…*

•Keep your hands and feet warm. When you're outside in the cold, wear thick gloves and thick socks. Dress in layers and always wear a hat.

•Keep your feet dry. Because peripheral neuropathy reduces sensation, it's sometimes hard to know if your feet are damp and cold. As soon as you get home from being outside in winter weather, remove your shoes and socks, dry your feet and put on a fresh pair of socks and warm slippers.

•Wear sheepskin gloves and sheepskin slippers to bed to help keep hands and feet warm during a long, cold winter night.

•Exercise regularly—indoors. Use a treadmill or stationary bicycle to exercise regularly. Regular aerobic exercise will improve your circulation, and core-strengthening exercises will help prevent falls. *Helpful:* Get an exercise prescription from a physical therapist.

•**Chronic obstructive pulmonary disease (COPD).** The number of COPD "exacerbations"—worsening symptoms such as breathlessness, requiring corticosteroids, antibiotics and/or hospitalization—double during winter, according to research published in *European Respiratory Journal.*

COPD sufferers take a hit for several reasons. For example, up to 70% of COPD exacerbations are triggered by bacterial or viral infections, which tend to peak in the winter. Low blood levels of vitamin D in wintertime may worsen the disease.

How to protect yourself from wintertime COPD exacerbations…

•Wear a scarf or mask when outside in cold, dry air—and avoid exercising outside in excessively cold temperatures.

•Wash your hands several times a day. It's the number one way to minimize your risk for infections from a cold or flu virus. Use warm water and soap. An alcohol-based hand sanitizer is fine if you don't have access to water.

•Get a flu shot. Protection is a must if you have COPD, which makes you far more susceptible to the flu and pneumonia. You should also get vaccinated for pneumonia. Talk to your doctor about the appropriate vaccination schedule for you.

•Boost your immunity. Load up on whole foods (phytochemicals in vegetables, fruits, beans and other whole foods strengthen the immune system)…and limit processed foods. Consider taking a multivitamin mineral supplement, with immune-strengthening vitamin C and zinc.

•Take vitamin D. A team of international researchers found that daily or weekly supplementation with vitamin D was safe and significantly reduced respiratory infections in people with COPD. Daily doses in research have ranged from 300 IU to 4,000 IU daily. Consult your doctor for the dose that's right for you.

Important: Cold, dry air can trigger asthma attacks, too. If you have a history of asthma, wear a mask or scarf when outdoors and avoid temperatures below 10°F when you're active.

Daily Steroid Inhaler Useless for Many Asthmatics

Stephen Lazarus, MD, professor of medicine at University of California, San Francisco, and director of the university's training program in pulmonary and critical care medicine. UCSFHealth.org

Doctors often instruct patients suffering from mild persistent asthma to use a steroid inhaler every day—but nearly half of those patients receive no noticeable benefit from doing so, according to a recent study published in *The New England Journal of Medicine.*

The study divided asthmatics into two groups—those who had high levels of a type of white blood cell called *eosinophils* in their sputum (phlegm) and those who did not. High levels of eosinophils are an indicator of a specific type of inflammation, and for patients suffering from this inflammation, the study confirmed that daily steroid use is beneficial. But 73% of the mild persistent asthma sufferers who participated in the study did not have indications of this type of inflammation—and for two-thirds of this larger group, daily steroid use was no more effective than a placebo. What's more, daily steroid use is expensive and can have adverse side effects—including increased risk for bone loss, cataracts and glaucoma.

If a daily steroid is not providing any noticeable improvement, ask your health-care provider…

"Can you confirm I'm using my inhaler properly?" Improper inhaler use is more common than people realize. If this fails to solve the problem, ask…

"Is it worth trying a different treatment option, such as a *long-acting muscarinic antago-*

Ozone-Safe Inhaler Not So Safe

Primatene Mist, the metered-dose epinephrine inhaler that was recalled in 2011, is now ozone safe, newly FDA-approved and available over-the-counter. However, respiratory health groups, including the American Lung Association, point out that epinephrine inhalers, such as Primatene Mist, are not recommended for asthma by any expert guidelines…and may tempt patients to self-treat rather than get proper medical care. Prescription albuterol and corticosteroid inhalers are safer, more effective and longer lasting.

Michael Blaiss, MD, executive medical director, American College of Allergy, Asthma & Immunology, Atlanta. ACAAI.org

nist (LAMA)?" LAMA is traditionally used for COPD. A LAMA inhaler can be effective for some asthma sufferers, with few side effects (notably, dry mouth).

Note: As yet, there is no easy and accurate way to test eosinophil levels—you may just have to try a LAMA and see if it works.

Asthma Alert Sticker

University of California, Irvine.

A "smart" sticker that adheres to an asthma patient's body may be able to detect breathing changes that signal an impending attack.

Hookah Smoke High in Toxins

American Heart Association statement on hookah use, published in *Circulation.*

About 5% of high school students and almost 14% of 18-to-24-year-olds in the US report using hookahs, often mistakenly believing that smoking tobacco from a hookah is less harmful because the tobacco is filtered through water. In addition to nicotine, hookah smoke contains other potentially harmful chemicals, particulate matter, volatile organics, lead, cadmium and arsenic—at levels that usually are higher than in cigarette smoke.

Vaping May Increase Susceptibility to the Flu

Meghan Rebuli, PhD, is a postdoctoral research associate at Center for Environmental Medicine, Asthma and Lung Biology, University of North Carolina at Chapel Hill.

E-cigarette users' immune response to a dose of FluMist (a vaccine that contains a live attenuated flu virus) was more suppressed than that of cigarette smokers and nonsmokers, suggesting that the immune response to the live virus in the vaccine was less effective for e-cigarette users. Preliminary findings show female response was more affected than male, though researchers still are investigating why.

This "Silent" Sleep Problem Stumps Even Some Doctors

Steven Y. Park, MD, assistant professor of otolaryngology at Albert Einstein College of Medicine in New York City. Dr. Park's research has been published in *Journal of Sleep Research* and other professional journals. He is author of *Sleep, Interrupted*. DoctorStevenPark.com

Ask people to name a disorder that interferes with a good night's shut-eye, and chances are obstructive sleep apnea (OSA) is what you'll hear.

But a little-known condition—often referred to as OSA's "silent sister"—also leads to unexplained daytime fatigue and can even contribute to seemingly unrelated health problems (see below). The problem is, the typical red flags that patients—and doctors—look for when zeroing in on a sleep disorder, such as loud snoring and gasping during sleep, often are missing.

This mysterious sleep saboteur is called upper airway resistance syndrome (UARS). Like

OSA, it causes multiple, micro-awakenings that occur when the sufferer unconsciously senses difficulty breathing while sleeping. The person will soon fall back to sleep only to awaken again, seconds or minutes later. This cycle can continue throughout the night—without the sufferer (or bed partner) even realizing it. But there are subtle differences between OSA and UARS. *What you need to know...*

HOW TO DETECT THIS "SILENT" DISORDER

No one knows exactly how many people have UARS. However, in a study of 527 subjects in a military hospital who had daytime fatigue, the prevalence was 8.4%, according to research published in the journal *Chest.*

Unlike OSA, in which breathing completely stops for tens of seconds at a time, breathing is merely impaired with UARS. The condition can be caused by a naturally narrowed airway (as may occur in a person who is thin)...an ill-positioned tongue (if it relaxes and partially covers the airway)...or loose throat tissues that interfere with breathing.

Some people with UARS go on to develop OSA, but many do not. As a result, these individuals can have UARS for years (or even a lifetime) without it being diagnosed and treated.

When UARS goes undetected, the repeated micro-awakenings cause sufferers to become not only tired and stressed in the daytime but may also make them highly sensitive to emotional triggers, light, sounds and weather changes.

The ongoing anxiety that so often accompanies UARS also can lead to tension headaches and depression. In research published in *Respiration*, the continual stress and lack of restorative sleep that mark UARS have been linked to the development of digestive symptoms, such as irritable bowel disease, and increased cardiovascular risks due to blood pressure spikes that can occur with the repeated micro-awakenings.

DO YOU HAVE THIS DISORDER?

If you have daytime fatigue, with or without the health problems that can accompany UARS, consider seeing a dentist or a sleep specialist who is familiar with the disorder—not all physicians are. Before scheduling an appointment, call the physician's office and ask whether he/she treats UARS.

A knowledgeable specialist will inspect the back of the mouth, nose and jaw to see whether the person's airway appears unobstructed to the eye.

A surprising clue: Crooked teeth or a "scalloped" tongue, in which ridges or indentations on the sides of the tongue indicate where it pushes against the molars, can indicate a crowded jaw and partially obstructed airway.

If UARS is suspected, the next step is a sleep study, in which the number and frequency of *respiratory effort-related arousals* (RERAs) are monitored. These arousals from sleep do not technically meet the definition of *apneas* (pauses in breathing) or *hypopneas* (periods of shallow breathing), both of which occur with OSA.

Note: A sleep study performed in a lab is more sensitive to the subtle obstructions that accompany UARS than in-home studies.

If apneas and hypopneas last for more than 10 seconds, they qualify as a sleep breathing event, and more than five such events an hour points to OSA if you have other symptoms such as daytime sleepiness, cognitive dysfunction or high blood pressure. When the patient does not have OSA, a high number of RERAs may suggest UARS.

Recent development: A procedure called drug-induced sleep endoscopy has emerged as a useful technique for diagnosing UARS. With this procedure, which is performed with the patient under sedation, a surgeon will insert a small camera through the nose into the airway to view any blockages that affect breathing during sleep.

3 SELF-CARE MEASURES

Even without an official diagnosis, people who suffer from unexplained daytime fatigue and suspect that they may have UARS can take steps to improve the disorder. *For example...*

•**Don't eat within three hours of bedtime.**

Here's why: When a person with UARS has difficulty breathing, stomach juices get sucked up into the throat causing swelling and more obstruction. Meal timing helps prevent this.

•**Choose the right sleep position.** Sleeping on your side or stomach (though this can trigger back pain in some people) helps many individuals with UARS. When sleeping on your back, it's easy for the tongue to fall back into the throat area and partially block the airway.

•**Try simple oral exercises.** Strengthening your airway muscles will help prevent UARS by reducing the odds that the muscles will collapse and impair breathing.

What to do: With an exercise called the "tongue slide," you push the tip of your tongue against the roof of your mouth and slide your tongue backward and forward, repeating the motion 20 times. Do this several times daily while working or watching TV.

WHEN MORE HELP IS NEEDED

If the steps above aren't adequate, you may need one of the following...*

•**Mouth guard.** If your dentist thinks you may have UARS due to a misaligned jaw, you can be fitted with a personalized mouth guard—known as a *mandibular advancement device* (MAD)—that slightly pushes the lower jaw and tongue forward to hold the airway open when the throat muscles relax. This prevents the airway from collapsing during deep sleep.

•**Bone-growth appliance.** Some dentists can fit an orthodontic device (known as an *anterior growth guidance appliance*), which can stimulate bone growth by allowing the jaw to expand outward, ultimately providing more space to breathe while sleeping. It is usually worn all day and night for up to two years.

•**CPAP.** Continuous positive airway pressure (CPAP) devices send a constant flow of air pressure into the throat to ensure that the airway stays open during sleep. CPAP is usually used for OSA but also helps relieve UARS.

•**Surgery.** The most definitive treatment for UARS is surgery to physically alter the anatomy of the breathing airway. This may involve, for example, stiffening of loose palate tissue and/or the placement of an implant.

The good news is that people who have been successfully treated for UARS report waking up

*Most insurers do not cover these treatments unless UARS progresses to OSA.

refreshed, as well as having a better quality of life and a reduced risk for the health problems related to this disorder.

You're Never Too Old for a New Allergy

Neeta Ogden, MD, an allergist in private practice in Edison, New Jersey. She is a member of the Medical-Scientific Council of the Allergy and Asthma Foundation of America and a spokesperson for the American College of Allergy, Asthma and Immunology. NeetaOgdenMD.com

You're sniffling. You're sneezing. You're itching. Is it a cold? A rash? You're too old for it to be an allergy, right? Wrong. Kids aren't the only ones who develop new allergies. In fact, adult-onset allergies are more common than you think.

A study published recently in *JAMA Network Open* found that among people who have food allergies, nearly half developed at least one of their allergies during adulthood. Researchers who study allergies are not certain what is to blame for this general trend of growing allergies in both kids and adults. Some have speculated that it could be related to changes in our habits, such as the overuse of hand sanitizers and antibiotics…as well as changes in our diets.

Adult-onset environmental allergies are more common as well, possibly because rising temperatures are leading to larger amounts of pollen in the air. Those pollen rates also are believed to be responsible for increasing rates of environmental allergies among children.

Here's what you need to know about adult-onset food and environmental allergies…

FOOD ALLERGIES

If you have a bad reaction to shellfish (hives, itching, breathing problems)—even if it has never happened to you before—odds are that you are allergic. In fact, the most common adult-onset food allergy is to shellfish.

Other likely allergens: Seafood, tree nuts, soy and peanuts, among other foods.

Potential symptoms: Food allergy sufferers typically experience itching and/or hives within minutes or up to an hour and a half to two hours after consuming the food. Sufferers also might experience coughing, difficulty breathing, abdominal pain, nausea, vomiting, light-headedness and/or swelling of the lips, face, throat and/or tongue.

Some exceptions…

Recently, an allergy to red meat including beef and pork has been reported—the allergy is to a carbohydrate called alpha-gal, which can enter the body from a Lone Star tick bite. When someone who has been bitten subsequently eats red meat, he/she can suffer an allergic reaction that is atypical because it occurs several hours after consuming the red meat.

It's also important to distinguish between an intolerance and an allergy. Symptoms such as cramps, gas, diarrhea and bloating that occur several hours after eating, without itchiness or hives, may suggest an intolerance or your body's inability to digest that food, but you are not allergic to it. Unlike allergies, these digestive issues do not occur because your immune response has misidentified a molecule in the food as something harmful.

Example: Many adults who have consumed dairy products without any issues for their entire lives suddenly start to experience cramping or gas after drinking milk or eating ice cream. These people have not developed a dairy allergy—they have developed lactose intolerance. Their digestive systems no longer produce enough of the lactase enzyme needed to digest a sugar found in dairy foods.

If you experience mild tingling or itching in your lips, tongue and/or throat after consuming certain fruits and vegetables, you might have a condition known as oral allergy syndrome, a very mild form of food allergy that actually suggests that you have a pollen allergy (see next page for more about pollen allergies). A protein in the fruit or vegetable is so similar to a protein in pollen that your body is misidentifying it. Causes of common oral allergies include apples, carrots, celery, corn, kiwis, lettuce, oranges, peaches, peppers and tomatoes. *What to do…*

•**If you have a reaction that includes difficulty breathing,** seek immediate medical attention. Many people don't realize that they can fall victim to allergies as adults and may try to convince themselves that it is something else, such as a stomach bug or flu. That can be a dangerous mistake. Call 911. A person having a serious allergic reaction needs epinephrine right away to ensure that his airways stay open.

After experiencing any allergic reaction, write down everything you had consumed in the 90 minutes before symptoms appeared, as well as any meats you ate in the five hours prior to symptoms. Do this even if it was a relatively mild reaction that did not require immediate medical attention. If possible, write down not just the names of the food products consumed, but a complete list of ingredients in those products. If appropriate, take digital photos of the ingredients lists on food packaging.

•**Schedule an appointment to see an allergist approximately one month after your allergic response.** Bring your list of suspect foods and ingredients to this appointment. Why wait a month to see an allergist? The allergist likely will conduct tests to determine what you are allergic to, and the odds of inaccurate test results increase during the weeks following an allergic reaction. In the meantime, avoid foods that you suspect might be the cause of your reaction—particularly the most likely culprits, such as shellfish and other seafood, nuts and soy.

Note: An initial mild allergic reaction does not guarantee that future reactions also will be mild—your next response could include potentially fatal anaphylaxis, which can constrict airways and cause a rapid drop in blood pressure.

Warning: Do not try to confirm whether you have the allergy by consuming suspect foods again.

If you do have a food allergy, the allergist likely will recommend that you avoid the food and carry an EpiPen Auto-Injector, a device that can be used to self-inject epinephrine if you were to have a severe allergic reaction in the future. Continued follow-up with your allergist—and yearly blood work—will help confirm if your allergy is persisting or has gone away.

ENVIRONMENTAL ALLERGIES

It's no secret that pollen, dust mites, mold spores and pet dander can trigger environmental allergies. But many adults are taken off guard when they suddenly develop environmental allergies, also called seasonal allergies or nasal allergies, in the years following a move to a different part of the country. There might be higher pollen levels in this new place…or different types of pollen than they have been exposed to in the past. Many people are allergic to certain types of pollen but not others. Similarly, their new home might harbor more dust or animal dander.

Potential symptoms: People who have environmental allergies often feel as though they have colds that they can't seem to shake, complete with runny noses, watery eyes and sneezing. But allergy sufferers typically also experience an itchy feeling in the throat and, potentially, in the eyes, nose and/or skin as well. If the allergy is to pollen, there likely will be a seasonal predictability to the symptoms—these people might believe they "come down with colds" every spring or fall, for example.

What to do: Adult-onset environmental allergies are far less likely than food allergies to be life-threatening, though they can be very uncomfortable. People who experience them rarely require emergency medical attention or an EpiPen. It sometimes is possible to control the symptoms of environmental allergies on one's own with over-the-counter medications such as antihistamines or steroid nasal sprays, but speak with your doctor before using these.

Important: If you know that your environmental allergies appear predictably at a certain time of year, start taking these medications approximately two weeks before then. If you wait until the full-blown season to start medications, your allergy symptoms may be harder to get under control.

Resource: Pollen.com gives local allergy forecasts on its national allergy map.

•**If over-the-counter medications fail to provide relief, see an allergist.** The allergist might be able to fine-tune your use of over-the-counter medications or prescribe allergy shots or oral allergy immunotherapy. An allergist also can perform skin tests or blood tests to determine precisely which allergens are causing your problems, and he could suggest other solutions.

Example: Perhaps you are allergic to dust mites, not pollen. If so, your symptoms might be dramatically reduced if you use allergen-proof bedding or a mattress cover, wash it frequently in water heated to at least 130°F, dust your home frequently using a damp rag, remove carpeting and/or install a HEPA filter air purifier.

Best Ways to Minimize Dust to Beat Allergies

Gabriel Filippelli, PhD, professor of earth sciences and director of the Center for Urban Health at Indiana University–Purdue University Indianapolis. He is a researcher with 360 Dust Analysis, a new project in which scientists are analyzing the contents of consumers' vacuums and gaining insight into the health dangers of dust, and editor in chief of GeoHealth. 360DustAnalysis.com

---

Scientists define dust as fine particulate matter that is made up of dirt, organic material, pollen and human and animal skin cells. Dust is also produced by mold spores and cigarette smoke. Although dust can enter your home when you open a window, about one-third of household dust is created inside your home.

It's no surprise that a major cause of dust is pets. Dogs and cats shed dander from their skin, which causes allergies for many people. And dust mites, another well-known allergen, feed off pet dander and skin cells shed by people. *Other sources of dust in the home…*

•**Textiles.** Carpets, bed linens and clothing are common sources of dust. The fabrics these items are composed of break down over time and give off chemicals that get absorbed into the dust we breathe. The routine use of flame retardants and surface protectants on textiles stopped when researchers demonstrated that these chemicals made their way into human blood and tissue. But other harmful chemicals, such as Teflon, are still used in textiles and can end up in household dust.

•**Lead.** The federal government banned consumer use of lead-containing paint in 1978. But lead paint is still present in millions of homes, under layers of newer paint, contributing to lead in house dust. Children exposed to lead can experience behavioral and learning problems, slowed growth, hearing problems and anemia.

•**Chemicals tracked in from outside.** Shoes worn outdoors pick up cancer-causing toxins from asphalt road residue, lawn chemicals that can disrupt the endocrine system (glands that produce hormones that regulate many functions in the body) and much more. Also, researchers find that 96% of shoes have traces of feces on their soles.

Other problems: We all know that dust can cause eye irritation, sneezing and coughing. But for people with asthma or chronic obstructive pulmonary disease (COPD), even small increases in dust can worsen symptoms.

BEST WAYS TO MINIMIZE DUST

Sweeping with a broom or using a feather duster just stirs up dust and spreads it around. *To reduce dust…*

•**Vacuum at least once a week using a vacuum with a high-efficiency particulate air (HEPA) filter,** which mechanically forces air through a fine mesh that traps harmful particles such as pollen, pet dander, dust mites and tobacco smoke particles. A HEPA vacuum filter will also trap harmful metals, such as lead, and chemicals in dust. A stand-alone HEPA air purifier is helpful, too.

•**Run an air conditioner.** Central air-conditioning can filter the entire home, and window air conditioners can help as well. Filters for a central system should be changed at the frequency recommended by the manufacturer. Filters for window units should be washed monthly and thoroughly dried.

•**Before entering your home, take off your shoes.** Change into slippers reserved for indoor use.

•**Make cleaning simple.** Mix one-part white vinegar with nine-parts water, dip a cloth in the mixture and wipe down surfaces. This is one of the most effective ways to get rid of dust, including lead dust, and helps to eliminate bacteria. And it's chemical-free.

•**Don't use antimicrobial cleaning products and hand soaps.** A recent study found that the antimicrobial chemical triclosan, which the FDA banned in antibacterial soaps in 2016 after discovering dangerous side effects, including possible impact on the endocrine system, is abundant in dust, resulting in organisms that can cause antibiotic-resistant infection. Triclosan is still used in consumer products that may not list it on the label. Plus, other antibacterial chemicals are used instead and may have the same impact on dust as triclosan.

•**Wash hands with plain soap and water,** and use vinegar (see above) to clean.

•**Be sure to use dust-blocking covers on your mattresses and pillows,** and when possible, replace carpets with hardwood flooring or tile.

IV Nutrient Therapy for Asthma and Allergy Relief

Laurie Steelsmith, ND, LAc, licensed naturopathic physician and acupuncturist in private practice in Honolulu. She writes Bottom Line's "Natural Healing Secrets for Women" blog and is coauthor of three books—*Natural Choices for Women's Health, Great Sex, Naturally* and *Growing Younger Every Day.* DrSteelsmith.com

---

The patient: "Stephanie," a 40-year-old nurse and avid cyclist.

Why she came to see me: Stephanie was clearly keyed up when she walked into my office for the first time. While originally from Hawaii—where my natural health center is based—she'd spent the last decade working at a hospital in Portland, Oregon. Shortly after returning to Oahu a year earlier, her body, as she put it, "went haywire." High stress was overwhelming her from morning to night. A rash had been breaking out on her face intermittently; the rest of her body felt relentlessly itchy, even her ears. Her eyelids were often swollen. She'd also been struck by either a cold or the flu every two to three months. And while she'd suffered from asthma and allergies for as long as she could recall, they had reached unbearable levels upon her return to the islands. In short, she was exhausted, anxious, itchy, constantly coughing—and incredibly frustrated.

How I evaluated her: I began our work together by striving to get a complete picture of Stephanie's medical history and lifestyle.

Stephanie had worked as a nurse in Honolulu for several years before a chance encounter with a fellow cyclist compelled her to try out a new life in Portland. There, she enjoyed a respite from the asthma and allergies she'd been diagnosed with in her teens, in part by leading a healthy lifestyle with her partner. When she and her partner amicably split, she wanted to be closer to her family and friends in Hawaii. She secured a work transfer, scored a great apartment and came home to start anew.

But the stress of relocating—no matter that she was returning "home"—seemed to have upset her "entire system," she said. Her asthma returned with a vengeance, as did her allergies. Her new primary care physician prescribed at least a year's worth of nasal steroids, inhalers and oral *prednisone* (a corticosteroid medication commonly used to treat allergies, skin diseases, immune system disorders and more).

They proved to be ineffective: Her symptoms only seemed to worsen, and she loathed the idea of relying on a series of medications to merely make it through the day. She had also seen an allergist, who provided "symptomatic relief" but not a cure.

Lastly, Stephanie had seen a dermatologist, who was concerned she may have an autoimmune condition such as lupus. To this end, the dermatologist had done a biopsy of the skin on her forehead. (Fortunately, the pathology report only revealed what appeared to be an allergic response.)

Meanwhile, Stephanie claimed she was getting sicker and sicker—so much so she frequently canceled on friends, called in sick to work, relied upon her mother for assistance and tried to find relief for her consistently-itchy skin and asthma attacks by watching Netflix and eating take-out and ice cream inside her air-conditioned apartment—dietary "snags" she tried to undo with copious glasses of lemon-infused water and short sessions on her apartment complex's indoor bike. "I came back to Hawaii to enjoy the beautiful outdoors and restart my life," she said unpityingly, just factually. "And now

I'm too uncomfortable and afraid to spend time outdoors. This is no life at all."

To get to the bottom of Stephanie's litany of symptoms, I did a full physical exam. This was followed by a blood test that would evaluate for food allergies and her levels of copper and zinc. I also ordered a stool culture to assess for yeast, bacteria and parasites.

What my evaluation revealed: Stephanie's results demonstrated that she was allergic to a number of foods and compounds, many of which she regularly consumed. These included gluten, dairy, beef, MSG, several food colorings and that lemon she ingested daily.

Her blood test demonstrated that she had a surplus of copper relative to zinc, which can contribute to inflammation and anxiety. She also had low vitamin D levels, which arrived as no surprise, given that she'd spent 10 years in rainy Portland and had willfully sequestered herself inside in Hawaii. (As I told Stephanie, low vitamin D levels impact immunity and the body's ability to fight off infection. It can also exacerbate anxiety and contribute to the health and metabolism of skin.) Finally, her stool culture revealed an imbalance in her intestinal flora: too much yeast, too little "friendly" gut bacteria and a slight overgrowth of a potentially-pathogenic flora. In sum, the foods Stephanie was consuming and the products she was using—from sausage on her pizza to her favorite face wash—were triggering a full-body inflammatory response, leaving her with aggravated asthmatic symptoms, anxiety and atopic dermatitis.

Note that Stephanie did not change her diet when she came back to Hawaii. She simply couldn't tolerate certain foods and chemicals anymore. Probably her detoxification systems were overwhelmed, and she most likely had leaky gut leading to excess allergy, increased systemic inflammation and an overwhelmed liver. The stress of the move was probably her tipping point.

How I addressed her problem: To restore Stephanie to the health she'd enjoyed for most of her life, we began with dietary treatment, as it was inarguable that she needed to eliminate any and all potential allergens. In addition to ridding herself of the foods mentioned above—gluten, dairy, lemon, beef, MSG and any food that contained food colorings (to be on the safe side)—I asked her to toss or donate her facial and body care products and start fresh with organic items that were comprised of natural ingredients. (Even the toothpaste she'd begun buying in Hawaii contained a dye that has been linked to hypersensitivity.) I also advised her to be especially careful of tartrazine. Also known as FD&C Yellow #5—and found in many brands of that ice cream she loved—it's been shown to result in hives, swelling, skin rashes and asthma.

Additionally, I prescribed Stephanie a set of dietary supplements to help decrease her allergic reactivity. *These included…*

• **Quercetin,** a flavonoid that has potent anti-inflammatory capacities

• **Zinc,** to help lower her copper levels

• **Vitamin A** to naturally support her immune system and mucous membranes.

• **Vitamins B5 and B1,** which organically promote adrenal health and the breakdown of histamine

• **SAMe (S-adenosyl-L-methionine),** a sulfur-based compound, to support hormone and cell function (and, thus, overall health).

I further suggested she take a probiotic to re-establish a healthy ratio of intestinal flora, and weekly acupuncture sessions to help her strengthen her qi (or life force).

Perhaps the biggest step I asked Stephanie to take was to sign up for intravenous (IV) nutrient therapy. Presently gaining a great deal of attention for its rapidity and efficacy, intravenous nutrient therapy is favored in hospitals and beyond to treat patients whose immune systems have been compromised. Administered directly into the blood, the nutrients used in these therapeutic cocktails bypass the intestines, which allows for direct and immediate access to cells. What's more, high doses of nutrients that would not be tolerated if ingested can be used, thereby accelerating the healing process and providing profound biochemical shifts that foster healthy change. An example is magnesium—an IV of high dose magnesium doesn't cause diarrhea but taking it orally could have this side effect. Also, glutathione, which is not very stable when taken orally but IV administration allows for therapeutic doses to be administered.

Now used in a variety of settings, the therapy has been shown to be beneficial in a variety of ways, including detoxification, sports recovery (such as pre and post marathon running, or high intense sports like Iron Man competitions), inflammatory conditions, allergies, supportive cancer care, eczema, chronic fatigue syndrome, autoimmune conditions, chronic tick infections and chronic viral conditions. I personally use it for jet lag and any time I'm in a weakened immune state and I feel like I'm about to come down with a cold. IV nutrient therapy is also used to "pre-condition" patients before surgery or an intense sports event. And it's recommended to expedite healing after a stressful occurrence, such as chemotherapy. I have found IV nutrient therapy has been key towards helping many of my patients restore *homeostasis* (balance in the body).

In Stephanie's case, the IV bag she would receive during treatments would include high doses of Vitamin C and magnesium with cofactor minerals and B-complex vitamins. This therapy has been shown to be particularly effective against asthma attacks and other disorders. I also added intravenous glutathione. While naturally produced in the body, high doses of this powerful antioxidant help shield the body from free radical damage and clear toxins like heavy metals from the blood and liver.

The patient's progress: Six weeks later, Stephanie was a changed woman. She'd found the dietary changes I'd recommended easier than imagined, exchanging traditional pizza for pies made with gluten-free cauliflower crusts, antioxidant-rich vegetables and dairy-free "cheese"…and swapping milk-heavy ice cream for dairy-free Coconut Bliss. While she still suffered from the occasional bout of atopic dermatitis, her skin was otherwise glowing, thanks in large part to the synthetic-free skincare brand she'd discovered.

Her real breakthrough—as we both noted—arrived with the sixth intravenous glutathione therapy I gave her. At that point, we'd increased her dosage of glutathione from 200 mg to 2,000 mg, which made a tremendous difference in terms of her symptoms. (In tradi-

tional naturopathic medicine, treating the liver is the golden chalice to healing from allergies and asthma, and glutathione is famed for its impact on this fundamental organ.) Her eyes had stopped swelling, the rash on her face had completely disappeared and her asthma attacks were far less frequent and destabilizing.

"I feel like my old self again, only even better than before," she said, stating that her fatigue was gone and her vitality had announced itself again. The first thing she planned to do with all that energy? To get outdoors on her bike, of course, and savor the paradise she'd missed.

Beware of Sesame Allergy

Ruchi Gupta, MD, MPH, director, Science and Outcomes of Allergy and Asthma Research, Northwestern University and Lurie Children's Hospital, both in Chicago.

More than 1.5 million adults and children in the US are allergic to sesame—and the condition is often undiagnosed.

Problem: Because the seeds are not included among the eight allergens that the FDA mandates for listing on food labels, consumers could be at risk for potentially serious allergic reactions. Sesame is found in many foods such as ethnic dishes (including sushi) and sauces (including tahini).

Note: Sesame-related ingredients are often identified with unfamiliar terms, such as "benne," "gingelly" or "simsim."

Cat Allergy Vaccine in the Works

The Journal of Allergy and Clinical Immunology

Swiss scientists are developing a vaccine that would neutralize an allergen that affects nearly 10% of humans in the Western population. The vaccine, which is administered to the animal, was found in a study involving 54 cats to be well tolerated and effective in protecting allergic patients.

Plants May Be Better Than Technology for Reducing Air Pollution

Bhavik Bakshi, PhD, professor of chemical and biomolecular engineering, The Ohio State University, Columbus, and leader of a study published in *Environmental Science & Technology*.

They could be cheaper and more effective at cleaning the air near industrial sites, roadways, power plants and oil and gas drilling areas. Restoring plants and trees to landscapes near pollution sources could reduce pollution by an average of 27%. The effect would occur in urban and rural areas, with real-world success rates depending on how much land was available for plant growth and how much pollution was already present. But there was only one specific sector studied—industrial boilers—in which technology would be cheaper for cleaning the air than extensive ecosystem upgrades.

How to Stop Choking on Your Own Saliva...

Murray Grossan, MD, ear, nose and throat specialist, Cedars-Sinai Medical Center, Los Angeles. GrossanInstitute.com

Choking and coughing from inhaling our own saliva has happened to most of us. And in most cases, the embarrassment while red-faced, spluttering and trying to catch a breath is the worst thing to worry about.

If you're otherwise healthy, the most common cause of choking on saliva is just being in a rush. We are all automatically swallowing our saliva all day. But actions such as talking too quickly, laughing too hard or turning your head quickly while swallowing can cause the normal automatic swallowing to turn into an inhalation—with the obvious result. You've probably already figured out the helpful tip here: Slow down!

On the other hand, your mouth may be too dry. Normally, salivary glands produce two to four pints of saliva daily. If you have dry mouth, not only do you not produce enough saliva but the saliva you do produce is thick and stringy—and easier to choke on.

Dry mouth can be caused by a number of things, including dehydration, mouth breathing, antihistamines, blood pressure drugs and certain other medications.

What helps: Mouthwashes and oral rinses made especially for dry mouth help stimulate the flow of saliva. Good brands to try are Biotene and ACT. Chewing gum also can get your salivary juices flowing. Sipping water frequently throughout the day also helps. Ask your doctor whether a medication you're taking causes dry mouth and, if so, whether switching to an alternative makes sense.

Another cause of thick saliva is having too much mucus in your nasal passages, possibly because of postnasal drip from a cold or allergies. Using a saline nasal spray, a neti pot or a pulsating water nasal irrigation device can thin mucus and open clogged sinuses—as can drinking hot beverages.

If these remedies don't help, or you if you seem to be choking on saliva frequently—especially if choking happens not just from saliva but also when you try to swallow foods or drinks—you should talk to your regular doctor or an otolaryngologist to rule out another health problem. There are many conditions ranging from mild to serious that can affect swallowing—examples include Sjögren's syndrome, an autoimmune disorder that causes the mouth and eyes to dry out...Parkinson's disease, which weakens muscles including those in the throat...and gastroesophageal reflux disease (GERD), which can cause choking when stomach acid backs up into the throat.

CHAPTER 18

Women's Health

Dangers of an Ill-Fitting Bra

Even though an ill-fitting bra may sound like a trivial problem, it has been linked to a range of health complaints. Yet research has found that up to 85% of women wear the wrong size bra. The harms related to a misfitted bra tend to occur in large-breasted women most often, but women of all breast sizes can be affected. *For example...*

***PROBLEM #1:* Neck and back pain.** Even though the lion's share of a bra's support comes from the bra band, which wraps around the torso just below the bust, many women find it more comfortable to opt for a larger band measurement than what they need. Without adequate support, however, large breasts fall forward, pulling the neck, shoulders and upper back with them, triggering or exacerbating neck and back pain.

To avoid it: Go down a size in the band but up a cup size—for example, from 36C to 34D—to increase support in the band while ensuring adequate space for your breasts.

Helpful: Always use the outermost hooks when trying on bras. A bra is guaranteed to stretch out with wear, so you want it to fit well—snug, but not uncomfortably so—in the loosest position. This will add several months of life to your bra. As it stretches, move to the next hook, until you get to the first.

Note: A too-loose bra band also can lead to painful shoulder grooves. That's because a band that's not snug forces the straps to do all of the work. If the band rides up in the back, the straps dig in, creating painful grooves in the shoulders of full-breasted women and uncomfortable indentations in smaller-breasted women. Shoulder grooves also can be avoided by going down a band size and up a cup size.

Elisa Lawson, a certified prosthesis specialist and certified mastectomy fitter (CMF) who operates the Women's Health Boutique at Mercy Medical Center's Weinberg Center for Women's Health & Medicine in Baltimore. Lawson has fit bras for more than 40 years.

PROBLEM #2: Heartburn. An overly tight band can aggravate heartburn—especially in fuller-figured women who already suffer from this condition. The problem happens mainly when sitting, which pushes the stomach upward, constricting the band and pressing on the diaphragm, the muscle that separates the chest and abdomen.

Because the diaphragm is positioned where the esophagus and stomach meet, pressure there can make it easier for stomach acid to move into the esophagus, causing discomfort and exacerbating heartburn.

To avoid it: Try a bra extender. These are small strips of fabric—roughly two inches in length—with hooks on one side and loops on the other. They lengthen the circumference of your bra to give some extra breathing room and cost far less than a new bra (you can find three-packs on Amazon.com for $8).

A bra extender isn't meant to be worn for months on end—think of it as a stopgap solution. If you use one and your indigestion improves, that's a sign you need to purchase a new bra with a looser band.

Also helpful: Try bumping up the band size and downsize the cup size—for example, go from a 36D to 38C.

PROBLEM #3: Rashes and skin irritation. A poorly fitting underwire is often the culprit here. The problem typically stems from the wire resting on breast tissue and the chest wall. Additionally, breasts that rest on the torso can trap perspiration, possibly causing rashes or even fungal infections.

To avoid it: Consider a bra without an underwire. Many women think a wire lifts, but a good-fitting bra—with or without a wire—is what lifts and shapes. If you prefer an underwire bra, go up a cup size so that all breast tissue fits within the frame of the wire. Underwire bras shouldn't rub against your skin, and your breasts shouldn't be touching your torso.

If you notice redness, irritation or itchiness underneath your breasts, see your health-care provider. He/she may prescribe an antibacterial or antifungal cream. And switch to a bra that holds your breasts up!

How to Get the Right Size Bra

Elisa Lawson, a certified prosthesis specialist and certified mastectomy fitter (CMF) who operates the Women's Health Boutique at Mercy Medical Center's Weinberg Center for Women's Health & Medicine in Baltimore. Lawson has fit bras for more than 40 years.

To get the correct bra size, the first step is to measure before shopping.
What to do…

Step #1: To calculate your band size, snugly wrap a tape measure around your rib cage just beneath your bust, where the bra band would normally rest.* If the number is odd, add five inches to the band size—for example, if you measure 33 inches add five inches, and your band is 38 inches. If the number is even, add four inches—for example, if you measure 32 inches add four inches, and your band size is 36 inches.

Step #2: Then loosely measure your chest at the level of your nipples.

Step #3: To determine your cup size, subtract the band measurement from the bust measurement. For example, if your bust is 38 inches and the band 35, then the difference is 3. Refer to the chart below. That corresponds to a "C" cup size, or a 38C.

FINDING YOUR CUP SIZE				
The difference in inches	0	1	2	3
Your cup size is:	AA	A	B	C
The difference in inches	4	5	6	7
Your cup size is:	D	DD	DDD, F	G

Important: Measurements are a good starting point. But bras are as irregular as jeans in sizing, so they should always be tried on. Sometimes a particular style is just not right for you. Also, it's important to remember that the size you arrive at through measuring may not apply to all bras.

*For both measurements here, round up to the next whole number in inches.

Note: Good-fitting bras can be found in all price points. The longevity of the bra, however, depends on quality and care. To extend the life of a bra, wash it in a lingerie bag with a mild detergent that contains no bleach and hang it to dry. Professional bra fitters typically can be found in lingerie shops or women's clothing stores.

More Women Should Get BRCA Screening

Douglas Owens, MD, chair, US Preventive Services Task Force and professor of medicine, Stanford University, California.

Previously, only women with a family history of a BRCA-related cancer (such as breast, ovarian, fallopian tube or peritoneal, a malignancy of the thin layer of tissue that lines the abdomen) were advised to undergo a risk assessment for the gene mutation that raises risk for these cancers.

Now: Women with a personal history of any breast, ovarian, fallopian tube or peritoneal cancer or those whose ancestry puts them at higher risk for BRCA-related breast cancer, such as Ashkenazi Jewish women, should be assessed and may consider BRCA gene testing if indicated after consulting a genetic counselor.

Dense Breasts and Breast Cancer Risk: What You Need to Know

Erin Hofstatter, MD, associate professor of medicine and codirector of the Smilow Cancer Genetics and Prevention Program at Yale School of Medicine in New Haven, Connecticut. Dr. Hofstatter is a medical oncologist with clinical and research expertise in breast cancer and clinical breast cancer genetics. She also serves as director of the Breast Cancer Prevention Clinic at Yale New Haven's Smilow Cancer Hospital.

When a woman gets her mammogram results, what she's most interested in hearing from her doctor is, "Every-thing looks fine." But even if the test doesn't show anything suspicious, there's another piece of information that women need to know.

In addition to showing breast changes—such as small white spots (known as calcifications) and/or lumps or tumors (called masses), mammograms indicate a woman's breast density, a measure of fibrous and glandular tissue versus fatty tissue in the breasts.

Why breast density matters: About half of women ages 40 to 74 have dense breasts, which can't be felt when a woman does a self-exam or when a doctor palpates her breasts. This is vital information because dense breasts make it harder to find malignancies on a mammogram.

Even more important, women with dense breasts are four to six times more likely to develop breast cancer than women without dense breast tissue. In fact, high breast density surpasses other known risk factors for developing breast cancer, such as family history or later-in-life childbirth, according to research published in *JAMA Oncology*.

Another important finding: In women with dense breasts, tumors tend to be larger when detected compared with women without dense breasts, according to a study of women ages 50 to 69 published in *Radiology*.

THE DETECTION CHALLENGE

On mammograms, the fibrous and glandular tissue that indicates breast density appears white. To distinguish the degree of breast density, radiologists use four categories—extremely dense (75% or more of the mammogram appears white)…heterogeneously dense (50% to 75% appears white)…scattered areas of density (25% to 50%)…and mostly fatty (0% to 25%). If a woman's mammogram falls within one of the first two categories, her breasts are considered dense.

Even though dense breasts can make mammograms more difficult to read, the test is crucial because many cancers may still be visible. Breast density, along with other risk factors, including personal and family history of breast cancer, should be taken into account when determining mammogram frequency. Women should talk to their doctors to come up with a personalized screening schedule—for both the frequency and types of tests performed.

For women with dense breasts, screening may include one or both of these tests…

•**3-D mammography.** A traditional mammogram is printed on film and is two-dimensional, with two X-ray images taken of each breast—top-to-bottom and side-to-side. With 3-D mammography, also called digital tomosynthesis, the machine takes multiple X-rays, or "slices," and combines them into a 3-D image that the radiologist reads on a computer screen, where breast tissue can be viewed one layer at a time. The resulting images are finer and clearer, showing abnormalities that might otherwise be difficult—or impossible—to see. Both types of mammography require the use of plates that compress the breasts.

3-D mammography delivers only very slightly more ionizing radiation than traditional mammography, but it's still considered safe by the FDA. There are about 40% fewer false positives with 3-D mammography compared with 2-D, preventing unnecessary anxiety in patients and repeated testing to confirm results.

•**Ultrasound.** This technology uses high-frequency sound waves to identify breast cysts or masses. A layer of gel is applied to each breast, and a handheld device called a transducer is placed directly on the skin, transmitting ultrasound waves into the body. A mass will block the sound waves' pathway, signaling a potential cancer. Ultrasound is noninvasive, creates no ionizing radiation and is typically used as a follow-up to any abnormal mammogram.

Important finding: When 3-D mammography and/or ultrasound was given to more than 3,200 women with "dense" or "extremely dense" breasts whose conventional screening mammograms had found no cancer, the additional tests found 24 breast cancers, according to a study published in *Journal of Clinical Oncology.*

One of these cancers was detected by 3-D mammogram alone…11 were detected by ultrasound alone…and 12 were detected by both 3-D mammogram and ultrasound.

Caveats: As part of the same study, there were 53 false-positive results for 3-D mammograms…and 65 false positives for ultrasound.

However, researchers considered this disparity to be statistically insignificant.

But do these additional tests actually save lives? That's debatable. Even though the additional screenings have been shown to identify breast cancers that would have otherwise been missed, modern breast cancer treatment is so effective that even if the cancer is detected a bit later, it's still often curable. Even so, the earlier a cancer is detected, the less likely a woman will need chemotherapy. So while an ultrasound may not save lives, it could minimize treatment…or make a treatment regimen less taxing.

The screening decision: This can be a challenging question because professional medical groups have no established screening guidelines based on breast density. These groups do not consider the additional cancers that are detected by ultrasound to be numerous enough to warrant the additional monetary—and potential emotional—cost.

Insurance coverage also has been spotty for both 3-D mammography and ultrasound, so consult your insurer before getting these tests. For those paying out of pocket, a 3-D mammogram costs about $100 more than a 2-D mammogram (about $380 versus $290). An ultrasound can cost several hundred dollars. But if you're one of the women whose cancer is detected with additional testing, it's money well spent.

Note: Women with a strong family history of a BRCA mutation, which increases breast cancer risk, are often advised to also get an MRI, but this scan is typically not recommended for women with dense breasts. For that reason, I usually do not recommend MRI for breast density alone.

OTHER BREAST CANCER FACTORS

You can't change certain risk factors, such as your family history of breast cancer, but other risk factors are under your control.

Most important steps to take: Strive for a healthy weight, achieved through 150 minutes of moderate-intensity physical activity a week plus a diet rich in plant-based foods and with less than 10% of calories from saturated fat.

There's strong evidence supporting the benefits of these strategies. For instance, nearly a quarter of breast cancers could be avoided by obese and overweight women attaining a body mass index under 25 (for example, a body weight of 140 pounds for a 5'4" woman). That's because fat cells produce estrogen—and an excess of this hormone increases risk for certain types of breast cancer.

Also: Don't smoke…limit alcohol use (to one drink a day or, even better, less)…and be judicious about using hormone replacement therapy, avoiding it if possible or taking it for the shortest course possible if you need it to alleviate menopausal symptoms. Fortunately, most women's breasts become non-dense after menopause.

---

6 Signs That DCIS Is Likely to Become Invasive Breast Cancer

Study titled "Predictors of an Invasive Breast Cancer Recurrence after DCIS: A Systematic Review and Meta-Analyses" by researchers at the Netherlands Cancer Institute, Amsterdam, published in *Cancer Epidemiology, Biomarkers & Prevention.*

Most *ductal carcinoma in situ* (DCIS) breast cancer will never become life-threatening, even if left untreated. However, there hasn't been a good way to tell when DCIS should be treated and when treatment can be safely skipped—until now. A new study has identified six factors that determine when DCIS is most likely to become invasive breast cancer.

DCIS is cancer that starts in a milk duct and has not spread outside the duct. Often called "stage 0," it's such an early stage of cancer that some experts believe it's actually a precancerous condition rather than actual cancer. DCIS has become increasingly common—possibly because women are living longer, more women are getting screening mammograms, and mammograms have become better at finding these small breast cancers. About 20% of all breast cancers are DCIS.

Most women with DCIS have a lumpectomy, and some also have radiation. The risk for DCIS recurrence after lumpectomy alone is about 25%

to 30%…adding radiation therapy drops the risk to about 15%. Only half of recurrences are invasive cancer—the rest are DCIS again.

However, as there hasn't been a way to reliably predict which women with DCIS will develop invasive breast cancer, guidelines call for all women with the condition to be treated with either surgery alone or surgery and radiation…and frequently hormonal therapy as well. Doctors are coming to believe that this is overtreatment for the majority of women.

Now: Researchers from the Netherlands Cancer Institute in Amsterdam reviewed 17 studies and identified 26 unfavorable prognostic factors associated with invasive breast cancer developing after DCIS. Six factors in particular emerged as the most significant indicators, with risk for invasive breast cancer after DCIS diagnosis ranging from 36% to 84%. *They were…*

•**Feeling a lump (84% risk).** DCIS does not cause symptoms and 80% of the time is found only by mammography. However, when DCIS causes a palpable lump (one that can be felt), it is likely to be aggressive.

•**Involved margins (63% risk).** When the tumor is removed, if tumor cells are found to extend out to the edge of normal breast tissue, the risk for recurrence increases—because surgery may leave some cells behind.

•**Diagnosed before menopause (59% risk).** Younger women produce more estrogen, which may stimulate tumor growth. They also have more of their lives still ahead, allowing more time for recurrence to occur.

•**High p16 (51% risk).** Overexpression of p16, a protein involved in regulating tumor-cell growth that is detected during biopsy, has been linked to more aggressive tumor growth.

•**Being African-American (43% risk).** For reasons that are not clearly understood, African-American women have higher rates of all types of breast cancer recurrence.

•**High histologic grade (36% risk).** Histologic grade refers to how different from normal cells tumor cells look when studied under a microscope. The more abnormal, or poorly differentiated (meaning that it is hard to tell if the cells are normal or cancer), the higher their grade—and, not surprisingly, the greater their risk for becoming aggressive cancer.

The researchers hope that their findings will be independently validated and help to inform new guidelines…and that future studies will continue to look for other factors that might play a role. In the meantime, if you have been diagnosed with DCIS, it's a good idea to include these six factors in the conversation you have with your doctor to determine the best next steps.

Pungent Way to Fight Breast Cancer

Gauri Desai, MPH, is a PhD candidate in epidemiology and environmental health at University at Buffalo, The State University of New York, and lead author of the study published in *Nutrition and Cancer*.

There's 49% lower risk for breast cancer among women who eat high amounts of onions and garlic than among women who don't.

Likely reason: The anti-cancer flavonols in garlic and onions. The study was done in Puerto Rico where garlic and onions are diet staples for many people. Enjoy them often, both cooked and raw.

Sleeping with Light Linked to Weight Gain

Yong-Moon "Mark" Park, MD, PhD, epidemiologist, National Institute of Environmental Health Sciences, Research Triangle Park, North Carolina.

Women who slept while exposed to light—either from a lamp or the TV—were 17% more likely to gain 11 pounds or more over an average of five-and-a-half years, according to a study of nearly 44,000 women ages 35 to 74.

Theory: Artificial light suppresses production of the sleep hormone melatonin and may affect metabolic processes that contribute to weight gain. A small night-light did not affect weight. Researchers believe the findings would be similar in men.

Beware This Fracture Risk

Sarang Latif Qazi, MBBS, MPH, researcher, Kuopio Musculoskeletal Research Unit, University of Eastern Finland.

Among 1,568 peri- and postmenopausal women, those with the greatest postural sway (the tendency to sway side-to-side and/or forward-backward while standing still) had twice the risk for bone fracture as women with the least postural sway. A five times higher overall fracture risk was associated with high postural sway and low bone-mineral density.

Watchful Waiting Might Be Best for Ovarian Cysts

Dirk Timmerman, PhD, professor in obstetrics and gynecology, Catholic University of Leuven, Belgium, and lead author of a study published in *The Lancet Oncology*.

For low-risk ovarian cysts, watchful waiting may be better than surgery. In a two-year study, 2,000 women who had ovarian cysts diagnosed by ultrasound to be at low risk for cancer, rupture or torsion (twisting and cutting off blood supply) had ultrasounds and clinical exams at three and six months. About 20% of cysts disappeared…0.2% had a rupture…0.4% had torsion…16% of the women needed surgery, and of those, less than 1% had ovarian cancer.

Preeclampsia Linked to Cardiovascular Disease

Pradeep Natarajan, MD, is director of Preventive Cardiology at Massachusetts General Hospital, Boston, and author of a study of more than 220,000 women published in *Journal of the American College of Cardiology*. MassGeneral.org

Women who had preeclampsia during pregnancy were significantly more likely to eventually develop hardened arteries, aortic stenosis, mitral regurgitation and heart failure. Women should tell their doctors about this history…obtain blood pressure screening at least once a year…and ask about lifestyle strategies to reduce risk.

Alert: Pregnancy Strokes Are on the Rise…and They're Preventable!

Larry B. Goldstein, MD, FAAN, FANA, FAHA, spokesperson for the American Heart Association and American Stroke Association. Study titled "Stroke and Cerebrovascular Disease in Pregnancy," led by researchers at the Centre for Surveillance and Applied Research, Public Health Agency of Canada, published in Stroke.

Stroke doesn't happen just to "old people." Young women are also at risk, particularly if they are pregnant—and the weeks just before and right after giving birth are especially dangerous. Alarming as this sounds, most of these strokes don't have to happen if pregnant women and new mothers—and their doctors—take the right preventive measures.

Stroke is the fourth-leading cause of death for women, in part because even a seemingly healthy pregnancy can raise the risk for stroke. Levels of the hormone estrogen increase dramatically during pregnancy, and estrogen helps blood to clot. Pregnancy also increases the risk for two conditions that can lead to stroke—preeclampsia (characterized by high blood pressure and protein in the urine)…and eclampsia (characterized by high blood pressure, protein in the urine and seizures). Women who become pregnant after age 40 are at highest risk for both these conditions.

According to a recent study led by researchers at the Centre for Surveillance and Applied Research in Canada, stroke during the postpartum period (42 days after delivery) rose almost six percentage points in a little more than a decade—from 10.8 out of every 100,000 pregnancies to 16.6 out of every 100,000 pregnancies. Data from the US Nationwide Inpatient Sample from 1994 to 1995 and from 2006 to 2007 showed a 47% increase for hospitalizations during pregnancy and an 83% increase for postpartum hospitalizations associated with stroke. And a more recent Centers for Disease Control and Prevention (CDC) study published in *Obstetrics and Gynecology* found a 62% increase in strokes during pregnancy or after childbirth over a 17-year period.

Risk for the deadliest form of stroke, hemorrhagic, is highest during the third trimester of pregnancy through 12 weeks after giving birth, according to an American Heart Association study that looked at 3.3 million births over a 10-year period.

WHAT YOU CAN DO

Among the factors that might be driving the increase in pregnancy-related stroke is that more women are having children at older ages, and older age is a stroke risk factor in itself. But while it may not be an option to choose pregnancy at a younger age, other factors—primarily, high blood pressure—that can make a pregnant women stroke-vulnerable are preventable.

Stroke-prevention steps to take during and after pregnancy…

•**Prioritize pre- and postnatal care.** The American College of Obstetricians recommends that women have a follow-up visit with their doctors within three weeks postpartum. This is an update from their previous recommendation that a follow-up visit should happen six weeks postpartum. If you're at high risk for stroke, you may need to check in even earlier than that.

•**Check your blood pressure at least several times a week.** Even if your numbers stay in the normal range, if there's a significant increase—20 points or more in the systolic (upper) number—you should call your doctor. It's especially important to check your blood pressure regularly if you were diagnosed with preeclampsia or eclampsia during or after pregnancy.

Best type of blood pressure monitor: The American Heart Association (AHA) recommends an automatic upper-arm cuff-style monitor.

•**Make time for your own health.** Now that your baby is in your arms rather than your belly, it may seem as though, along with breast milk, your little bundle of joy sucks up all your time and energy. But you need to find time to take care of your own health, too. Eat a healthful diet (both Mediterranean and DASH diets are excellent for stroke prevention)…exercise regularly…take steps to manage stress…don't smoke and avoid environmental tobacco smoke exposure…and avoid or limit alcohol.

Also, if you have been diagnosed with diabetes, or pregnancy caused your blood sugar to go into the diabetic range, take steps to keep your blood sugar at a healthy level. And if you're overweight, discuss with your doctor safe, healthy ways to control your weight during pregnancy and shed pounds once your baby is born.

•**Be alert to stroke symptoms.** The acronym F-A-S-T, developed by the AHA, makes it easy to recognize the signs and get help immediately. It stands for **F**acial drooping…**A**rm weakness…**S**peech difficulty…and **T**ime to call 911 right away! Also realize that stroke symptoms in women can be different from those in men.

•**Discuss with your doctor whether you should take aspirin.** Low-dose aspirin (81 mg/day) may have cardio-protective benefits for women at high risk for preeclampsia. However, aspirin can also increase risk for bleeding complications, so discuss the pros and cons with your obstetrician.

•**Know your health history.** Preexisting conditions, such as diabetes, heart disease, lupus, rheumatoid arthritis, blood-clotting disorders, atrial fibrillation (A-Fib) and irregular heartbeat, can increase risk for stroke. So can a history of multiple miscarriages. Be sure to discuss your whole health history during prenatal and postpartum checkups.

Breastfeeding Boosts Heart Health

Irene Lambrinoudaki, MD, is professor of endocrinology at National and Kapodistrian University, Athens, Greece, and leader of a study of 283 postmenopausal women presented at the European Society of Endocrinology annual meeting in Lyon, France.

Moms who breast-feed get a heart-health bonus later in life.

Recent finding: Just six months of breast-feeding led to reduced arterial stiffness and plaque and a lower risk for heart disease. The longer women nursed, the greater the benefit. Breast-feeding also helps prevent postpartum depression and certain cancers and can help regulate blood sugar. Nursing women have high levels of prolactin, a hormone that lowers the risk for diabetes.

Trying to Get Pregnant? Here's the Best Season to Conceive

The study "Seasonal Patterns in Fecundability in North America and Denmark: A Preconception Cohort Study," led by researchers at Boston University School of Public Health and published in *Human Reproduction*.

It's been said that timing is everything. But does that also apply to getting pregnant?

Apparently so, according to recent research led by scientists at the Boston University School of Public Health (BUSPH).

The study, which involved more than 14,000 women in the US, Canada and Denmark who were trying to get pregnant, analyzed data that included details on intercourse frequency, menstruation, smoking, diet, income and education.

Described as a first-of-its-kind study, the researchers focused on *fecundability,* which is the women's probability of becoming pregnant during a single menstrual cycle. The women were tracked with detailed surveys until they either conceived, initiated fertility treatment or had tried to conceive unsuccessful for 12 menstrual cycles.

"There are a lot of studies out there that look at seasonal patterns in births, but these studies don't take into account when couples start trying, how long they take to conceive or how long their pregnancies last," explained Amelia Wesselink, PhD, a postdoctoral associate in epidemiology at BUSPH.

North Americans in the study were more likely than Danes to begin trying to conceive in the fall (perhaps so the birth would occur in the summer when their work schedules may be less demanding).

Results of the study, which was published in *Human Reproduction*, suggest that seasonal variability does play a role in pregnancy...

•**In the US and Canada,** the probability of becoming pregnant in late fall and early winter was 16% higher than in the spring.

•**In Denmark,** the probability of becoming pregnant in the fall was 8% higher than in the spring.

•**In all countries,** the probability of becoming pregnant was lowest in the spring.

The researchers controlled for other factors that might play a role in fecundability, including frequency of sexual intercourse, frequency of menstruation, smoking, consumption of sugar-sweetened beverages and medication use. These factors did not appear to explain the seasonal variation in fertility.

Even though the researchers do not know why the season appears to affect fecundability, they have some hypotheses that they would like to explore. These include temperature, humidity and vitamin D exposure.

Beware of Smoking Pot During Pregnancy

Ryan Bogdan, PhD, associate professor of psychological and brain sciences, Washington University in St. Louis, and senior author of a study of 4,361 children born to mothers between 2005 and 2008, including 201 exposed to marijuana in the womb, published in *JAMA Psychiatry*.

Pot smoking during pregnancy may raise the child's risk for psychosis. Children exposed to marijuana after their mothers knew they were pregnant had a slightly increased risk for psychosis in middle childhood, around age 10. The study did not prove cause and effect, and the association was not found in mothers who used marijuana before they knew they were pregnant—possibly because the *endocannabinoid system*, which responds to cannabis, may not be fully developed early in pregnancy. More research is needed.

Pregnancy Exercises That Don't Put Abdominal Muscles at Risk

Stefanie Gordon, Pilates Method Alliance–certified Pilates teacher (PMA-CPT), National Academy of Sports Medicine–certified personal trainer, corrective exercise specialist and STOTT Pilates certified instructor, based in Short Hills, New Jersey. Ms. Gordon is also a pre/postnatal Pilates specialist with The Center for Women's Fitness in Chicago.

It's important to stay fit while you're pregnant. But you need to make sure that how you exercise won't cause *diastasis recti*—a common condition that can leave you with pelvic muscles that don't work properly. You might also be at risk for this common condition because of other factors. The good news is that strengthening the right muscles can help you avert diastasis recti. Below are three exercises that help.

Diastasis recti is the abnormal separation of abdominal muscles. The outer muscle of the abdominal wall is the *rectus abdominis*, two columns of muscle that run vertically down the abdomen. Between these two columns is the *linea alba*—a long strip of connective tissue that is an extension of the fascia that covers the rectus abdominis. During pregnancy, pressure from the expanding uterus against the abdominal wall causes the linea alba to widen. Diastasis recti occurs when the space widens more than it should.

Pregnancy is the most common cause of diastasis recti, especially for successive pregnancies, pregnant women over age 35 and pregnancies with multiple births. Genetic tendency and/or excessive abdominal fat can also put you at greater risk...as can rapid changes in weight and intense weight-lifting. The condition can affect men as well as women. Diastasis recti prevents core and pelvic floor muscles from functioning properly and, besides giving you a loose, saggy belly, can cause back pain, constipation and urinary leakage.

DO YOU HAVE A DIASTASIS?

There is a simple way to check for a diastasis...

•**When you are not pregnant (or for men).** Lie on your back on the floor, knees bent and feet flat on the ground, and place your index finger and middle finger about two inches above your navel. Curl your head, neck and shoulders off the ground while gently pressing down with your fingers to feel for the sides of your rectus abdominis muscles. If you feel a gap that is more than two fingertips wide, you probably have a diastasis. (A gap greater than four fingertips is typically considered severe.)

•**When you are pregnant.** When lying on your back and flexing up, a diastasis may look like a visible bulge down your midline where the muscles should be together—often described as "coning." (Your pregnant belly should look rounded…coning looks like a peak.)

MOVES TO AVOID…AND EXERCISES THAT HELP

While your abdominal wall is already under stress as a result of pregnancy, you don't want to put any more pressure on it. So, avoid crunches, planks, push-ups and other spinal flexion exercises that is, curling up of the upper torso from a supine position).

What you want to do instead is strengthen your transverse abdominis, the deepest layer of your abdominals. Pilates exercises are one great way to safely work these weakened muscles. But not all Pilates exercises are OK to do during pregnancy, so look for an instructor who has experience with prenatal clients. If you already have a diastasis, perhaps from a previous pregnancy, it's best to consult a qualified physical therapist who has postpartum therapy experience before doing any kind of exercises.

MOVES THAT SAFELY STRENGTHEN ABDOMINAL MUSCLES…

•**Transverse abdominis engagement.** Lie on your back with your knees flexed and feet flat on the floor, about six inches away from your sit bones (the part of the pelvis under your glutes). Place your hands on your navel. Inhale through your nose….then exhale through your mouth as you pull your navel toward your spine without tucking your pelvis underneath you. Do ten reps.

•**Heel drops.** Besides strengthening the transverse abdominis, this exercise also works spinal-stabilizer muscles. Lie on your back with your arms at your sides and both legs in tabletop position (knees bent, legs together and lower legs in the air and parallel to the floor). Inhale and drop your right heel about halfway toward the ground. Exhale while lifting your foot back to starting position. Do the same with your left heel. Do ten reps for each leg, alternating sides. Make sure to keep your shoulders relaxed and your abdominals engaged and avoid arching your back.

•**Bridging with articulation.** This exercise increases spinal mobility while working the abdominals. Lie on your back, knees bent and feet flat on the ground about six inches away from your sit bones. Inhale…then exhale while slowly lifting your hips towards the ceiling, peeling your vertebrae off the mat until you are supported on your upper back. Avoid putting stress or pressure on your head or neck. Hold the position as you inhale…then exhale while slowly rolling back down to starting position. Do five to 10 reps.

Exercise in Pregnancy Is Good for Infants

Study of 60 healthy women and their newborns by researchers at East Carolina University, Greenville, North Carolina, published in *Medicine & Science in Sports & Exercise.*

Newborns whose mothers did supervised, moderate-intensity, 50-minute exercise sessions three times a week had more advanced motor skills than infants whose mothers did not do the exercise sessions. The effect was more noticeable in girls, who at this age tend to have lower motor-skill levels than boys. The differences were not large, but researchers suggest they could be enough to encourage growing children to be more active in the future. Researchers have speculated that the release of hormones during exercising as well as improved blood flow due to aerobic exercise may contribute to the difference found.

Vaginal Birth Is Good for Baby's Health

Study of 18 babies born in San Juan, Puerto Rico, by researchers at New York University, New York City, published in *Nature Medicine*.

Exposure to their mothers' vaginal fluids may improve the health of babies born via C-section. Vaginal delivery transfers beneficial microbes to a baby during birth. But babies born through C-section are exposed only to environmental bacteria, not the helpful ones from their mothers—these babies may be more prone to immune and metabolic disorders, such as type 1 diabetes, obesity and asthma.

New technique: In vaginal microbial transfer, a mother's vaginal fluids are collected before the birth and swabbed all over the infant within a minute or two of delivery. A small initial study showed that this approach established bacterial colonies on C-section babies that were similar to those from vaginal births, although they still fell short in some areas. Further research is planned.

Sjögren's Syndrome Update

Alan Baer, MD, a professor of medicine and director of the Jerome L. Greene Sjögren's Syndrome Center at Johns Hopkins University School of Medicine in Baltimore. Dr. Baer, also an associate investigator at the Sjögren's Syndrome Clinic at the National Institutes of Health, is engaged in clinical research studies regarding Sjögren's syndrome.

Sjögren's (pronounced SHOW-grins) syndrome is far from a minor irritant for many of those affected. Chronic and progressive, it can cause a wide variety of symptoms. Because Sjögren's attacks glands that provide moisture, its symptoms can include dry eyes and mouth, eye pain, blurry vision, burning mouth, loss of taste, rampant tooth decay and difficulty swallowing.

Very often, the syndrome also causes fatigue, joint and muscle pain, rashes and brain fog. Plus, there can be complications, including lung or kidney inflammation. And those with Sjögren's can have a 15 to 20 times higher risk of developing lymphoma, a form of blood cancer, than those without it.

Striking up to 10 in 10,000 people—the vast majority of them women around menopause age—Sjögren's is not only frequently minimized, it's one of the most difficult autoimmune conditions to diagnose and treat.

Diagnostic challenges: An accurate diagnosis can help pinpoint how severely a patient is affected…and estimate the patient's risk for lymphoma. Unfortunately, the symptoms of Sjögren's often don't help with getting a proper diagnosis, as many are common to other health conditions. And no single test can diagnose it. *Useful diagnostic tests that can be underutilized…*

• **An array of antibody blood tests is the best starting point,** since the majority of patients have antibodies that support the diagnosis. However, the antibody tests alone are not sufficient.

• **An eye exam that includes special tests.** The Schirmer test measures tear flow. And the ocular surface stain test assesses damage to the surface of the eye due to dryness.

• **In-office biopsy of the tiny salivary glands inside the lip.** This is an essential test to confirm Sjögren's if the antibody tests are negative. The simple procedure, which involves a shallow incision to remove four to seven glands for analysis, is best done by an oral surgeon with experience in obtaining a good sample for Sjögren's diagnosis.

• **An ultrasound of the salivary glands uncovers changes in the glands caused by Sjögren's and helps define the severity of the syndrome.** For some, this can be a substitute for the lip biopsy.

Best treatments now: A patient with Sjögren's may be seeing multiple specialists, including an ophthalmologist, a dentist, a dermatologist and others, for treatment. A rheumatologist is the best type of doctor to serve as a quarterback of sorts to work collaboratively with all the specialists involved. *The most common Sjögren's treatments now include…*

•**Artificial tears and anti-inflammatory prescription eyedrops**—*cyclosporine* (Restasis) and *lifitegrast* (Xiidra).

•**Cholinergic agonist drugs,** including *pilocarpine* (Salagen) and *cevimeline* (Evoxac), for dry mouth.

•**Prescription-strength fluoride toothpaste** to mitigate tooth decay.

•**Antifungal medications or mouthwashes** to treat thrush.

•*Hydroxychloroquine* **(Plaquenil)** for arthritis, fatigue and certain rashes.

•**Immunosuppressant drugs,** like *methotrexate* (Trexall), *mycophenolate mofetil* (CellCept) and *azathioprine* (Azasan)…the biologic *rituximab* (Rituxan)…and corticosteroids, to reduce inflammation in the body.

•**Pain relievers,** including *acetaminophen* (Tylenol), *gabapentin* (Neurontin) and *duloxetine* (Cymbalta), for joint, nerve and muscle pain. Topical diclofenac can relieve pain in large joints.

Sjögren's patients often find that various natural treatments, such as massage, acupuncture and stress-reduction techniques, help their symptoms. An anti-inflammatory diet that includes plenty of whole fruits and vegetables, healthy fats, fiber and moderate amounts of organic meat…and eliminates or reduces trans fats, processed foods, preservatives and red meat may help as well.

Latest research: It's hoped that new clinical trials will discern if existing *disease-modifying antirheumatic drugs* (DMARDs), used successfully for other autoimmune disorders, might also work for Sjögren's. Arresting inflammation in the moisture-producing glands is the next big goal. To find clinical trials focusing on new treatments, go to info.Sjogrens.org/clinical-trials.

Smart Tampon for Fertility

Forbes

A "smart" tampon that collects endometrial tissue during menstruation can help evaluate a woman's fertility. The tampon, in development, would be used for about two hours, then sent to a laboratory for testing.

Next step: Clinical trials.

Migraines Can Lower Diabetes Risk for Women

Guy Fagherazzi, PhD, senior research scientist of diabetes epidemiology, Center of Research in Epidemiology and Population Health, University of Paris-Saclay, France, and corresponding author of a study of more than 74,000 women, published in *JAMA Neurology*.

Migraines may have protective effects. The intense headaches have been linked to stroke, heart attack and psychiatric disorders.

But they also seem to have some positive impact: Women with active migraines were 20% to 30% less likely to develop type 2 diabetes during a 10-year study than women with no history of migraine. And if their migraine status improved, their risk for diabetes went up.

Binge Drinking May Be Worse for Women

Shivendra D. Shukla, PhD, Margaret Proctor Mulligan Professor of medical research, University of Missouri School of Medicine, Columbia, and leader of a study published in *The Journal of Pharmacology and Experimental Therapeutics*.

According to a recent study, female rats were more sensitive to alcohol and had higher levels of alcoholic liver injury than comparable male rats. A protein that enables tumor growth and cancer increased 20% in male rats given alcohol equivalent to the amounts binge-drinking humans take in…but the protein level went up 95% in female rats.

Reason: Unknown—further research is necessary.

What if You Have a Pelvic Mesh Implant?

Cheryl B. Iglesia, MD, director, Female Pelvic Medicine and Reconstructive Surgery (FPMRS), MedStar Washington Hospital Center, and professor, departments of obstetrics/gynecology and urology, Georgetown University School of Medicine, both in Washington, DC.

Now that the FDA has halted use of transvaginal pelvic mesh for repair of *pelvic organ prolapse*—stating that the risks of serious health problems outweigh the benefits—women who already have these pelvic mesh implants are understandably concerned. If you have a pelvic mesh implant, you need to talk to your surgeon. What you should do about it depends on how the mesh was surgically put into place.

Pelvic organ prolapse (POP) is caused by muscles, ligaments and connective tissue supporting the pelvic organs becoming damaged, such as through childbirth or injury...or weakening as a result of age and menopause...allowing the uterus, rectum or bladder to drop (prolapse) into the vagina. The usual repair for POP has been to restore anatomy by shoring up the torn ligaments. This is done using sutures...or by surgically implanting permanent (pelvic) mesh, a netlike medical device typically made from polypropylene, to permanently support the torn ligaments and muscles and help hold these organs in place.

THE PROBLEM WITH MESH IMPLANTS

The surgical procedure to repair prolapse can be done using mesh placed either through the vagina or through an abdominal incision. Mesh placed through the vagina carries more risk than mesh placed abdominally for prolapse.

Reason: The vaginal approach requires a larger piece of mesh and is placed through incisions made inside the vagina. Mesh placed this way is more likely to lead to infection or contraction, or it and can move out of place and/or damage tissues that attach to it—for instance, it can perforate the vaginal tissues or erode into nearby organs.

In 2018, the FDA decided that surgery using polypropylene mesh was unsafe for repair of rec-

tum prolapse (rectocele). In 2019, the FDA said that synthetic mesh repair of bladder prolapse (cystocele), the most common type of pelvic organ prolapse, was also unsafe—saying that they have not "received sufficient evidence to assure that the probable benefits of these devices outweigh their probable risks" and concluding that "these products do not have reasonable assurance of safety and effectiveness." The companies that sell the mesh were told to stop.

Note: The FDA action does not apply to surgical mesh slings to support the urethra for stress urinary incontinence or synthetic polypropylene mesh implanted abdominally or with laparoscopic/robotic surgery. No direct incisions are made on the vagina for these procedures, and the mesh used is much smaller and lighter weight compared with transvaginal mesh products.

IF YOU HAVE PELVIC MESH

If your repair is working and you don't have any problems, the mesh can stay. But do continue regular check-ups annually with your gynecologist or surgeon. *Also be alert to signs of trouble, such as...*

- **Vaginal bleeding or discharge**
- **Pelvic or groin pain, discomfort or pressure**
- **Pain during sexual intercourse**
- **Pain for a partner during intercourse** (could indicate exposed mesh protruding into the vagina)
- **Frequent urinary tract infections**
- **Leaking of urine (incontinence)**
- **Bulge inside or protruding from your vagina.**

If you are having health problems caused by your pelvic mesh, you may need to have it removed and a new POP repair done. This is a challenging procedure and should only be done by a specialist in female pelvic medicine and reconstructive surgery called a urogynecologist. Check the American Urogynecologic Society website, AUGS.org, to find one near you.

SAFER POP OPTIONS

If you have been diagnosed with POP but have not had surgery, you should work with a pelvic medicine specialist to determine the most appropriate treatment for you. Surgery is usually not the first option. *A specialist may advise…*

- **Kegel exercises to strengthen your pelvic muscles**

- **A pessary,** a soft, flexible device that can be inserted (and removed) into the vagina to support prolapsed organs

- **Losing weight if you are overweight.**

If you do need surgery, there are options other than using the synthetic mesh. These include transvaginal surgery using your own (native) tissue and sutures…laparoscopic and robotic procedures…abdominal surgery with light-weight mesh mostly attaching to your tailbone…or a new technique that uses incisionless suture devices. Clinical trials are currently under way with new innovations for making grafts using your own tissues or other biologic tissues.

New Libido-Enhancer for Women

Anita H. Clayton, MD, is chair of the department of psychiatry and neurobehavioral sciences, University of Virginia School of Medicine, Charlottesville.

The FDA-approved a libido-enhancer for premenopausal women with *hypoactive sexual desire disorder* (HSDD)—low desire that causes distress and that is not due to medications or health conditions. The drug *bremelanotide* (Vyleesi) excites sexual interest in about 50% of HSDD sufferers. It's self-administered by injection 45 minutes before intimacy. Do not use if you have high blood pressure or cardiovascular disease because it can raise blood pressure for up to 12 hours.

Index